Retinoid Therapy

Retinoid Therapy

A review of clinical and laboratory research

Edited by W. J. Cunliffe and A. J. Miller

The Proceedings of an International Conference
held in London,16-18 May 1983

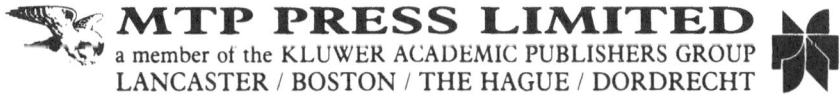

MTP PRESS LIMITED
a member of the KLUWER ACADEMIC PUBLISHERS GROUP
LANCASTER / BOSTON / THE HAGUE / DORDRECHT

Published in the UK and Europe by
MTP Press Limited
Falcon House
Lancaster, England

British Library Cataloguing in Publication Data

Retinoid therapy.
  1. Skin–Diseases–Congresses
  2. Retinoids–Congresses
  I. Cunliffe, W.J.   II. Miller, A.J.
616.5'061   RL110

ISBN-13: 978-94-011-6351-4   e-ISBN-13: 978-94-011-6349-1
DOI: 10.1007/ 978-94-011-6349-1
Published in the USA by
MTP Press
A division of Kluwer Boston Inc
190 Old Derby Street
Hingham, MA 02043, USA

Library of Congress Cataloging in Publication Data

Main entry under title:

Retinoid therapy

"Proceedings of an international conference held in London,
16–18 May 1983."
  Bibliography: p.
  Includes index.
  1. Retinoids–Therapeutic use–Congresses.
2. Skin–Diseases–Chemotherapy–Congresses.
3. Etretinate–Testing–Congresses.   4. Isotretinoin
Testing–Congresses.   5. Dermatologic agents–Congresses.
I. Cunliffe, W.J. (William James), 139–
II. Miller,, A.J. (Allan John). 1936–   [DNLM:
1. Vitamin A–Therapeutic use–Congresses.   2. Vitamin A–
Analogs and derivatives–Congresses.   3. Skin diseases–
Drug therapy–Congresses.   WR. 650 R438 1983]
RL 120.R48R48 1983   616.5'061   83–22255

Redwood Burn Ltd   Trowbridge, Wiltshire

Contents

CONTENTS

Preface

The impact of the retinoids in clinical practice has primarily been in dermatology. When Dr Werner Bollag began his basic research and screening programme in the early 1960's, the expectation was that the retinoids would have a major impact on oncology. However, the laboratory and clinical experiences of Bollag and his colleagues in Switzerland, Stuttgen and Orfanos in Germany, led to publications on both etretinates (Tigason) and isotretinoin (Roaccutane) in the years between 1972 and 1976 in the field of dermatology. In fact the first symposium on retinoid research held in Berlin in 1981 was almost entirely dermatological. A year later a retinoid workshop in Iowa was designed to provide a forum for dermatologists from the USA involved in specific protocols investigating oral retinoids.

In the UK, research into the retinoids began rather later than in Continental Europe or in the USA, although Tigason was first marketed here. It was felt in late 1982 that as many dermatologists had relatively little experience with these compounds it would be appropriate to hold an International Symposium on retinoid therapy in the UK.

Thus on 16–18 May 1983 in London, 37 speakers from 11 countries addressed an audience of 300, aminly UK, dermatologists. The scientific organizing committee consisted of but two persons Dr William Cunliffe of Leeds General Infirmary, representing the European Society of Dermatological Research, and myself from Roche Clinical Research. The Symposium was held under the auspices of the ESDR and of Roche Products Limited.

The structure of the Symposium was based around the safety and efficacy of two retinoids, etretinate and istotretinoin.

Concern in the UK exists over the safety and management of etretinate in some of those disorders in which it has undoubted efficacy such as severe refractory psoriasis and inherited disorders of keratinization. The first section of the Symposium evidences both European and UK overall clinical experience and highlights safety of use in children with ichthyoses, pharmacokinetics of etretinate and the combination of etretinate with PUVA therapy in palmo-plantar psoriasis and psoriasis vulgaris.

The remarkable results achieved with isotretinoin in severe nodulo-cystic acne in the USA, where the first trials took place, are confirmed by studies in the UK and in Continental Europe. At the time of the Symposium, isotretinoin was not approved by the Committee on Safety of Medicines and it was felt appropriate to consider in depth various aspects of therapy including: a dose response study in cystic acne, the relapse rate and duration of remission following cessation of therapy, the lack of an interaction with oral contraceptive drugs, and comparative studies with standard and other new therapies for severe refractory acne.

Although the major sections of the Symposium concentrate on the clinical aspects of both compounds, a part of each is devoted to new basic research. The inhibition by etretinate of both polymorph migration and response to chemotactic stimuli may account for some of the efficacy in active forms of psoriasis. Isotretinoin is shown to beneficially affect the four major factors in the pathogenesis of acne, viz. sebum production, ductal hyperkeratinization, surface and ductal bacterial colonization and mediation of inflammation.

The role of retinoid therapy in neoplasia has yet to be determined. Section 3 of the proceedings gives hints to effective chemophylaxis of high risk cancer patients with pre-cancerous bronchial and skin conditions.

The last sections cover the use of retinoids in other conditions such as isotretinoin in rosacea and the arotinoid (Ro 13–6298) in psoriate arthropathy. On this latter point research workers in Roche Welwyn demonstrate anti-inflammatory activities of three retinoids, that not only may contribute to the efficacy of these compounds in dermatology, but may also lead to other therapeutic fields such as rheumatic diseases.

It is always exciting to be involved in the development of new therapeutic tools as it was to be associated with Bill Cunliffe in his early and continuing work with isotretinoin. I must here pay compliment to Dr Cunliffe without whose clinical studies, advice, help and industry neither the Symposium nor these proceedings would have taken place. Appreciation is also due to Mr Jack Harrison and his colleagues from Roche and finally to my own secretary Miss Sarah Chapman.

A.J. Miller

List of Contributors

Dr H. AL-BAGHADI
Department of Anatomy
University of Leeds
Leeds 2, UK

Mrs W.L. ALLEN
Department of Pharmacology &
  Therapeutics
New Medical School
Ashton Street
Liverpool L69 3BX, UK

Dr D.J. ATHERTON
Department of Dermatology
The Hospital for Sick Children
Great Ormond Street
London WC1N 3JH, UK

Dr D.J. BACK
Department of Pharmacology &
  Therapeutics
New Medical School
Ashton Street
Liverpool L69 3BX, UK

Mr S. BARTON
Department of Medicine
Welsh National School of Medicine
Heath Park
Cardiff CF4 4XN, UK

Professor R. BAUER
Department of Dermatology
University Medical Center
  Steglitz
The Free University of Berlin
Hindenburgdamm 30
D-1000 Berlin 45, West Germany

Dr B. BERRETTI
Department of Dermatology
Polyclinique D'Aubervilliers
55 rue Henri Barbusse
F-93300 Aubervilliers, France

Dr W. BOLLAG
Department of Pharmaceutical
  Research
F.Hoffman-La-Roche & Co Ltd
Grenzacherstrasse 124
CH-4002 Basle, Switzerland

Dr D. BRADSHAW
Department of Pharmacology
Roche Products Ltd
Welwyn Garden City, Herts,
  AL7 3AY, UK

Dr L. BRUMMITT
Department of Dermatology
Leeds General Infirmary
Great George Street
Leeds, LS1 3EX, UK

Dr S.M. BURGE
Department of Dermatology
Slade Hospital
Headington, Oxford OX3 3JH, UK

Dr A. BUSSLINGER
Department of Pharmaceutical
  Research
F.Hoffmann-La-Roche & Co Ltd
Grenzacherstrasse 124
CH-4002 Basle, Switzerland

Mr C.H. CASHIN
Department of Pharmacology
Roche Products Ltd
Welwyn Garden City, Herts,
   AL7 3AY, UK

Dr T.P. CHORZELSKI
Department of Dermatology
Warsaw Academy of Medicine
PL-02-008 Warsaw, Poland

Dr P.R. COBURN
Department of Dermatology
Charing Cross Hospital
London W6 8RF, UK

Dr R. CÖRLIN
Universitats-Hautklinik
Liebermeisterstrasse 25
D-7400 Tubigen, West Germany

Dr W.J. CUNLIFFE
Department of Dermatology
Leeds General Infirmary
Great George Street
Leeds LS1 3EX, UK

Dr W.J. CUNNINGHAM
Department of Medical Research -
   Dermatology
Hoffmann-La Roche Inc
340 Kingsland Street
Nutley, NJ 07110, USA

Dr D.C. DICK
Department of Dermatology
University of Glasgow
Anderson College Bldg
56 Dumbarton Road
Glasgow, G11 6NU, UK

Dr M.M. FERGUSON
Department of Oral Medicine and
   Pathology
Glasgow Dental Hospital and
   School
378 Sauchiehall Street
Glasgow, G2 3JZ, UK

Dr M. FRACZYKOWSKA
Department of Dermatology
Warsaw Academy of Medicine
PL-02-008 Warsaw, Poland

Professor P. FRITSCH
Department of Dermatology
University of Innsbruck
Anichstrasse 35
A-6020 Innsbruck, Austria

Dr R.A. FULTON
Department of Dermatology
Royal Infirmary
Castle Street
Glasgow, G4 OSF, UK

Dr H., GAGET
Service des Maladies Sanguines et
   Tumorales et ICIG (INSERM)
Hôpital Paul-Brousse
14-16 avenue Paul-Vaillant-   Couturier
F-94804 Villejuif Cédex, France

Dr J.M. GEIGER
Department of Clinical Research
F. Hoffmann-La Roche & Co Ltd
Grenzacherstrasse 124
CH-4002 Basle, Switzerland

Dr J. GOUVEIA
Service des Maladies Sanguines et
Tumorales et ICIG (INSERM)
Hôpital Paul-Brousse
14-16 avenue Paul-Vaillant-Couturier
F-94804 Villejuif Cédex, France

Dr R. GREENWOOD
Department of Dermatology
Leeds General Infirmary
Great George Street
Leeds, LS1 3EX, UK

Dr F. GROS
Service des Maladies Sanguines et
Tumorales et ICIG (INSERM)
Hôpital Paul-Brousse
14–16 avenue Paul-Vaillant-Couturier
F-94804 Villejuif Cédex, France

Dr Ch. GRUPPER
Department of Dermatology
Polyclinique D'Aubervilliers
55, rue Henri Barbusse
F-93300 Aubervilliers, France

Dr S. GUTSCHMIDT
Department of Internal Medicine
and Gastroenterology
University Medical Center Steglitz
The Free University of Berlin
Hindenburgdamm 30
D-1000 Berlin 45, West Germany

Dr N. HAMMERSLEY
Department of Oral Medicine and
Pathology
Glasgow Dental Hospital and
School
378 Sauchiehall Street
Glasgow, G2 3JZ, UK

Dr T. HASHIMOTO
Department of Medicine
Welsh National School of Medicine
Heath Park
Cardiff, CF4 4XN, UK

Dr M. HAZELL
Department of Medicine
Welsh National School of Medicine
Heath Park
Cardiff, CF4 4XN, UK

Dr K.T. HOLLAND
University of Leeds
Old Medical School
Leeds, UK

Dr J.P. HOMASSON
Service des Maladies Sanguines et
Tumorales et ICIG (INSERM)
Hôpital Paul-Brousse
14-16 avenue Paul-Vaillant-Couturier
F-94804 Villejuif Cédex, France

Dr S. JABLOŃSKA
Department of Dermatology
Warsaw Academy of Medicine
PL-02-008 Warsaw, Poland

Dr D.H. JONES
Department of Dermatology
Leeds General Infirmary
Great George Street
Leeds LS1 3EX, UK

Dr M.J. KAMIŃSKI
Department of Dermatology and
Department of Histology
Medical School
Koszykowa 82A
PL-02008 Warsaw, Poland

Dr A.J. KENNEDY
Department of Pharmacology
Roche Products Ltd
Welwyn Garden City
Hertfordshire AL7 3AY, UK

Dr B. KIM
Service des Maladies Sanguines et
Tumorales et ICIG (INSERM)
Hôpital Paul-Brousse
14-16 avenue Paul-Vaillant-Couturier
F-94804 Villejuif Cédex, France

Dr K. KING
Department of Microbiology
Leeds Polytechnic
Leeds, UK

Dr T. KINGSTON
Department of Medicine
Welsh National School of Medicine
Heath Park
Cardiff, CF4 4XN, UK

Dr I. KNIPPEL
Department of Dermatology
University Medical Center Steglitz
The Free University of Berlin
D-1000 Berlin 45, West Germany

Dr A. LANGNER
Department of Dermatology
Warsaw Academy of Medicine
PL-02-008 Warsaw, Poland

Dr C.M. LAWRENCE
Department of Dermatology
Royal Victoria Infirmary
Queen Victoria Road
Newcastle-upon-Tyne
NE1 4LP, UK

Dr G. LEMAIGRE
Service des Maladies Sanguines et
Tumorales et ICIG (INSERM)
Hôpital Paul-Brousse
14-16 avenue
  Paul-Vaillant-Coutureir
F-94804 Villejuif Cédex, France

Dr F. LYONS
Department of Dermatology
The Mercy Hospital
Cork, Ireland

Professor R.A. MacKIE
Department of Dermatology
University of Glasgow
Anderson College Bldg
56 Dumbarton Road
Glasgow, G11 6NU, UK

Dr B. MAAS
Universitäts-Hautklinik
Moorenstrasse 5
D-4000 Dusseldorf 1,
West Germany

Dr A. MACK
Department of Clinical Research
Hoffmann-La Roche AG
D-7889 Grenzach-Wyhlen,
West Germany

Dr S. MAJEWSKI
Department of Histology
Medical School
Chalubinskiego 5
PL-02-004 Warsaw, Poland

Dr J.M. MARKS
Department of Dermatology
University of Newcastle-upon-Tyne
Newcastle-upon-Tyne
NE1 7RU, UK

Professor R. MARKS
Department of Medicine
Welsh National School of Medicine
Heath Park
Cardiff, CF4 4XN, UK

Dr J.R. MARSDEN
Department of Dermatology
University of Newcastle-upon-Tyne
Queen Victoria Road
Newcastle-upon-Tyne,
NE1 4LP, UK

Professor G. MATHÉ
Service des Maladies Sanguines et
Tumorales et ICIG (INSERM)
Hôpital Paul-Brousse
14-16 avenue Paul-Vaillant-Couturier
F-94804 Villejuif Cédex, France

Dr S. MILLARD
University of Leeds
Old Medical School
Leeds 1, UK

Dr A.J. MILLER
Department of Clinical Research
Roche Products Ltd
Welwyn Garden City, Herts
AL7 3AY, UK

Dr J.L. MISSET
Service des Maladies Sanguines et
Tumorales et ICIG (INSERM)
Hôpital Paul-Brousse
14-16 avenue Paul-Vaillant-Couturier
F-94804 Villejuif Cédex, France

Dr J. NEUHOFER
Department of Dermatology
University of Innsbruck
Anichstrasse 35
A-6020 Innsbruck, Austria

Professor C.E. ORFANOS
Department of Dermatology
University Medical Center Steglitz
The Free University of Berlin
Hindenburgdamm 30
D-1000 Berlin 45, West Germany

Dr M. ORME
Department of Pharmacology and
  Therapeutics
New Medical School
Ashton Street
Liverpool L69 3BX, UK

Dr U. PARAVICINI
Department of Biopharmaceutical
Research
Hoffmann-La Roche & Co Limited
CH-4002 Basle, Switzerland

Dr S. PARKER
Department of General Medicine
The General Hospital
Ashington, Northumberland, UK

Dr M. PAWIŃSKA-PRONIEWSKA
Department of Dermatology
Medical School
PL-02-008 Warsaw, Poland

Mr A D. PEARSE
Department of Medicine
Welsh National School of Medicine
Heath Park
Cardiff CF4 4XN, UK

Dr W. RAUSCHMEIER
Department of Dermatology
University of Innsbruck
Anichstrasse 35
A-6020 Innsbruck, Austria

Dr H.J. van der RHEE
Department of Dermatology
Leyenburg Hospital
Leyweg 275
2545 CH The Hague,
The Netherlands

Dr O. ROLLMAN
Department of Dermatology
University Hospital
University of Uppsala
S-75185 Uppsala, Sweden

Dr G. SANTELLI
Service des Maladies Sanguines et
Tumorales et ICIG (INSERM)
Hôpital Paul-Brousse
14-16 avenue Paul-Vaillant-Couturier
F-94804 Villejuif Cédex, France

Dr J.G. van der SCHROEFF
Department of Dermagology
University Hospital
Rijnsburgerweg 10
2333 AA Leiden, The Netherlands

Dr A.R. SHALITA
Department of Dermatology
SUNY Downstate Medical Center
450 Clarkson Avenue
Brooklyn, NY 11203, USA

Professor S. SHUSTER
Department of Dermatology
The University
Newcastle-upon-Tyne
NE1 7RU, UK

Dr N. SIMPSON
Department of Dermatology
Glasgow Royal Infirmary
84 Castle Street
Glasgow G4 OSF, UK

Dr M.C. SUDRE
Service des Maladies Sanguines et
Tumorales et ICIG (INSERM)
Hôpital Paul-Brousse
14-16 avenue Paul-Vaillant-Couturier
F-94804 Villejuif Cédex, France

Dr A.J. SZMULRO
Department of Histology
Medical School
PL-02-004 Warsaw, Poland

Dr J. SZYMAŃCZYK
Department of Dermatology
Warsaw Academy of Medicine
PL-02-008 Warsaw, Poland

Dr L. TÖRÖK
Department of Dermatology
County Hospital
Nagykörösi u 15
6000 Kecskemét, Hungary

Dr D. TSAMBAOS
Department of Dermatology
University Medical Center Steglitz
The Free University of Berlin
Hindenburgdamm 30
D-1000 Berlin 45, West Germany

Mr J. TSIA
Department of Pharmacology &
Therapeutics
New Medical School
Ashton Street
Liverpool L69 3BX, UK

Dr A. VAHLQUIST
Department of Dermatology
University Hospital
University of Uppsala
S-75185 Uppsala, Sweden

Dr R.S. WELLS
Department of Dermatology
The Hospital for Sick Children
Great Ormond Street
London WC1N 3JH, UK

Dr J.D. WILKINSON
Department of Dermatology
Wycombe General Hospital
Wycombe, Bucks, UK

Dr H. WOKALEK
Oberarzt der
 Universitäts-Hautklinik
Hauptstrasse 7
D-7800 Freiburg/Breisgau,
West Germany

Dr B. ZIMMERMANN
Department of Dermatology
University Medical Center Steglitz
The Free University of Berlin
Hindenburgdamm 30
D-1000 Berlin 45, West Germany

1
The Development of Retinoids in Dermatology

W. BOLLAG and J.-M. GEIGER

The retinoids are a class of compounds comprising both the natural forms and the synthetic analogues of vitamin A.

Vitamin A is essential to certain functions such as vision, growth and reproduction. Furthermore, it also plays a major role in the proliferation and differentiation of epithelial structures, particularly those of the skin. Vitamin A has been in use as a therapeutic agent in dermatology for over 40 years.

Vitamin A as Therapy in Dermatology

Research in animals has demonstrated that a lack of vitamin A results in modifications of the epithelial structure such as increased epidermal keratinization and squamous metaplasia of the mucous membranes.[1] Since administration of vitamin A in the form of retinol or retinyl esters is capable of correcting these defects, it has come to be known as an 'anti-keratinizing factor'. In vitamin A deficiency states in man, similar manifestations have been observed: dry skin with follicular hyper-keratosis.[2] This finding led various authors in the forties to postulate an essential role of vitamin A in the pathogenesis and treatment of Darier's disease[3] and other cutaneous disorders characterized by disturbances of keratinization, such as the ichthyoses.[4] The role of vitamin A rapidly evolved from that of a nutritional element to become, in non-physiological doses, an agent for the treatment of conditions for which previously no therapy had existed. Vitamin A has also been tested in two dermatological indications which are important by virtue of the frequency of their occurrence, namely acne and psoriasis. Given the key role of follicular hyperkeratosis in the pathomorphogenesis of acne, this condition has also been treated with vitamin A since 1943.[5] Good results have been reported in mild and moderate forms of acne after 4 months' treatment with daily doses of 100,000 –300,000 IU vitamin A.[6,7]

The idea of using vitamin A in psoriasis emerged as a result of observations in the rat made in the Roche laboratories by Studer and Frey in 1949. It was found that, in sub-toxic doses, vitamin A can induce 'peeling' of the horny layer.[8] Three years later, Frey and Schoch[9] reported the first findings on the effects of vitamin A in psoriasis: daily doses of 400,000 IU were completely without effect whereas administration of between 2 and 4 million IU, while slightly improving the disease symptomatology, led to a hypervitaminosis A syndrome with dryness of the mucous membranes, desquamation of healthy skin, and nervous disturbances. Megadoses of vitamin A of this order were for a long time considered an interesting treatment for psoriasis[10] and for various other disorders of keratinization, despite the frequency and intensity of the side-effects, notably the signs of intracranial hypertension.

In addition, retinol and its esters have also been used with positive results in the treatment of premalignant lesions such as actinic keratoses[6,7,11] and basal cell carcinomas.[11]

Vitamin A Acid

In 1962, Stüttgen[12] demonstrated that the acid derivative of vitamin A, all-*trans*-retinoic acid, can be used as a therapeutic agent in dermatology, and that the topical application is of particular interest in the treatment of different conditions characterized by disorders of keratinization: ichthyoses, pityriasis rubra pilaris and actinic keratoses. In the same year, Beer[13] confirmed the keratolytic activity of vitamin A in ichthyosis vulgaris but did not observe any beneficial effect in psoriasis or in palmo-plantar keratosis. Some years later, Frost and Weinstein[14] made a contradictory claim, establishing the marked efficacy of topically applied retinoic acid in psoriasis and lamellar ichthyosis, and finding an absence of effect in ichthyosis vulgaris. Kligman and co-workers[15] were the first to report that topically applied retinoic acid is very effective in the treatment of acne vulgaris and that this effect is associated with an inhibition of comedo formation owing to the increased production of non-coherent horny cells in the follicular orifice.

Having shown that, in mice, retinoic acid has a favourable effect in the prevention and the treatment of chemically-induced skin papillomas and carcinomas[16,17] we studied the effects of this substance on premalignant and malignant cutaneous lesions in the clinic.[18] Applied topically, retinoic acid induced a partial or complete regression of actinic keratoses and of basal cell carcinomas of the skin.[18] Oral administration of all-*trans*-retinoic acid had provided promising results in the treatment of certain disorders of keratinization.[19] This notwithstanding, its use had to be abandoned because of the serious side-effects of the hypervitaminosis A type resulting when therapeutically effective doses were used.

Selection of New Retinoids

The therapeutic effects of orally administered vitamin A and all-*trans*-retinoic acid were insufficient. For this reason, in 1968, we initiated a research programme in our laboratories with the aim of finding synthetic analogues of vitamin A which would be both superior in terms of therapeutic efficacy and better tolerance. Structural chemical modifications of the three building units of vitamin A – the initial cyclic group, the polyene side-chain and the terminal polar group – yielded a series of more than 1,500 products. Selection of compounds for clinical use in both oncology and dermatology was based on the 'therapeutic index' determined for each product in animal testing. This index is calculated on the basis of two criteria: the efficacy on chemically-induced papillomas in the mouse and the toxicity as measured by a grading system of different signs and symptoms of hypervitaminosis A.[20–22]

The papilloma model was chosen because it was suitable for screening of both the antitumour and the antipsoriatic/antikeratinizing properties of retinoids. Since the chemically-induced papilloma shows a high proliferation rate in the basal cell layer and increased keratinization – both features shared by several disorders of keratinization – this model seemed to meet investigational needs in certain dermatological diseases.

Following this procedure since 1970, we have prepared for clinical investigation the derivatives listed in Table 1.

Clinical Investigation of Synthetic Retinoids

The first clinical evaluation of these retinoids was reported in 1973 by Runne and co-workers[23] who observed a slight therapeutic response to an ethylamide derivative of retinoic acid (Ro 8-4968) and to 13-*cis*-retinoic acid (Ro 4-3780) in psoriasis patients.

13-*cis*-retinoic acid, or isotretinoin, had been studied in Europe since 1971 in acne. Oral doses of 5–20mg daily had yielded good results in comedonic, papulo-pustular and cystic forms of acne (Eichenberger, H., Meyer-Latzke, E., Stüttgen, G. and Vollrath, W., unpublished data on file, F. Hoffmann-La Roche & Co. Ltd, Basle). However, at that time, in the psychological climate engendered by the thalidomide tragedy, it would have been inconceivable to develop an agent with teratogenic properties for the treatment of such a common complaint as acne. In 1976 in the USA, Peck and Yoder[24] reported the beneficial effects of isotretinoin in lamellar ichthyosis and certain other disorders of keratinization. Shortly afterwards, the remarkable results of this treatment in cystic and conglobate acne were observed and reported by the same authors and their co-workers.[25] It was found that this effect in severe acne could be largely explained by the compound's capacity to inhibit the activity of the sebaceous glands.[26]

With a therapeutic index 10 times more favourable than that of all-*trans*-retinoic acid, the aromatic retinoid etretinate (Ro 10-9359) was tested for the first time in patients with psoriasis. The first results, reported in 1975 by Ott and ourselves[27] showed the very marked activity of etretinate in severe generalized psoriasis vulgaris and particularly in the erythrodermic and pustular forms. Other cutaneous disorders were soon to benefit from this new therapeutic agent, such as Darier's disease,[28,29] lichen planus[30] and other conditions characterized by disturbed keratinization.[31] Thus, within a period of a few years, etretinate proved an important therapeutic tool in dermatology, particularly as a treatment for a large number of previously untreatable skin disorders.

Two other aromatic retinoids have been undergoing clinical investigation. A dichloro analogue of etretinate, Ro 12-7554, has been shown by animal studies[32] to have a therapeutic index identical to that of etretinate. In clinical studies in man, a pilot study in patients suffering from psoriasis or

Table 1. Chemical structures of the synthetic retinoids investigated in dermatology.

	Chemical structure	Roche number	Trade marks
13-*cis*-Retinoic acid (Isotretinoin)		Ro 4-3780	ROACCUTANE ACCUTANE (USA)
Ethyl retinamide		Ro 8-4968	–
Trimethylmethoxyphenyl analogue of retinoic acid ethyl ester (Etretinate)		Ro 10-9359	TIGASON
Trimethylmethoxyphenyl analogue of retinoic acid ethyl amide (Motretinid)		Ro 11-1430	TASMADERM
Dichloromethylmethoxy-phenyl analogue of retinoic acid ethyl ester		Ro 12-7554	–
Arotinoid ethyl ester		Ro 13-6298	–

different congenital disorders of keratinization[33] confirmed the similarity of Ro 12-7554 and etretinate in terms of clinical efficacy and overall safety.

An ethyl amide analogue of etretinate, Ro 11-1430, has been tested with some success in the topical treatment of acne vulgaris.[34] Ro 11-1430 has demonstrated an efficacy equivalent to that of retinoic acid, but is better tolerated.[35]

The arotinoid Ro 13-6298 belongs to a new class of retinoids whose chemical structure containing three cyclic groups is rather remote from the original structure of vitamin A. This compound is active in our animal model at doses 500 times lower than those of etretinate but possesses an identical therapeutic index.[32,36] In the light of the results obtained by Ott and ourselves[37] in 17 patients with severe psoriasis receiving a dose of only 1 μg/kg/day, Ro 13-6298 showed a slightly lower overall therapeutic usefulness than etretinate. More favourable results, however, have been reported by Tsambaos and co-workers,[38] in a variety of typical indications for retinoids such as psoriasis vulgaris and arthropathica, congenital ichthyosis, lichen planus, Darier's disease, lichen mucosae erosivus and palmo-plantar keratoderma.

Conclusions

All the above-mentioned synthetic retinoids have therapeutic effects in cutaneous disorders showing very different clinical and pathophysiological aspects such as acne, psoriasis, congenital disorders of keratinization or preneoplastic and neoplastic lesions of the epidermis. Activities on cell proliferation and differentiation, keratinization, sebum production and inflammation are involved to a different degree in these therapeutic effects. The great drawback of the retinoids is their relative toxicity which to some extent limits their clinical use.

Thus, the retinoids possess a variety of biological properties some being therapeutically advantageous and others unwanted. In the future, our pharmacological research will concentrate on developing retinoids that are better tolerated, possess greater selectivity of action and have potential for clinical application in dermatology as well as in other fields of medicine.

References

1. Wolbach, S.B. and Howe, P.R. (1925). Tissue changes following deprivation of fat-soluble A-vitamin. *J. Exp. Med.*, **42**, 753
2. Frazier, C.N. and Hu, C.K. (1931). Cutaneous lesions associated with a deficiency in vitamin A in man. *Arch. Intern. Med.*, **48**, 507

3. Peck, S.M., Chargin, L. and Sobotka, H. (1941). Keratosis follicularis (Darier's disease), a vitamin A deficiency disease. *Arch. Derm. Syph.*, **43**, 223
4. Rapaport, H.G. (1942). The treatment of ichthyosis with vitamin A. *J. Pediatr.*, **21**, 733
5. Straumfjord, J.V. (1943). Vitamin A: its effects on acne. *Northwest Med.*, **42**, 219
6. Savitt, L.E. and Obermayer, M.E. (1950). Treatment of acne vulgaris and senile keratoses with vitamin A: results of a clinical experiment. *J. Invest. Dermatol.*, **14**, 282
7. Kalkoff, K.W. and Conraths, H. (1956). Zur peroralen Vitamin-A-Therapie von Dermatosen. *Münch. Med. Wochenschr.*, **89**, 1129
8. Studer, A. and Frey, J.R. (1949). Ueber Hautveränderungen der Ratte nach grossen oralen Dosen von Vitamin A. *Schweiz. Med. Wochenschr.*, **17**, 382
9. Frey, J.R. and Schoch, M.A. (1952). Therapeutische Versuche bei Psoriasis mit Vitamin A, zugleich ein Beitrag zur A-Hypervitaminose. *Dermatologica*, **104**, 80
10. Hoefer-Janker, H., Scheef, W. and Blumenberg, F.W. (1969). Ueberraschende Wirkung subtoxischer Vitamin-A-Dosen auf die Psoriasis. *Aerztl. Prax.*, **21**, 5238
11. Scherber, G. (1943). Zur Wirkung von Vitaminen auf Hyperkeratosen der Haut. *Wien. Med. Wochenschr.*, **93**, 273
12. Stüttgen, G. (1962). Zur Lokalbehandlung von Keratosen mit Vitamin-A-Säure. *Dermatologica*, **124**, 65
13. Beer, P. (1962). Untersuchungen über die Wirkung der Vitamin-A-Säure. *Dermatologica*, **124**, 192
14. Frost, P. and Weinstein, G.D. (1969). Topical administration of vitamin A acid for ichthyosiform dermatoses and psoriasis. *J. Am. Med. Assoc.*, **207**, 1863
15. Kligman, A.M., Fulton, J.E. and Plewig, G. (1969). Topical vitamin A acid in acne vulgaris. *Arch. Dermatol.*, **99**, 469
16. Bollag, W. (1971). Effects of vitamin A acid on transplantable and chemically induced tumours. *Cancer Chemother. Rep.*, **55**, 53
17. Bollag, W. (1972). Prophylaxis of chemically induced benign and malignant epithelial tumours by vitamin A acid (retinoic acid). *Eur. J. Cancer*, **8**, 689
18. Bollag, W. and Ott, F. (1971). Therapy of actinic keratoses and basal cell carcinomas with local application of vitamin A acid. *Cancer Chemother. Rep.*, **55**, 59
19. Schumacher, A. and Stüttgen, G. (1971). Vitamin-A-Säure bei Hyperkeratosen, epithelialen Tumoren und Akne. Orale und lokale Anwendung. *Dtsch. Med. Wochenschr.*, **96**, 1547
20. Bollag, W. (1974). Therapeutic effects of an aromatic retinoic acid analog on chemically induced skin papillomas and carcinomas of mice. *Eur. J. Cancer*, **10**, 731
21. Bollag, W. (1981). From vitamin A to retinoids: chemical and pharmacological aspects. In Orfanos, C.E. *et al.* (eds.). *Retinoids: Advances in Basic Research and Therapy*. pp. 5–11. (Berlin, Heidelberg, New York: Springer-Verlag)
22. Bollag, W. and Matter, A. (1981). From Vitamin A to retinoids in experimental and clinical oncology: achievements, failures and outlook. *Ann. N.Y. Acad. Sci.*, **359**, 9
23. Runne, U., Orfanos, C.E. and Gartmann, H. (1973). Perorale Applikation zweier Derivate der Vitamin-A-Säure zur internen Psoriasis-Therapie. 13-cis-beta-Vitamin A-Säure und Vitamin-A-Säure-aethylamid. *Arch. Dermatol. Forsch.*, **247**, 171
24. Peck, G.L. and Yoder, F.W. (1976). Treatment of lamellar ichthyosis and other keratinising dermatoses with an oral synthetic retinoid. *Lancet*, **2**, 1172
25. Peck, G.L., Yoder, F.W., Olsen, T.G., Pandya, M.D. and Butkus, D. (1978). Treatment of Darier's disease, lamellar ichthyosis, pityriasis rubra pilaris, cystic acne and basal cell carcinoma with oral 13-cis-retinoic acid. *Dermatologica*, **157** (Suppl.), 11
26. Strauss, J.S., Peck, G.L., Olsen, D.T., Downing, D.T. and Windhorst, D.B. (1978) Sebum composition during oral 13-cis-retinoic acid administration. *J. Invest. Dermatol.*, **70**, 228
27. Ott, F. and Bollag, W. (1975). Therapie der Psoriasis mit einem oral wirksamen neuen Vitamin A-Säure-Derivat. *Schweiz. Med. Wochenschr.*, **105**, 439
28. Schimpf, A. (1976). Zur systemischen Anwendung eines aromatischen Vitamin-A-Säure-Derivates (Ro 10–9359) bei Psoriasis und Keratosen. *Z. Hautkr.*, **51**, 265
29. Orfanos, C.E., Kurka, M. and Strunk, V. (1978). Oral treatment of keratosis follicularis with a new aromatic retinoid. *Arch. Dermatol.*, **114**, 1211
30. Schuppli, R. (1978). The efficacy of a new retinoid (Ro 10–9359) in Lichen planus.

Dermatologica, **157** (Suppl.), 60

31. Marks, R., Finlay, A.Y. and Holt, P.J.A. (1980). Skin changes in patients with congenital disorders of keratinization treated with Ro 10–9359. *Br. J. Dermatol.*, **103**, 11
32. Bollag, W. (1979). Retinoids and cancer. *Cancer Chemother. Pharmacol.*, **3**, 207
33. Ott, F. and Bounameaux, Y. (1983). Pilot study of a new retinoid Ro 12–7554, in psoriasis and in some congenital disorders of keratinization. *Dermatologica,* **167**, 52
34. Scherrer, A. and Ott, F. (1976). Die Lokaltherapie der Akne vulgaris mit einem aromatischen Retinoid. *Schweiz. Rundsch. Med. Praxis,* **65**, 453
35. Christiansen, J., Holm, P. and Reymann, F. (1976). Treatment of acne vulgaris with the retinoic acid derivative Ro 11-1430. A controlled clinical trial against retinoic acid. *Dermatologica,* **153**, 172
36. Bollag, W. (1981). Arotinoids: a new class of retinoids with activities in oncology and dermatology. *Cancer Chemother. Pharmacol.*, **7**, 27
37. Ott, F. and Geiger, J.M. (1983). Therapeutic effect of arotinoid Ro 13–6298 in psoriasis. *Arch. Dermatol. Res.* **9275**, 257
38. Tsambaos, D., Gollnick, H. and Orfanos, C.E. (1982). Orales Arotinoid bei Psoriasis kongenitaler Ichthyose, Lichen, Palmoplantar Keratosen, M. Darier (15 Patienten). Presented at the *33. Tagung der Deutschen Dermatologischen Gesellschaft*, September 30 – October 3, Vienna

Section 1

Etretinate – Clinical and Laboratory

2
Etretinate and Isotretinoin, Two Retinoids with Different Pharmacokinetic Profiles

U. PARAVICINI and A. BUSSLINGER

The development of vitamin A analogue compounds for use as therapeutic agents was mainly governed by the challenge to dissociate pharmacological effects from toxic side-effects, known as the hypervitaminosis A syndrome. According to groups of compounds with similar chemical structure within the general class of vitamin A analogues, Bollag[1] discriminates three generations of retinoids: (1) chemically modified molecules of retinoic acid (including isomeric compounds), (2) retinoids, in which the β-Ionone ring of retinoic acid is exchanged by various other ring systems (e.g. aromatic rings), and (3) analogues with different forms of cyclizations particularly of the polyene side chain.

Two retinoids which meet both properties of a high therapeutic index and a good therapeutic effect – representatives of the first and second generation – have reached particular importance in the therapy of certain dermatological diseases: etretinate (Tigason), an aromatic retinoid, showing excellent effect in severe, generalized psoriasis[2-4] and isotretinoin (Roaccutane, 13-*cis*-retinoic acid) which has dramatic effects in cystic acne.[5-7]

Both compounds are shown in Figure 1. Together with the endogenous metabolite of vitamin A, the all-*trans*-retinoic acid[8] and their main metabolites,[9-11] they have been both subject to extensive investigational effort, including clinical pharmacokinetics and metabolism.

In the light of new experimental data about tissue distribution of etretinate, it seems justifiable to summarize and discuss pharmacokinetic profiles of both drugs.

RETINOID THERAPY

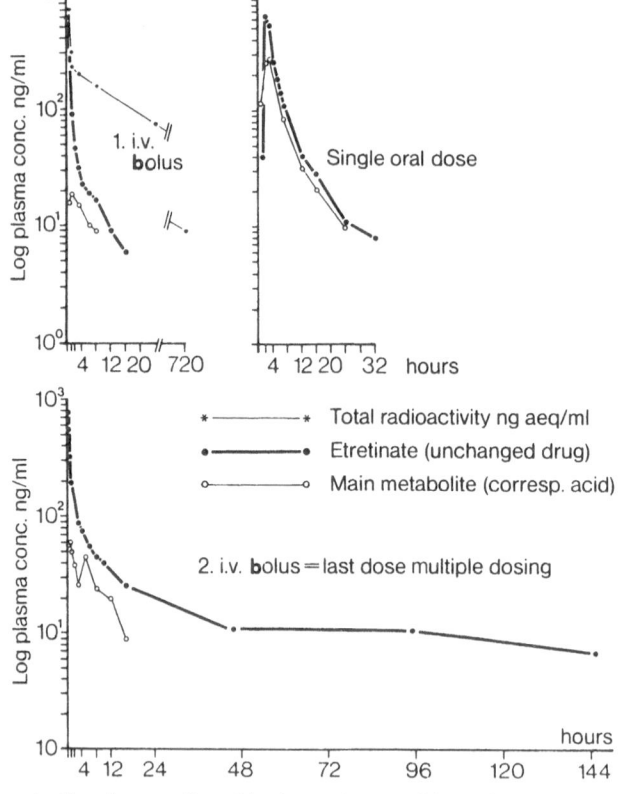

Retinoic Acid
(Vitamin A Acid)

Etretinate

Isotretinoin

RO 10-1670

4-oxo-Isotretinoin

Figure 1. Structures of retinoic acid and two of its analogues, etretinate and isotretinoin, with their main metabolites.

Figure 2. Concentration time profiles of both etretinate and its main metabolite following an i.v. bolus (10mg) before and after a multiple dose regimen of 2 weeks as well as after a single oral dose (100mg).

12

Etretinate

Early pharmacokinetic studies with single oral and intravenous doses to volunteers provided plasma concentration vs. time profiles for etretinate, which could be well described with a linear three compartment model.[9] Simultaneous fitting of oral and i.v. data was possible. The mean half-life of elimination was 7.3 h. Peak plasma concentrations between 400 and 1600 ng/ml were reached within 2–3 h.

Absolute bioavailability of the clinical formulation showed high variability ranging from 30 per cent to 70 per cent compared to an intravenous dose. Threshold of detection (5–10ng/ml) in plasma following a single 100mg dose to volunteers was generally reached at 24–36 h, using a HPLC-assay.[12-14] The concentration profile after an i.v. bolus at the end of a 2 – week daily oral dosing, however, was not predictable using the single dose data. Concentrations were measurable over more than 144 h compared to approximately 16 h after a single dose (Figure 2).

The suggestion, that the drug could slowly return from a deep peripheral to the central compartment, was confirmed by the slow decline of etretinate plasma concentrations after cessation of a chronic therapy to psoriatic patients. In Figure 3 the mean concentrations of etretinate and its main metabolite (Ro 10-1670) in plasma of three patients during the last 7 days of a chronic therapy and 140 days after discontinuation of the drug are plotted. It is noteworthy that 4 months after the last dose the threshold of detection was still not reached. A rigorous pharmacokinetic analysis was

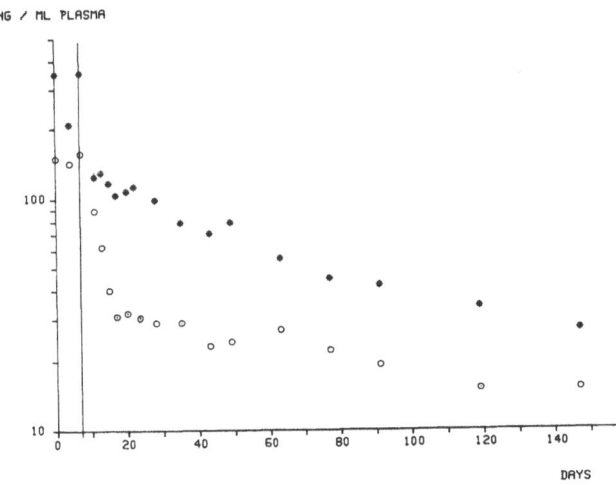

Figure 3. Mean concentrations of etretinate (*) and its main metabolite Ro 10-1670 (⊙) in the plasma of three patients who were on chronic etretinate therapy (cumulated dose 10–18g). The figure shows C_{min} values during the last 7 days of treatment and concentrations up to 140 days after cessation of therapy.

13

not possible, since it could not be decided whether or not the slope of the regression line through the concentration points of the last 3 months represented the half-life (80–100 days) of the very terminal elimination phase. In order to overcome this lack of information, a multicentre retrospective study was conducted, in which 197 patients on etretinate were involved.

Patients were chosen in such a manner that the time span between

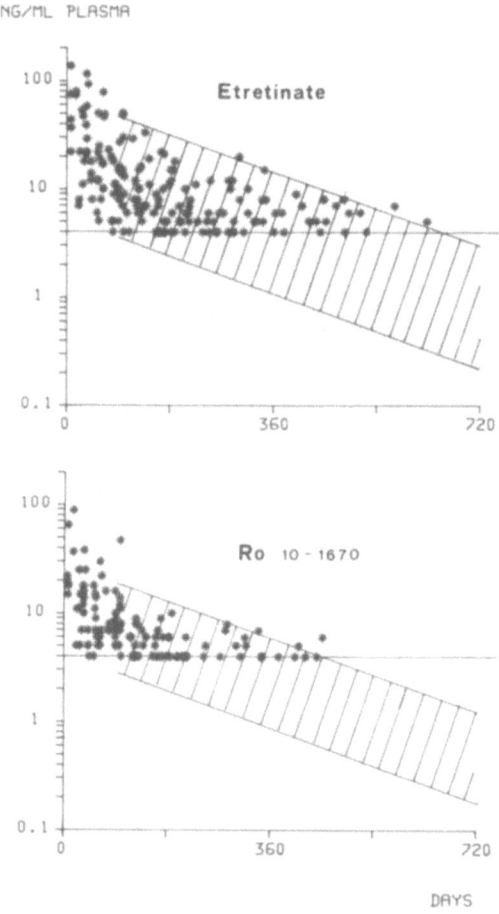

Figure 4. Concentrations of etretinate (upper part) and its main metabolite Ro 10-1670 (lower part) in the plasma of 197 patients who had terminated etretinate therapy at different times before blood samples were taken for analysis. The horizontal line at the 4ng/ml level indicates the threshold of detection. The hatched area is an arbitrary expansion of the measurable concentrations below the threshold of detection to give an idea of the distribution of all the concentration values. The number of concentration points in the figure represents only about 50 per cent and 35 per cent of the number of totally analysed samples for etretinate and Ro 10-1670 respectively. The slope of the decline curve is determined by visual assessment.

14

cessation of therapy and the etretinate determination in the plasma (1–2 points per patient) were evenly distributed over 2 years. In Figure 4 plasma concentrations are plotted against time.

50 per cent and 35 per cent of the total number of samples, which had been analysed for both parent drug and main metabolite (Ro 10-1670) respectively, are represented by the plotted points. The rest of the concentration values, which were below the theshold of detection, are indicated by the hatched area, which is drawn according to visual assessment. From 120 to 360 days 50 per cent of the etretinate concentrations were below the detection limit, and from the measurable values ($n = 144$) only 8 per cent were in the range of 15–33ng/ml. In the second year, 85 per cent of the values were below detection limit and measurable values did not exceed 9ng/ml.

For Ro 10-1670 both the number of detectable concentrations as well as the absolute values are considerably smaller.

From this study the following conclusions can be drawn:

(1) Within the first half-year after cessation of therapy with etretinate, its plasma concentrations are falling to levels which cannot be correlated to a pharmacological or toxic effect.

(2) After the first half-year, concentrations are steadily decreasing beyond the limit of detection. The parallel declining of Ro 10-1670 values on a lower level suggests formation limitation of the metabolite half-life of elimination.

(3) The elimination half-life, determined in the previous study (80–100 days) does not therefore represent the terminal elimination phase.

Although the available plasma data cannot be described with a rigorous pharmacokinetic model, that would in general allow predictions of plasma concentrations for any multiple dosing regimens, they strongly point to the existence of a deep compartment. Its physiological substrate, however, remained unknown. Vitamin A is physiologically stored in the liver.[15,16] We therefore speculated that this may be true for etretinate as well, although there are indications from rat studies that the drug is not stored in the liver lipocytes.[17]

In order to prove this hypothesis, liver biopsy samples from a group of patients, who were involved in a clinical trial for investigation of potential hepatotoxicity[18] of etretinate, were analysed for their concentration of etretinate and Ro 10-1670 at the end of a 6 months daily dosing.

Table 1 shows the mean values of two histological groups. It is apparent that normal liver tissue cannot be a specific storage site for etretinate, for concentrations on one hand are comparable to those observed in plasma (1.3μg/g) during therapy. On the other hand they are two to three hundred times smaller than those of vitamin A under physiological conditions.[15,16]

In fatty degenerated livers, however, etretinate concentrations are significantly higher ($5.4\mu g/g$), an indication for fat being a storage site. No Ro 10-1670 was found in the liver specimens.

The suggestion that etretinate may be stored in fatty tissue was confirmed by subsequent concentration measurements in pieces of fat from patients who were on etretinate therapy. Normal tissue samples from biopsy, autopsy and in one case from liposarcoma were analysed. In two cases of autopsy, additional samples from liver and brain were included. Blood samples were taken simultaneously as far as possible.

Table 2 shows the concentrations of etretinate and Ro 10-1670 for different organs together with the respective time which has elapsed between the last dose and the sample taking. Cumulated etretinate dose ranged from approximately 3 to 8g. Etretinate in general shows two orders of magnitude higher concentrations in different kinds of fatty tissue than in plasma. It was, therefore, not unexpected that even several months after cessation of therapy remarkably high concentrations of etretinate were still found.

This was the case not only in patients with a decreased liver function, where the values were very high, but also in a case of a normal liver. No etretinate was detectable either in the liver or in the brain of the patient who died 5 months after cessation of etretinate without any signs of disturbed liver functions, whereas etretinate was found in a patient with massive liver damage. Again Ro 10-1670 was not detectable in any of the tissue samples.

Assuming a total mass of body fat of 15kg with an etretinate concentration of $10\mu g/g$, the amount of etretinate in the body is approximately 150mg, corresponding to 2.5 per cent of the cumulated dose during an 8 months daily dosing with 25mg.

Although these data are insufficient to provide any information about the time course of etretinate in the fatty tissue, they strongly support the plasma concentration time profile data.

In the context of potential toxicity of this compound, the question arises

Table 1. Liver biopsy samples of patients undergoing etretinate therapy were analysed for etretinate and Ro 10-1670. Concentrations in fatty livers were significantly higher than in normals ($p < 0.0025$).

Degree of fatty degeneration	N	Liver tissue wet weight ($\mu g/g$)	
		Etretinate	Metabolite Ro 10-1670
Normal/mild	11	1.3 ± 0.8	0
Moderate/severe	6	5.4 ± 3.8	0

Table 2. Concentrations of etretinate and its main metabolite Ro 10-1670 in different kinds of tissue from patients who were on etretinate therapy. Tissue samples were either from biopsy or autopsy.

Liver function	Elapsed time since etretinate stop	Plasma		Fat		Liver		Brain	
		Etretinate	Metabolite Ro 10-1670	Etretinate	Metabolite Ro 10-1670	Etretinate	Metabolite Ro 10-1670	Etretinate	Metabolite Ro 10-1670
normal	under therapy	0.074	0.035	4	0	–	–	–	–
normal	under therapy	0.21	0.074	9 Liposarcoma 24	0	–	–	–	–
normal	under therapy	0.046	0.028	Subcutaneous 6	0	–	–	–	–
normal	5 months	–	–	7	0	0	0	0	0
	7 months	0.182	0.112	71	0	3.2	0	0.34	0
	6 days	–	–	42	0	–	–	–	–

μg/g tissue wet weight or μg/ml plasma

as to whether displacement from the fat may play a role. This question cannot be answered definitively without information about the binding in the fatty tissue. The high lipophilicity of the ethyl ester etretinate, however, speaks in favour of a non-specific binding. In this case a displacement by other drugs seems rather unlikely, because of the large capacity of the fat to bind lipophilic drugs. In the case of increased fat catabolism, one could, however, imagine that a higher rate of release into the plasma could take place, leading to higher plasma concentrations. Toxic levels could only be expected when the amount of totally stored etretinate is released into the systemic circulation within a very short time. This is unlikely to happen.

In plasma, etretinate is bound more than 98 per cent to proteins, to which lipoproteins contribute more than 75 per cent.[19-21]

Overall, the pharmacokinetic profile of etretinate is complex and prediction of plasma levels, in particular, during the time after long-term therapy remains unsatisfactory.

Simple linear pharmacokinetic models are not useful for the prediction of etretinate plasma levels at time points which lie several months or more than a year beyond the last dose and which are in general close to or below the threshold of detection.

Instead, more emphasis should be put on the fact that, under normal conditions, etretinate is released from its binding sites into the blood such that concentrations are far below values where any pharmacological or toxic effects have ever been observed.

An apparent elimination half-life of 80–100 days is acceptable as approximation for the practical clinical use of the drug. It must, however, be pointed out, that, in particular for late phases of etretinate elimination, the fact that concentrations in plasma are below detection limit does not mean that no drug is present any more in the body. The real half-life of elimination is still not known.

Isotretinoin

13-*cis*-retinoic acid (isotretinoin, Roaccutane), a retinoid from the first generation, has pharmacokinetically less problems than etretinate. In order to make a comparison of the pharmacokinetic profiles of the two retinoids possible, we shall briefly review the main points from the literature without going into details.[22,23]

The drug is well observed from its clinical dosage form after oral administration, leading to peak concentrations in the blood (after an 80mg single dose)[24] ranging from 180 to 459ng/ml at 1–6 h (Figure 5). The absolute bioavailability, estimated from dog studies, was 25 per cent. Biodegradation in the gut lumen and extensive presystemic first-pass clearance are suggested to be the reason for this apparently low value. 4-oxo-

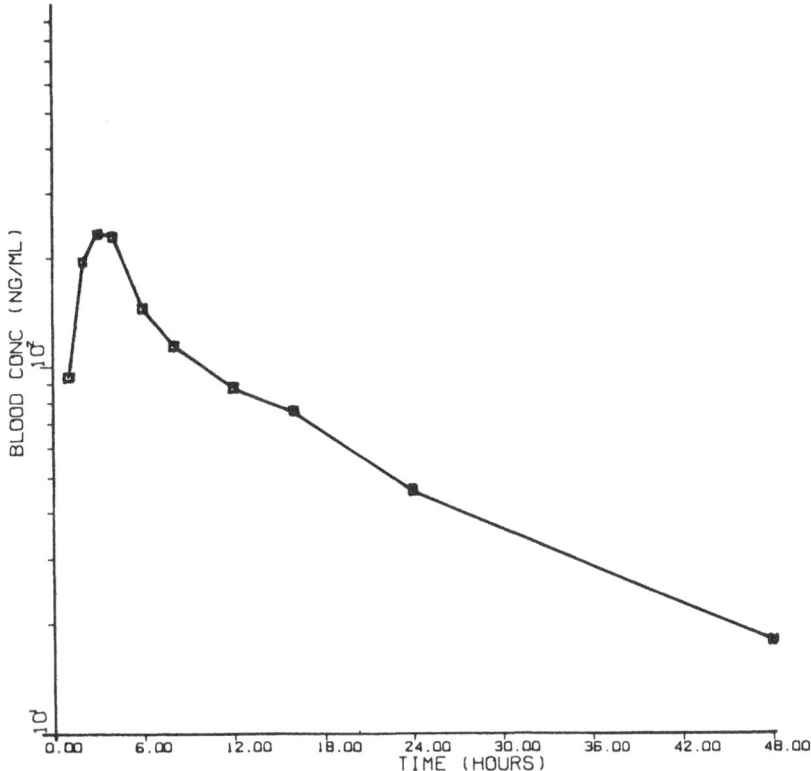

Figure 5. Mean blood concentrations of isotretinoin following the oral administration of 80mg isotretinoin as two 40-mg capsules to 15 normal volunteers. (From Brazzell, R.K. *et al.* (1982). *J. Am. Acad. Dermatol.*, **6**, 643.)

isotretinoin has been shown to be the main metabolite in human blood.[23] Tretinoin (retinoic acid) and its 4-oxo-metabolite have been detected in concentrations close to the threshold of detection in the blood of patients undergoing isotretinoin therapy. These compounds are possible metabolites of isotretinoin.

Isotretinoin is in the therapeutic concentration range linearly 99.9 per cent bound to plasma albumin. The blood concentration profile of isotretinoin after a single oral dose in man can well be described using a linear two-compartment model with first order absorption following a lag time of approximately 0.5 h. The terminal elimination half-life is in general between 10 and 20 h (Figure 5). The metabolite 4-oxo-isotretinoin shows a different blood concentration profile (Figure 6). Maximum concentrations ranging from 87 to 399μg/ml following a single oral 80mg dose of isotretinoin to patients occurred between 6 and 20 h after admini-

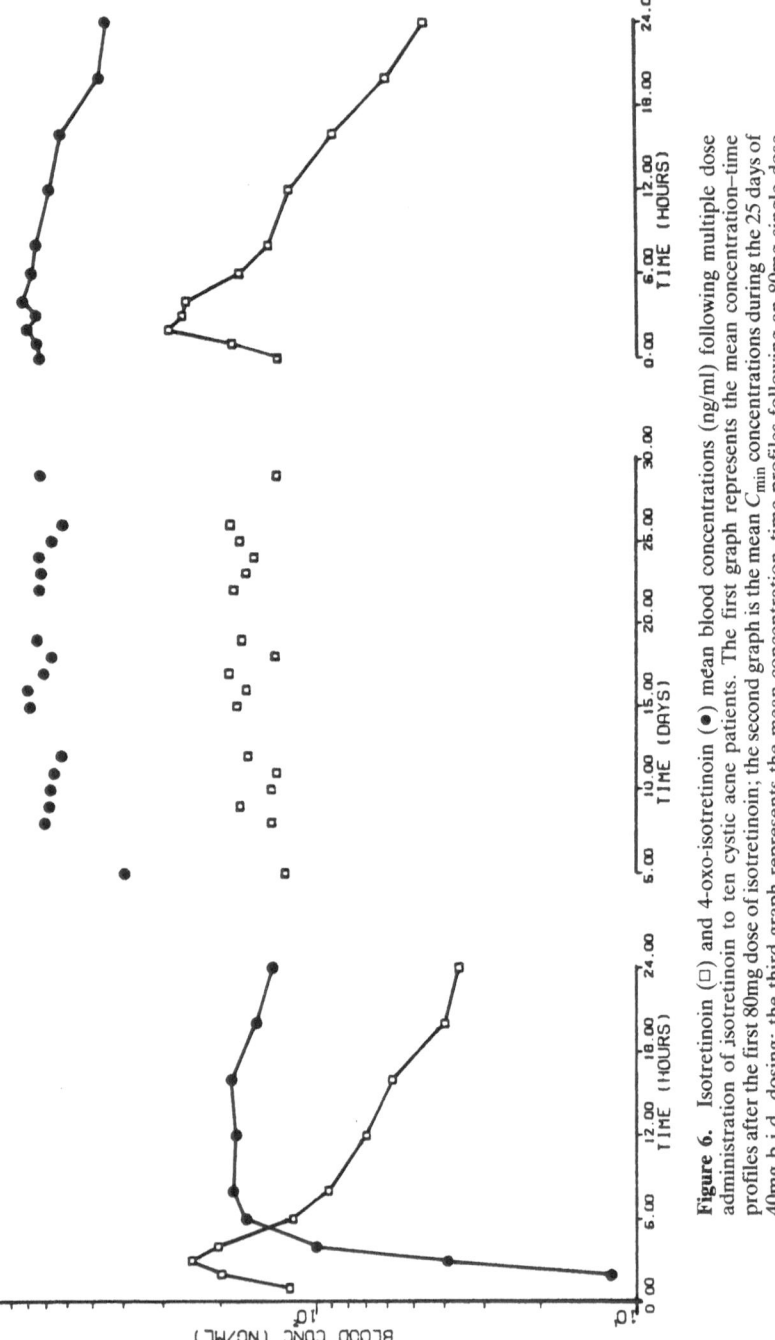

Figure 6. Isotretinoin (□) and 4-oxo-isotretinoin (●) mean blood concentrations (ng/ml) following multiple dose administration of isotretinoin to ten cystic acne patients. The first graph represents the mean concentration–time profiles after the first 80mg dose of isotretinoin; the second graph is the mean C_{min} concentrations during the 25 days of 40mg b.i.d. dosing; the third graph represents the mean concentration–time profiles following an 80mg single dose administered 12 h after the last 40mg b.i.d. dose. (From Brazzell, R.K. *et al.* (1982). *J. Am. Acad. Dermatol.*, **6**, 643)

stration.[23] Its blood concentrations were usually higher than those of the parent drug from the 6th hour on and declined more slowly with a half-life ranging from 11 to 50 h. On multiple dosing, the metabolite should accumulate more than the parent drug, but the AUC_0^∞ ratios between metabolite and parent drug after the first and the last dose of a multiple dosing regimen should be equal, if linear pharmacokinetic theory holds, which was confirmed by the results of multiple dose studies.

Biliary excretion, a common way of elimination for retinoids as well as enterohepatic recycling of isotretinoin, was studied comparing the blood concentration profiles for isotretinoin, the total ^{14}C blood data and the total ^{14}C excretion values for bile, urine and faeces following oral ^{14}C-isotretinoin doses to male volunteers with and without a biliary T-tube. From these studies it was suggested that enterohepatic circulation may take place.

In two clinical studies the multiple dose pharmacokinetics of isotretinoin was investigated. In one study cystic acne patients were dosed during 25 days with 40mg b.i.d., starting 5 days after a 80mg dose and ending with another 80mg dose. Figure 6 shows the corresponding mean blood concentrations of isotretinoin and its main metabolite. In another study patients who were on isotretinoin therapy for their dyskeratinizing diseases after a discontinuation for 2–3 weeks restarted therapy for 28 days with a subsequent final dose. The mean half-lives of elimination of isotretinoin after the first as well as after the last dose were in good agreement with those from single dose studies in normal people.

From both studies, which represented two groups of patients, it could be concluded that pharmacokinetics did not change during multiple dosing. The linear pharmacokinetic model, which was derived from single dose studies, allows us to predict plasma concentrations of both parent drug and metabolite during and after multiple dosing.

Concluding Comparative Remarks

Etretinate and isotretinoin, although vitamin A analogues and therefore suggestive of showing similar properties in many respects, are two quite different drugs. They are not only representatives of two different generations of retinoids, but they also show different therapeutic and pharmacokinetic profiles. The profiles of side-effects (hypervitaminosis A syndrome, teratogenicity), however, are similar.

Etretinate, an ethyl ester, is more lipophilic than its main metabolite, the analogue carboxylic acid or isotretinoin, another carboxylic acid. This property may be responsible for its high affinity to fatty tissue in the body and hence for the prolonged phase of elimination. This kind of pharmacokinetic behaviour coupled with potential teratogenicity clearly is a disadvantage in treatment of women who must avoid pregnancy during the year following discontinuation of etretinate therapy.

Linear pharmacokinetics of isotretinoin with the relatively short half-life of elimination and the lack of evidence for a deep compartment makes therapeutic handling easier.

References

1. Bollag, W. (1983). Vitamin A and retinoids: from nutrition to pharmacotherapy in dermatology and oncology. *Lancet*, 1, 860
2. Jablonska, S., Wolska, H., Dąbrowski, J., Haftek, M., Groniowska, M. and Jarząbek-Chorzelska, M. (1981). Aromatic retinoids in psoriasis: clinical, histological, histochemical, electron-microscopical and immunological investigations. In Orfanos, C.E. *et al.* (eds.). *Retinoids: Advances in Basic Research and Therapy.* pp. 165–173. (Berlin, Heidelberg, New York: Springer-Verlag)
3. van der Rhee, H.J. and Polano, M.K. (1981). Treatment of psoriasis vulgaris with a low-dosage Ro 10-9359 (Tigason) orally combined with corticosteroids topically. In Orfanos, C.E. *et al.* (eds.). *Retinoids: Advances in Basic Research and Therapy.* pp. 193–199. (Berlin, Heidelberg, New York: Springer-Verlag)
4. Lassus, A. (1980). Systemic treatment of psoriasis with an oral retinoic acid derivatic (Ro 10-9359). *Br. J. Dermatol.*, 102, 195
5. Peck, G.L., Olsen, T.G., Yoder, F.W., Strauss, J.S., Downing, D.T., Pandya, M., Butkus, D. and Arnaud-Battandier, J. (1979). Prolonged remission of cystic and conglobate acne with 13-*cis*-retinoic acid. *N. Engl. J. Med.*, 300, 329
6. Landthaler, M., Kummermehr, J., Wagner, A., Nikolowski, J. and Plewig, G. (1981). Effects of 13-*cis*-retinoic acid on sebaceous glands in humans. In Orfanos, C.E. *et al.* (eds.). *Retinoids: Advances in Basic Research and Therapy.* pp. 259–266. (Berlin, Heidelberg, New York: Springer-Verlag)
7. Jones, D.H., Cunliffe, W.J. and Cove, J.H. (1981). 13-*cis*-retinoic acid in acne (A double-blind study of dose response). In Orfanos, C.E. *et al.* (eds.). *Retinoids: Advances in Basic Research and Therapy.* pp. 255–258. (Berlin, Heidelberg, New York: Springer-Verlag)
8. De Luca, H.F. (1979). Retinoic acid metabolism. *Fed. Proc.*, 38, 2519
9. Paravicini, U., Stöckel, K., MacNamara, P.J., Hänni, R. and Busslinger, A. (1981). On metabolism and pharmacokinetics of an aromatic retinoid. *Ann. N.Y. Acad. Sci.*, 359, 54
10. Hänni, R., Bigler, F., Vetter, W., Englert, G. and Loeliger, P. (1977). Der Metabolismus des Retinoids Ro 10-9359. Isolierung und Identifizierung der Hauptmetaboliten aus Plasma, Urin und Faeces des Menschen sowie aus der Galle der Ratte. Synthese von drei Urinmetaboliten. *Helv. Chim. Acta*, 60, Fasc. 7, 2309
11. Vane, F.M. and Buggé, C.J.L. (1981). Identification of 4-oxo-13-*cis*-retinoic acid as the major metabolite of 13-*cis*-retinoic acid in human blood. *Drug Metab. Dispos.*, 9, 515
12. Paravicini, U. and Busslinger, A. (1983). Determination of etretinate and its main metabolite in human plasma using normal phase high performance liquid chromatography. *J. Chromatogr. Biomed. Applic.* (In press)
13. Palmskog, G. (1980). Determination of plasma levels of two aromatic retinoic acid analogues with antipsoriatic activity by high-performance-liquid chromatography. *J. Chromatogr.*, 221, 345
14. Besner, J.G., Meloche, S., Leclaire, R., Band, P. and Mailhot, S. (1982). High-performance-liquid chromatography of Ro 10-9359 (Tigason) and its metabolite Ro 10-1670 in human plasma. *J. Chromatogr.*, 231, 467
15. Hoppner, K., Phillips, W.E.J., Murray, T.K. and Campbell, J.S. (1968). Survey of liver vitamin A stores of Canadians. *Can. Med. Assoc. J.*, 99, 983
16. Smith, B.M. and Malthus, E.M. (1962). Vitamin A content of human liver from autopsies in New Zealand. *Br. J. Nutr.*, 16, 213

17. Jnouye, T., Minick, O., Grubbs, C., Moon, R. and Kent, G. (1978). Hepatic lipocytes and storage of vitamin A analogues. *Fed. Proc.*, 37, **299**, Abstr. No. 468
18. Roenigk, H.H. Jr., Sparberg, M., Yokoo, H. and Glazer, S. (1981). Ro 10-9359 in psoriasis prospective liver biopsy study of potential hepatotoxicity. In Orfanos, C.E. *et al.* (eds.). *Retinoids: Advances in Basic Research and Therapy.* pp. 375–381. (Berlin, Heidelberg, New York: Springer-Verlag)
19. Vahlquist, A., Michaëlsson, G., Kober, A., Sjöholm, J., Palmskog, G. and Pettersson, U. (1981). Retinoid-binding proteins and the plasma transport of etretinate (Ro 10-9359) in man. In Orfanos, C.E. *et al.* (eds.). *Retinoids: Advances in Basic Research and Therapy.* pp. 109–116. (Berlin, Heidelberg, New York: Springer-Verlag)
20. Gross, E.G., Zech, L.A., McClean, S.W., Ruddell M.E., DiGiovanna, J.J. and Peck, G.L. (1982). Differential binding of synthetic retinoids to beta-lipoproteins. *Clin. Res.*, **30**, 587
21. Lauharanta, J. (1981). Vitamin A transport complex during treatment with an oral aromatic retinoid (Ro 10-9359). *Acta Derm.-Venereol.*, **61**, 264
22. Brazzell, R.K. and Colburn, W.A. (1982). Pharmacokinetics of the retinoids isotretinoin and etretinate. *J. Am. Acad. Dermatol.*, **6**, 643
23. Vane, F.M., Stoltenberg, J.K. and Buggé, C.J.L. (1982). Determination of 13-*cis*-retinoic acid and its major metabolite, 4-oxo-13-*cis*-retinoic acid, in human blood by reversed-phase high-performance liquid chromatography. *J. Chromatogr.*, **227**, 471
24. Khoo, K.C., Reik, D. and Colburn, W.A. (1982). Pharmacokinetics of isotretinoin following a single oral dose. *J. Clin. Pharmacol.*, **22**, 395

3
Experience with Etretinate in the UK

M. HAZELL and R. MARKS

Etretinate has been in use in Cardiff since May 1978, and the aim of this study was to re-assess the use of etretinate based upon this experience and to determine whether our findings were similar to those in other centres in the UK. We were particularly interested to record the degree of acceptance of the drug by the patients, the toxic and side-effects experienced, and the comparison by dermatologists and patients of etretinate to other treatments. For this purpose we have reviewed our own patients and surveyed the experience of others.

The Cardiff Study

More than 100 patients have been treated with etretinate in Cardiff in the 5 years we have used the drug, and a special clinic was set up to review as many of these as possible. We were eventually able to interview and examine 66 patients. In addition, sufficient information was obtained for analysis in a further 14 patients by means of a detailed questionnaire, which was correlated with the clinical records of all patients. The conditions treated with etretinate are shown in Table 1.

In an attempt to evaluate the effectiveness of treatment, two methods were used. In the first, the patients were asked to indicate on 10cm analogue scales the state of the skin at the time of interview, immediately prior to treatment, and the state of their skin at its best whilst taking etretinate (Figure 1). Each patient acted as his own control in completing the analogue scales, as the limits of the scale were determined by the state of that patient's skin when completely clear at one end, and at its worst ever at the other. The degree of improvement was ascertained by measuring the

Table 1. Conditions treated with etretinate.

Psoriasis	Ichthyoses		Disorders of keratinization		Miscellaneous	
39	ADI	5	Darier's disease	4	Acne	2
	X-linked	2	PRP	2	Lichen planus	2
	Epidermolytic		Tylosis	2	Keloid	1
	hyperkeratosis	4	EKV	2	Solar keratoses	1
	Lamellar	3	Symmetrical			
	Follicular	2	progressive			
			erythrokerato-			
			derma	1		
	Undefined	5	Pachyonychia			
			congenita	1		
			Verrucous			
			naevus	1		
			Kyrle's disease	1		
39		21		14		6

0 cm   10 cm

Clear ————————————————————————— Worst ever

State of treated condition

(1) At time of assessment
(2) Prior to commencing etretinate
(3) At best whilst taking etretinate

Figure 1. Análogue scales.

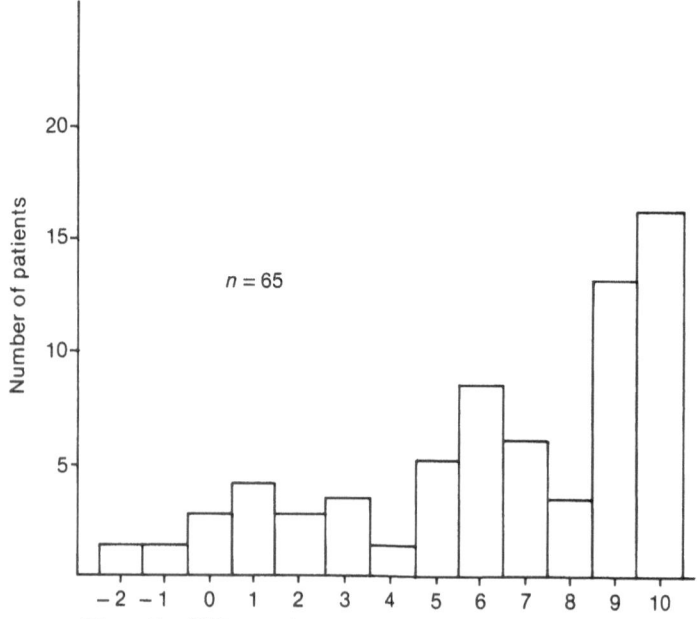

Figure 2. Difference between scales 2 and 3 on Figure 1.

Table 2. Effect of etretinate on treated condition: patient assessment.

		Number	Per cent
(1)	Cleared	10	14
(2)	Much improved	41	59
(3)	Moderate improvement	9	13
(4)	Unchanged	5	7
(5)	Worse	2	3
(6)	Much worse	3	4
Total		70	100

Table 3. Effect of etretinate on treated condition: investigator assessment.

		Number	Per cent
(1)	Cleared	14	20
(2)	Much improved	33	47
(3)	Moderate improvement	14	20
(4)	Unchanged	9	13
(5)	Worse	0	0
(6)	Much worse	0	0
Total		70	100

difference between the scores before and after treatment, giving the distribution shown in Figure 2. This was felt to be the most suitable means of assessing the improvements.

The second method of assessment was the completion of a simple questionnaire administered by the investigator, and the results are as shown in Table 2, most patients considering the treated condition to have cleared or improved. In order to verify this latter method, the investigator completed a similar assessment (Table 3), and the difference between the assessments made is shown in Figure 3. This demonstrates close agreement, with 64 of 70 paired statements being within one point on the assessment scale. These figures were broken down into the three main groups of conditions treated – psoriasis (Figure 4), the ichthyoses (Figure 5), and other disorders of keratinization (Figure 6), showing close agreement in psoriasis and the ichthyoses, but less with the other disorders of keratinization. With both the ichthyoses and the other disorders of keratinization there was a tendency for patients to overestimate the improvement with etretinate compared to the assessment of the investigator, possibly reflecting the ineffectiveness of previous treatments.

With regard to side-effects, we found the incidence shown in Table 4, which corresponds closely to the experience of others.[1,2] We found several unexpected side-effects, most notably gout in three patients (4 per cent – only one patient known to have the condition prior to treatment with etretinate) and an urticarial rash in two patients (3 per cent) (Table 5).

The laboratory parameters showing the most marked changes on treat-

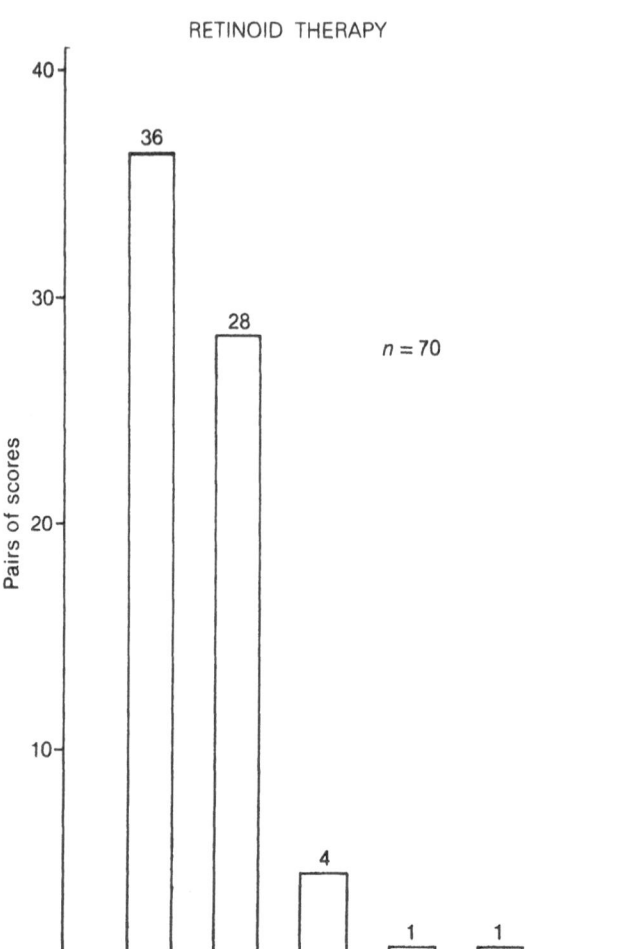

Figure 3. Difference between patient and investigator scores.

ment with etretinate were the liver function tests (Table 6) and fasting lipids (Table 7). Table 7 shows some overall increase in the post-treatment levels of fasting lipids but relatively few changes from the normal to the abnormal range. Most other investigators who have described their experience with oral retinoids have recorded similar findings with etretinate[3-5] but greater increases with isotretinoin.[2,4] Very few patients developed abnormal liver function tests while on treatment.

Patients were asked to make an overall assessment of the drug, taking into consideration both its effect on the condition being treated, and side-effects. The results are shown in Table 8, 79 per cent of patients classing the drug as good or excellent.

Although the numbers available for analysis were small, patients were

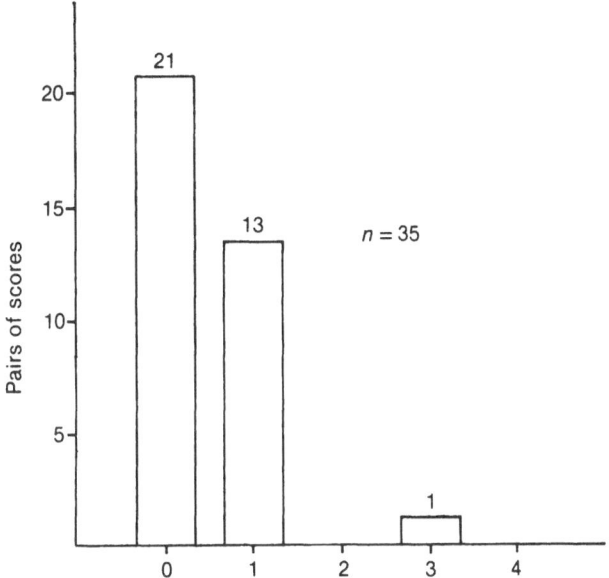

Figure 4. Difference between patient and investigator scores – psoriasis.

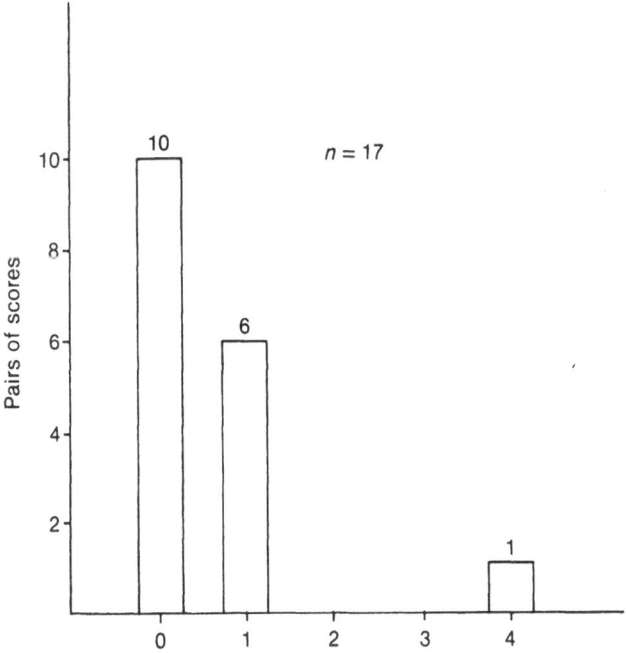

Figure 5. Difference between patient and investigator scores – ichthyoses.

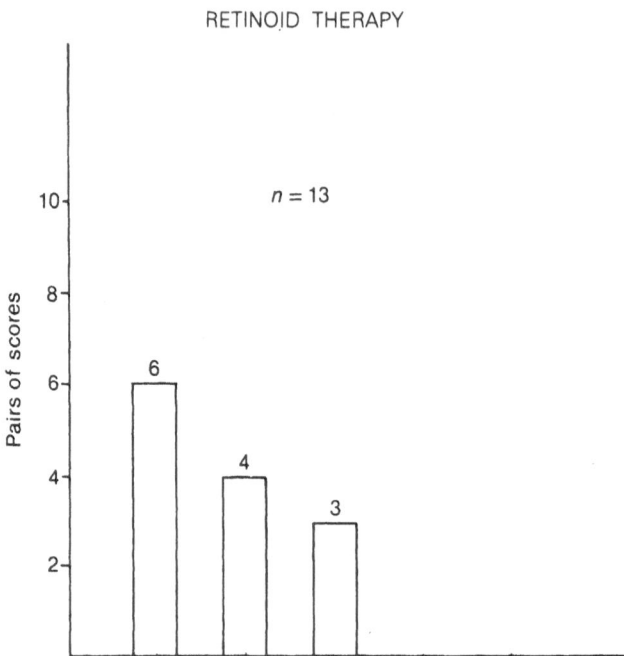

Figure 6. Difference between patient and investigator scores – other disorders of keratinization.

Table 4. Side-effects in 80 patients.

	Number	Per cent
Sore/dry lips	76	95
Sore/dry nose	44	55
Hair loss	43	54
Peeling palms/soles	29	36
Dry eyes	23	29
Paronychia	14	17.5
Epistaxes	9	11
Itching	6	7.5
Eczema	5	6
Nails affected	5	6
Sticky skin	4	5
Arthropathy	1	<1

Table 5. Uncommon side-effects ($n = 80$).

	Number of patients
Gout	3
Urticaria	2
Raynauds	1
Nausea/vomiting	1
Tinnitus	1

Table 6. Laboratory parameters: liver function tests $(n = 54)$.

	Alkaline phosphatase		AST	
	Number	Per cent	Number	Per cent
Increased >20 per cent	20	37	16	29.6
Increased >50 per cent	4	7.4	13	24
Increased >100 per cent	1	1.9	2	3.7
Changed from normal to abnormal	4	7.4	2	3.7

Table 7. Laboratory parameters: fasting lipids $(n = 45)$.

	Triglycerides		Cholesterol	
	Number	Per cent	Number	Per cent
Increased >20 per cent	8	17.8	12	26.7
Increased >50 per cent	12	26.7	7	15.5
Increased >100 per cent	4	8.5	1	2.2
Changed from normal to abnormal	9	20	3	6.7

Table 8. Overall assessment of drug by patient.

		Per cent	Number
(1)	Excellent	43	30
(2)	Good	36	25
(3)	Indifferent	13	9
(4)	Poor	8	6
(5)	Terrible	0	0
Total		100	70

Table 9. Treatment comparison. Etretinate vs. dithranol.

		Number
(1)	Much better	7
(2)	Better	1
(3)	No better	1
(4)	Worse	0
(5)	Much worse	0
Total		9

Table 10. Treatment comparison. Etretinate vs. MTX.

		Number
(1)	Much better	4
(2)	Better	1
(3)	No better	2
(4)	Worse	1
(5)	Much worse	0
Total		8

asked to compare etretinate to the most effective alternative treatment they had used, and Tables 9 and 10 show the results for the comparisons with dithranol and methotrexate respectively.

Survey

In October 1981, etretinate was licensed for use in hospitals in the UK, and to obtain a broader view of the use, and usefulness, of the drug, a questionnaire was sent to 65 per cent of the practising dermatologists in Great Britain. We were particularly interested in ascertaining the overall usage of the drug, the conditions being treated, the age of the patients being treated (especially its use in children) and the incidence of side-effects. Dermatologists were also asked to compare its usefulness to other available treatments.

Of the 130 questionnaires sent out, we received 106 replies, of which 102 contained numerical data – a gratifying compliance rate of 81.5 per cent! The majority of dermatologists replying (67 of 102: 66 per cent) had treated from four to 25 patients, the overall experience of each dermatologist being

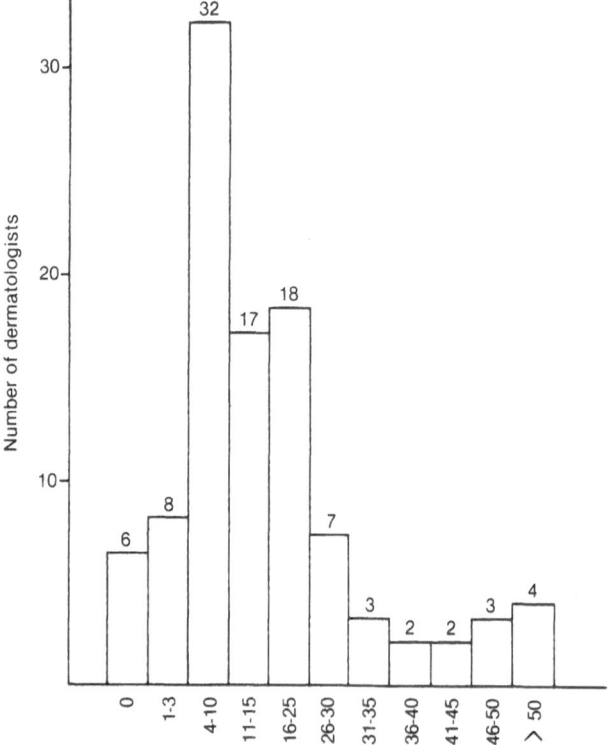

Figure 7. Number of patients treated.

Table 11. Treatment of different disorders as a proportion of each physician's experience (Mean ± SD) ($n = 74$).

	Per cent±SD
Severe plaque type psoriasis	36±23
Erythrodermic psoriasis	8±12
Pustular psoriasis	25±21
Autosomal dominant ichthyosis	1±3
X-linked ichthyosis	1±3
Bullous ichthyosiform erythroderma	3±6
Non-bullous ichthyosiform erythroderma	3±6
Other ichthyotic disorders	2±6
Erythrokeratoderma variabilis	1±2
Darier's disease	9±14
Pityriasis rubra pilaris	4±10

Table 12. Other diseases treated.

	Number of patients
All palmo-plantar keratodermas	37
Acne	31
Warts	14
All porokeratosis	6
Premalignant and malignant epidermal lesions	10
Bullous disorders	5
Lichen planus	6
MF and Sezary's syndrome	9

shown in Figure 7. The disorders treated most commonly, expressed as a proportion of each physician's total experience, are shown in Table 11, with disorders treated less commonly being listed in Table 12.

From the general comments made on the questionnaires, etretinate was considered useful in recalcitrant psoriasis (29 comments), in pustular psoriasis (18 comments), not useful in ordinary psoriasis (16 comments), but useful in combination with other treatments (14 comments). Referring to ichthyotic disorders and Darier's disease, etretinate was deemed excellent,

Table 13. Main advantages of etretinate.

	Number of times comment made
'Oral treatment', ease of treatment	28
Efficacy for Darier's disease	6
Efficacy for ichthyotic disorders	10
Efficacy for pustular psoriasis	8
Efficacy in combination treatments for psoriasis	10
Efficacy in intractable psoriasis	8
Relative absence of serious side-effects	5
General efficacy	6

(20 comments) or useful (16 comments) in the ichthyoses, and excellent, good or useful in Darier's disease (17 comments).

The stated main advantages of etretinate are shown in Table 13 and the main disadvantages in Table 14. Table 15 shows the incidence of the main side-effects reported. These are not very different from our own figures (Table 4) or the experience of others. Table 16 shows the less common side-effects reported.

Of 95 dermatologists replying to the question, 26 had stopped the drug in none of the patients under treatment, 53 in 6–30 per cent of patients in whom treatment had been started, and ten had stopped treatment in 31–50 per cent.

Table 14. Main disadvantages.

	Number of comments made
Mucosal side-effects	21
Teratogenicity	24
Hyperlipidaemia	20
Long-term safety	9
'Side-effects'	28
Cost	5
Loss of hair	2
Long half-life	2
Other side-effects	5
Lack of efficacy in psoriasis	5
'Lack of efficacy'	6
Unpredictable response	4

Table 15. Side-effects.

	Mean per cent±SD
Drying and cracking of lips	88.7±19.7
Loss of hair	20.3±20.8
Generalized pruritis	6.3±16.4
Abnormal skin sensitivity	7.1±11.3
Peeling of palms and soles	22.4±27.3
Abnormal skin stickiness	2.6±11.9

Table 16. Other side-effects.

	Number of replies
Nose bleeds	6
Eye complaints	8
Headaches, dizziness, lassitude, 'funny feeling'	7
Skin fragility	2
Facial redness or rash	4
Worsening of psoriasis or pain in lesions	4
'Hair like golliwog', 'eyebrows sticking out'	2
Gastrointestinal (nausea, diarrhoea)	3

Table 17. Comparison with other treatments.

Etretinate more or less useful than	More	Less	Equal	No. of replies
PUVA	7	49	16	34
Methotrexate	13	56	10	27
Tar regime	16	53	4	33
Dithranol	7	64	6	29

Comparing etretinate with other treatments, Table 17 shows the figures for PUVA, methotrexate, tar and dithranol, with etretinate being considered less useful than each by a majority of those replying. It is interesting to compare these figures to those in Tables 9 and 10, which relate to patient preferences.

The limitations of this type of investigation must be remembered when interpreting information obtained by means of a questionnaire. Inaccuracy of recall, the differing criteria for diagnosis and response, and the fact that incomplete compliance and response to the questionnaire may allow the formation of a biased group for analysis, may permit inaccuracies. However, there are also advantages to the technique, especially its ability to give an overall view of trends and experience by supplying a great deal of information rapidly. It may also be the only way of obtaining sufficient information concerning the relative prevalence of toxic side-effects and its use in less common disorders.

Based on the patients reviewed in Cardiff and the experience of many others in the United Kingdom, we believe that the following conclusions can be drawn.

In psoriasis, etretinate is most likely to find a place in the management of those patients with severe, extensive disease, relapsing rapidly after topical treatments. Furthermore, the results indicate that it is most appropriate for patients with pustular and erythrodermic psoriasis. It seems of particular use in patients with recalcitrant pustular psoriasis of the palms and soles. In addition, patients requiring systemic therapy, but who are unsuitable for, or unable to tolerate other drugs, may benefit from etretinate therapy.

In the ichthyoses and other disorders of keratinization, etretinate is the only effective treatement for severely affected individuals, but patients with bullous ichthyosiform erythroderma may experience an exacerbation of blistering when on the drug and may prefer a hard carapace to the tender skin beneath.

There appears to be a place for the use of maintenance treatment with etretinate, at lower doses, in patients with unstable or rapidly relapsing psoriasis who have been significantly improved by standard doses. If long-term therapy is contemplated the possibility of as yet unknown toxic side-effects must be kept in mind. Although our own experience is small, it does appear from the results of the survey that many dermatologists are struck by the usefulness of etretinate in combination with PUVA or dithranol. There appears to be an excellent therapeutic response from these 'combination regimens' and the dose of PUVA is much reduced. In addition, those patients substantially improved by etretinate, but experiencing troublesome side-effects on standard doses, may be able to continue on smaller doses, and maintain worthwhile improvement, with reduction in the severity of side-effects.

In summary, we have reported the effect of etretinate treatment in a number of disorders, as assessed by both the patient and the investigators, and compared our experience with that of nearly two thirds of the consultant dermatologists in the UK. We have found that the incidence of side-effects in our patients and in those of the dermatologists surveyed are similar in nature and incidence to those reported by others.[1,2] In addition we found a 4 per cent incidence of gout in our patients whilst taking the drug, and noted two patients who ascribed a persistent urticarial rash to the drug. The abnormal laboratory parameters we report also accord with those previously reported.[3-5]

Our conclusions concerning the use of etretinate are similar to those of others.[6,7] Etretinate is an important addition to the treatment of severe psoriasis and a striking advance in the management of patients with severe disorders of keratinization.

Acknowledgements

We would like to thank all those dermatologists who gave their time to reply to our questionnaire, and also our patients, who have often travelled long distances, and also given generously of their time, to attend our clinics.

References

1. Lassus, A. (1980). Systemic treatment of psoriasis with an oral retinoid acid derivative (Ro 10-9359). *Br. J. Dermatol.*, **102**, 195
2. Windhorst, D.B. and Nigra, T. (1982). General toxicology of oral retinoids. *J. Am. Acad. Dermatol.*, **6**, 657
3. Glazer, S.D., Roenigk, H.H., Yokoo, H. and Sparberg, M. (1982). A study of the potential hepatotoxicity of etretinate used in the treatment of psoriasis. *J. Am. Acad. Dermatol.*, **6**, 683
4. Gollnick, H., Schwartzkopff, W., Luley, G. and Orfanos, C.E. (1982). Alterations of lipid metabolism under treatment with oral retinoids (isotretinoin and etretinate). In Farber, E.M., Cox, A.J., Nall, L. and Jacobs, P.H. (eds.). *Psoriasis*. pp. 479–485. (New York: Grune & Stratton)
5. Orfanos, C.E., Mahrle, G., Goerz, G., Happle, R., Hofbauer, M., Landes, E. and Schimpf E. (1979). Laboratory investigations in patients with generalized psoriasis under oral retinoid treatment: a multicentre study of computerized data. *Dermatologica*, **159**, 62
6. Guilhou, J.J., Michel, B. and Meynadier, J. (1981). Treatment of severe psoriasis by

Ro 10-9359. In Orfanos, C.E. *et al.* (eds.). *Retinoids: Advances in Basic Research and Therapy.* pp. 483–486. (Berlin, Heidelberg, New York: Springer-Verlag)

7. Marks, R., Finlay, A. and Holt, P.J.A. (1981). Severe disorders of keratinization: effects of treatment with Tigason (etretinate). *Br. J. Dermatol.*, **104**, 667

4
The Treatment of Children with Etretinate

J.G. van der SCHROEFF and H.J. van der RHEE

Introduction

The synthetic retinoids etretinate and isotretinoin are widely applied in dermatology and it can be expected that these drugs will be administered to many children with disorders of keratinization or psoriasis. Despite the greater therapeutic index of these synthetic retinoids in comparison with vitamin A, many side-effects correspond to the features of vitamin A intoxication. Chronic hypervitaminosis A in children may cause several serious symptoms, among which are retardation of growth and premature closure of epiphyseal plates.[1,2] Recently, Milstone et al.[3] reported the case of a 10-year-old boy who developed abnormal bone remodelling and premature partial closure of the epiphyses during treatment with isotretinoin. To our knowledge, no such reports exist for etretinate. Only limited information is available on the safety of long-term treatment of children with synthetic oral retinoids. Van der Rhee et al.[4] regularly measured the height and urinary hydroxyproline excretion in five children during treatment with etretinate. No signs of growth retardation were found for the treatment periods studied (varying between 11 and 17 months). Tamayo and Ruiz-Maldonado[5] concluded from their experience with 30 children that long-term treatment with etretinate (up to 42 months) did not interfere with growth and development.

During the past 5½ years, 19 children with various skin disorders were treated at the outpatients clinic in Leiden with etretinate for prolonged periods. The clinical data with regard to therapeutic results, side-effects and growth are the subject of this report.

Patients and Results of Treatment

Between 1977 and 1983, 19 children (eight boys and eleven girls) with
psoriasis vulgaris, erythrokeratodermia variabilis, xeroderma pigmentosum, Sjögren-Larsson syndrome and lamellar ichthyosis were treated
with etretinate. The age at the onset of therapy ranged from 4 to 14 years
(mean 8.9 years). After a short initial treatment period, etretinate was
administered for maintenance treatment at an average dose of 0.6mg/kg
body-weight (range: 0.3–1mg/kg). The duration of treatment varies
between 8 and 66 months (mean 33.3 months). The patients with psoriasis
vulgaris received additional therapy with topical corticosteroids (patients
1, 3, 4, 5, 6, 8, 9 and 10) or anthralin (patients 2 and 7).

Detailed information about the patients and the results of treatment are
given in Table 1.

Side-Effects

The patients hardly complained about side-effects. Nevertheless, eight
patients suffered from mild cheilitis, one patient complained about pruritus
and one patient noticed transient hair loss. In particular, none of the
patients complained about painful bones or joints.

Laboratory Investigations

For four patients an abnormal but transient rise of serum alkaline
phosphatase levels was found. Determination of iso-enzyme patterns
revealed that the hepatic fraction was increased in these cases. Transient
elevations of serum lactic dehydrogenase and SGOT were observed in two
patients with elevated and in one patient with normal alkaline phosphatase
levels. Calcium and phosphate levels in serum showed no significant
alterations. Serum triglyceride and cholesterol levels remained within the
normal range during treatment.

Growth and Development

During etretinate therapy, height and body-weight were measured
regularly. Both height and weight remained in the respective percentile for
each patient. Patients 7 and 10 deserve special attention, since both
patients developed arrestment of growth due to topically applied corticosteroids before the onset of retinoid treatment. During treatment with
etretinate, however, growth was re-established at a practically normal rate
for these patients.

From 12 patients, roentgenograms of the left hand were examined at

Table 1. Clinical data from children treated with etretinate.

Patients	Sex/age (years)	Diagnosis	Maintenance dosage (mg/kg)	Duration of treatment (months)	Therapeutic results
1	F/11	psoriasis	0.5	23	moderate
2	M/8	psoriasis	1.0	26	excellent
3	F/12	psoriasis	0.7	37	good
4	F/7	psoriasis	0.5	34	good
5	F/10	psoriasis	0.7	8	good
6	F/9	psoriasis	0.3	66	good
7	M/5	psoriasis	1.0	48	moderate
8	M/13	psoriasis	0.3	16	excellent
9	F/12	psoriasis	0.6	53	good
10	F/4	psoriasis	1.0	33	good
11	F/4	EKV*	0.8	17	good
12	M/10	EKV*	0.5	61	excellent
13	F/10	EKV*	0.6	62	good
14	M/10	XP†	1.0	8	**
15	F/8	XP†	0.8	8	††
16	M/5	XP†	1.0	29	**
17	F/14	S–L‡	0.5	53	good
18	M/10	S–L‡	0.5	31	good
19	M/7	lamellar ichthyosis	0.7	19	good

*erythrokeratodermia variabilis
†xeroderma pigmentosum
‡Sjögren–Larsson syndrome
**Since onset of therapy no malignant skin tumours were observed.
††During etretinate therapy two squamous cell carcinomas and one basal cell carcinoma developed.

various stages during treatment for assessment of bone age. Except for patient 7, who developed a corticosteroid-induced growth inhibition prior to etretinate therapy, the bone age of all patients remained in accordance with the calendar age. No radiographic signs of osteoporotic changes were observed. Normal development of secondary sexual characteristics occurred for the patients at pubertal age during treatment.

Comments

Treatment with etretinate was successful for most of our patients. The advantage of combined therapy with etretinate and topical corticosteroids, namely reduction of both corticosteroid and retinoid dosage,[6] also applies to the treatment of children with psoriasis vulgaris. The efficacy of etretinate in the treatment of ichthyosiform skin disorders is well known.[5,7,8] Prevention of malignant skin tumours in patients with xeroderma pigmentosum is a promising aspect of etretinate therapy.[9] Nevertheless, one of our patients developed two squamous cell carcinomas and one basal cell carcinoma during therapy.

The treatment was well tolerated by the children. It is remarkable how infrequently side-effects of etretinate therapy are reported by the children. The transient disturbances of hepatic function tests occurring in some of the patients are part of the well-known features of retinoid therapy in adults.[10] The most reassuring finding was that growth and development of the children was not hampered by long-term treatment with etretinate. No discrepancies were found between bone age and calendar age, which indicates that skeleton maturation was not influenced by retinoid treatment. Since growth retardation by retinoids is only likely to occur at high dosage regimens, it is necessary to emphasize the need for low dosage therapy. It should be noted that probably one of the most important signs of damage to bone or cartilage by retinoids is pain in the extremities.[1-3] One cannot rely on elevations of alkaline phosphatase or calcium in serum, because serious skeletal deformities may occur at normal values.[3]

We conclude from the data reported thus far, and from the present results, that etretinate used in a relatively low dosage can be applied successfully and safely for the treatment of a variety of skin disorders in children. However, since the experience remains limited, regular performance of laboratory investigations and measurement of growth will be needed.

References

1. Pease, C.N. (1962). Focal retardation and arrestment of growth of bones due to vitamin A intoxication. *J. Am. Med. Assoc.*, **182**, 980
2. Ruby, L.K. and Mital, M.A. (1974). Skeletal deformities following chronic hypervitaminosis A. *J. Bone Jt. Surg.*, **56**, 1283
3. Milstone, L.M., McGuire, J. and Ablow, R.C. (1982). Premature epiphyseal closure in a child receiving oral 13-cis retinoic acid. *J. Am. Acad. Dermatol.*, **7**, 663
4. Van der Rhee, H.J., Van Gelderen, H.H. and Polano, M.K. (1980). Is the use of Ro 10-9359 (Tigason) in children justified? *Acta Dermato-Venereol. (Stockholm)*, **60**, 274
5. Tamayo, L. and Ruiz-Maldonado, R. (1981). Long-term follow-up of 30 children under oral retinoid Ro 10-9359. In Orfanos, C.E., Braun-Falco, O., Farber, E.M. Grupper, Ch., Polano, M.K. and Schuppli, R. (eds.). *Retinoids: Advances in Basic Research and Therapy.* pp. 287–294. (Berlin, Heidelberg, New York: Springer-Verlag)
6. Van der Rhee, H.J., Tijssen, J.G.P., Herrmann, W.A., Waterman, A.H. and Polano, M.K. (1980). Combined treatment of psoriasis with a new aromatic retinoid (Tigason) in low dosage orally and triamcinolone acetonide cream topically: a double-blind trial. *Br. J. Dermatol.*, **102**, 203
7. Van der Schroeff, J.G. and Suurmond, D. (1981). Treatment of erythrokeratodermia variabilis with oral retinoid (Ro 10-9359). In Orfanos, C.E., Braun-Falco, O., Farber, E.M., Grupper, Ch., Polano, M.K., and Schuppli, R. (eds.). *Retinoids: Advances in Basic Research and Therapy.* pp. 295–301. (Berlin, Heidelberg, New York: Sringer-Verlag)

8. Jagell, S. and Lidén, S. (1983). Treatment of the ichthyosis of the Sjögren–Larsson syndrome with etretinate (Tigason). *Acta Dermato-Venereol. (Stockholm)*, **63**, 89

9. Braun-Falco, O., Galosi, A., Dorn, M. and Plewig, G. (1982). Tumorprophylaxe bei xeroderma pigmentosum mit aromatischem retinoid (Ro 10-9359). *Hautarzt*, **33**, 445

10. Orfanos, C.E., Mahrle, G., Goerz, G., Happle, R., Hofbauer, M., Landes, E. and Schimpf, A. (1979). Laboratory investigations in patients with generalized psoriasis under oral retinoid treatment. *Dermatologica*, **159**, 62

5
Austrian Experience with Etretinate

P. FRITSCH

Etretinate has been used by our group as an experimental drug since 1976 in more than 500 patients suffering from a spectrum of hyperkeratotic skin conditions and a few disorders of the dermal collagen. Our clinical experience has been presented in several reports;[1-12] it is largely in agreement with the numerous clinical studies which have been published in the past years by many, particularly European, groups. Today, the extraordinary therapeutic effects, the posology and side-effects of etretinate appear to be well known and accepted; in this paper, we therefore wish to express a few general views concerning the indications and limitations of etretinate, which have emerged from our experience with this drug.

Therapeutic Effects of Etretinate

Etretinate, being a synthetic aromatic retinoid, obviously shares a large part of the biological action spectrum of the whole class of compounds. Etretinate acts as well on epithelial as on mesenchymal tissues and may also be a potent modulator of immune and inflammatory functions. The understanding of the molecular events underlying its complex actions somewhat lagged behind the rapidly expanding clinical experience with etretinate; to characterize the therapeutic effect of this drug we still have to use wholesale terms, such as 'anti-keratinizing', 'differentiation promoting', 'anti-neoplastic', etc. In a number of disorders, e.g. pityriasis rubra pilaris or psoriasis, the therapeutic effect cannot be adequately explained on theoretical grounds. In others, e.g. pustular psoriasis, the rather unexpected excellent effectiveness promoted the detection of hitherto unknown properties of the compound (inhibition of chemotaxis). We feel that, by

45

using etretinate as a mere systemic keratolytic agent, we exploit but a restricted fraction of its potential uses and anticipate that more indications will arise in the future.

Non-specificity of the 'Anti-keratinizing' Properties of Etretinate

Etretinate induces complex changes of epidermal morphology and function including acanthosis, hyperproliferation, pertubation of epidermal cell glycosylation, dyshesion and premature shedding of the horny cells and impairment of the barrier function.[6,7,10] Horny cell dyshesion appears to be the major factor underlying the anti-keratinizing effect of this drug. As a rule, excessive horny material is removed by systemic administration of etretinate irrespective of the underlying cause, as demonstrated by the response of as different disorders as psoriasis, lichen planus, chronic discoid lupus erythematosus, actinic keratoses, ichthyoses, etc. Disorders bearing specific histological markers, such as Darier's disease or epidermolytic hyperkeratoses, invariably continue to exhibit their histological hallmarks despite clinical remission. Etretinate thus represents a powerful but – in this context – symptomatic and non-specific systemic keratolytic agent with little or no impact on the basic defect itself; substantial benefit can be clearly expected in disorders where excessive horn formation represents the major clinical feature; conversely, the net effect in conditions which express hyperkeratosis only as an associated feature depends on the underlying defect and can in fact be adverse.

Main Indications of Etretinate ('Drug of Choice')

For several hereditary hyperkeratotic skin diseases, etretinate emerged as the first dramatically effective therapeutic modality and has remained the drug of choice: erythrokeratodermia figurata variabilis,[1] Darier's disease,[2] lamellar ichthyosis (Figure 1) and a spectrum of ichthyosiform disorders. With appropriate doses, most patients can be brought to and kept in close to symptom-free states for as long as etretinate medication is continued. After withdrawal hyperkeratosis begins to reappear immediately. Patient compliance is usually excellent in severe cases, since the substantial benefit clearly outweighs the sometimes bothersome side-effects. In less severe cases, it may prove difficult to maintain a satisfactory equilibrium between the desired therapeutic effect and the symptoms of drug toxicity. For this reason, treatment should be considered only in instances where adequate relief cannot be attained with topical remedies alone. Therefore ichthyosis vulgaris, X-linked ichthyosis and milder forms of Darier's disease will rarely form an indication for etretinate therapy. The same strategy should be pursued in hereditary palmo-plantar keratoderma: substantial relief of

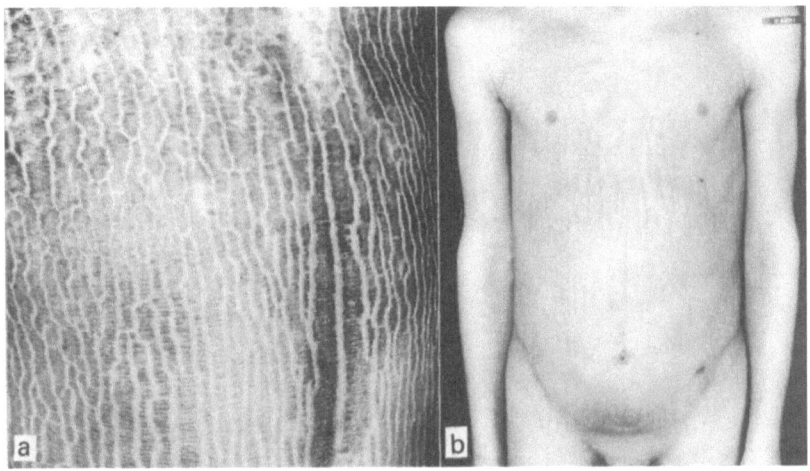

Figure 1. Lamellar ichthyosis is one of the principal indications of etretinate. This 12-year-old boy (a) acquired an almost normal appearance of his skin after 2 weeks of treatment (b).

subjective symptoms can be achieved in the papular and striate forms and mutilating palmo-plantar keratoderma (Figure 2), whereas little can be gained in the rather symptomless diffuse varieties.

Pityriasis rubra pilaris, particularly the juvenile form, is another 'ideal' indication for etretinate. In our experience, this notoriously recalcitrant condition responds to etretinate completely within a few weeks. Apparently, long-term treatment is not necessary since the defect is not genetically determined; up to now, relapses were not observed in three cases followed by us (observation period 1-3 years).

Psoriasis and Etretinate

Etretinate represents a major achievement in the treatment of psoriasis although the average case responds far less readily than the aforementioned dermatoses. In general, the response of psoriasis to etretinate monotherapy is somewhat disappointing and usually inferior to conventional topical therapy or photochemotherapy. After a rapid initial response in terms of disappearance of scaling, the lesions tend to persist for many months in most instances. Complete clearing after long-term treatment has been reported in approximately a quarter of the cases.[12,13] Despite this, etretinate represents an invaluable tool in psoriasis therapy since it transforms the psoriatic plaques to become exquisitely sensitive to most conventional treatment modalities. Oral photochemotherapy, initiated 1-2 weeks after onset of etretinate administration, leads to rapid clearing; etretinate reduces the UV-A energy requirements to achieve clearing by approximately

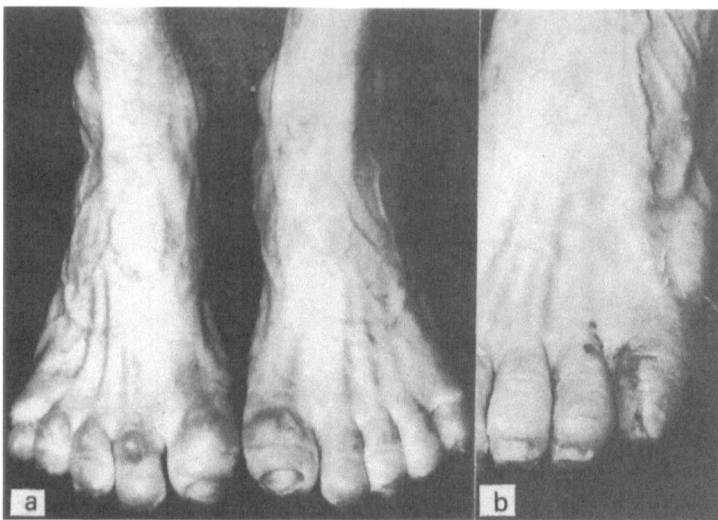

Figure 2. Removal of hyperkeratotic masses by etretinate may serve other than cosmetic purposes. This young man suffers from the mutilant type of hereditary palmo-plantar keratoderma. Note painful hyperkeratotic rings strangling both fifth toes which led to ischaemia and interfered with walking (a). After 3 weeks of etretinate treatment, the ring had disappeared and unimpaired function was restored (b).

50 per cent and permits to maintain the cleared state at lower energy requirements.[4,5,9] Similar augmentation can be achieved by combination of etretinate with UV-B therapy as well as with topical dithranol, tar and even corticosteroid preparations. The augmenting effect of etretinate is particularly advantageous in psoriasis of the scalp. The mechanism of etretinate augmentation is not fully understood but is likely to be, at least in part, related to the reduction of the horny layer.

Obviously, different mechanisms of action are operative in the often dramatic response of pustular psoriasis to etretinate, both of the generalized (Zumbusch) and localized types (Barber, Hallopeau). In our experience, the eruption of pustules ceases within 2–3 days after etretinate administration and a close to symptom-free state can be maintained with adequate maintenance doses. These, however, are not infrequently unacceptably high (>1mg/kg/day) necessitating additional photochemotherapy treatment. Etretinate has also been used as an adjunctive agent in psoriatic arthropathy with some success,[15,16] but appears significantly inferior in this indication to the third generation retinoid arotinoid.[17]

Factors Limiting the Use of Etretinate in Hyperkeratotic Skin Conditions

Functional Impairment

Removal of excessive horny material by etretinate can be more or less easily achieved in any hyperkeratotic skin disorder; this aesthetic benefit may, on the other hand, be linked to functional disadvantage, depending on the underlying basic defect. The skin of patients with epidermolytic ichthyosis, e.g., is less hyperkeratotic but much more fragile after etretinate therapy. This is even more obvious in the rare condition of epidermolytic palmo-plantar keratoderma. We treated four members of a family with this disorder[3] (Figure 3); in all patients, smooth, thin, almost normal appearing skin developed after 3 weeks of treatment, the patients being capable of perceiving sensation of touch and of temperature for the first time in their lives. Nevertheless, the drug had to be withdrawn in all patients due to easy blistering of their palms and soles which interfered with walking and working.

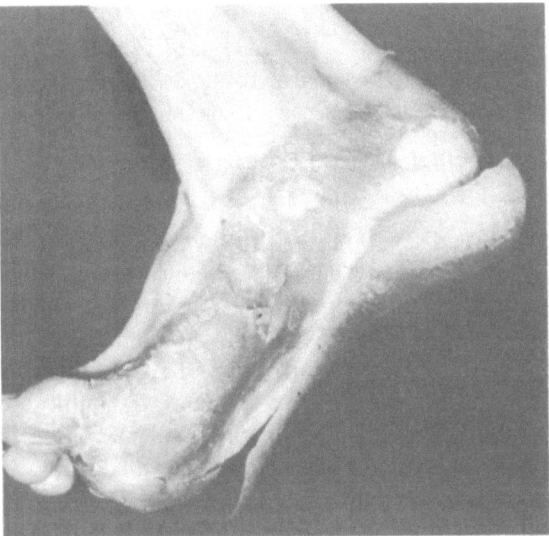

Figure 3. Removal of hyperkeratotic masses by etretinate may lead to functional impairment: in this patient with hereditary epidermolytic palmo-plantar keratoderma, the hyperkeratotic masses detached in one piece after 2–3 weeks of etretinate treatment. Increased blistering activity of the newly formed, seemingly normal sole skin necessitated withdrawal of the drug.

Enhancement of Inflammation and Ulceration

In a number of hyperkeratotic skin conditions with associated features of inflammation or a propensity to erosions and ulcers, the net effect of etretinate may in fact be adverse in face of successful keratolysis. In a case of generalized inflammatory linear verrucous naevus, etretinate improved the hyperkeratotic component of the disorder, but substantially worsened inflammation; the drug had to be withdrawn for severe pruritus (Figure 4). Erosive lichen planus of the mucous membranes may respond well to

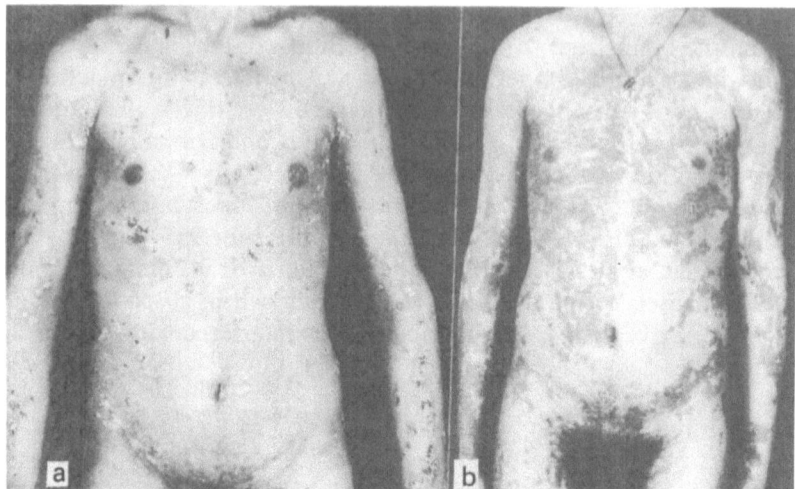

Figure 4. Etretinate may accentuate inherent inflammatory features of hyperkeratotic skin conditions. This patient with generalized linear verrucous inflammatory naevus (a) was cleared of his scaling but, at the same time, underwent considerable deterioration of inflammation (b).

etretinate; we observed several cases, however, in which the erosions rapidly became more extensive and painful. Initially minor mucosal and plantar erosions in one girl with pachyonychia congenita worsened considerably while finger and toe nails began to grow in an almost normal manner.

The most dramatic deterioration observed so far by us occurred in a case of Netherton's syndrome (ichthyosis linearis circumflexa, trichorrhexis invaginata, atopy). Following administration of etretinate (1mg/kg/day), the patient became erythrodermic within 4 days and developed burning and oozing erosions of his face and chest (Figure 5). The same occurred at a second try after an exposure to 10mg etretinate and, at a later date, an exposure to 10mg isotretinoin. Similar, if less severe, deterioration was noted in a second case. The mechanism underlying this unexpected reaction pattern is unclear: we suspect that it may be linked to the atopic disposition since atopic patients, as a rule, undergo flare-ups if treated with retinoids for unrelated causes.

Long-term versus Short-term use of Etretinate

Long-term application of etretinate is obviously necessary in genetically determined dermatoses. In these instances, benefits and long-term risks and disadvantages of this drug, particularly with regard to liver function, triglyceridaemia and bone remodelling (danger of premature epiphyseal closure in prepubertal children)[18] have to be carefully weighed. In contrast, short-term administration of etretinate can be performed more liberally

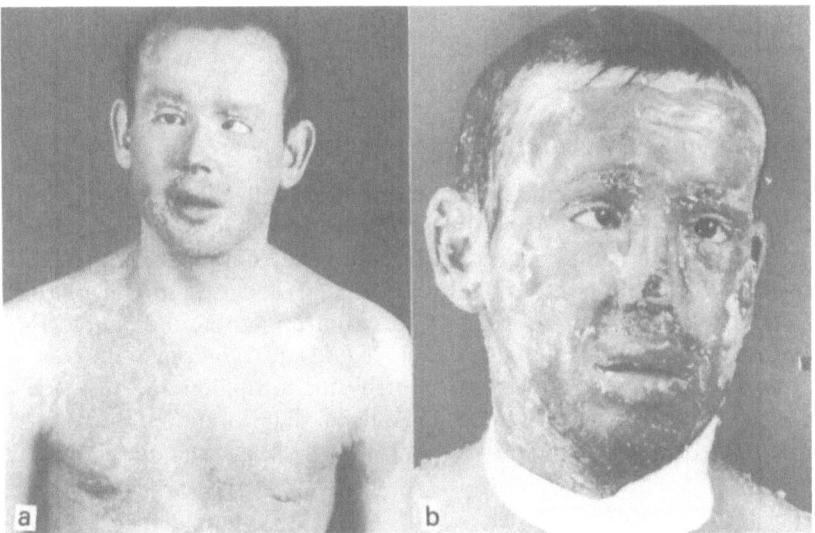

Figure 5. Atopic patients should not be treated with etretinate. This 23-year-old patient with Netherton's syndrome (a) experienced a dramatic flare-up following etretinate administration (b).

(doses at up to 1.5mg/kg for 2–3 weeks). Short courses of etretinate as an addition to conventional therapeutic measures can be of considerable help in the treatment of hyperkeratotic eczema, tylosis and even plane and plantar warts.

Anti-neoplastic Properties of Etretinate

This most fascinating and – in *in vivo* and *in vitro* models – extensively studied[19,20] activity of the retinoids has as yet found little clinical application. For obvious reasons, retinoids can hardly compete with conventional surgical treatment in the management of skin cancer. Keratoacanthomas may be an exception to this rule in certain instances because they usually respond readily[21] and pose lower risks in case of treatment failure.

In contrast, tumour prophylaxis appears to be an important and promising field for the the employment of retinoids. Emergence of new lesions can be prevented or at least slowed down in basal cell naevus syndrome,[22] Ferguson–Smith type keratoacanthomas[21] and xeroderma pigmentosum.[23] We have been currently treating a patient with xeroderma pigmentosum with relatively low doses of etretinate (25mg/kg/day) for almost 3 years. Before onset, she had developed more than 200 different skin tumours, mostly keratoacanthomas and actinic keratoses; after onset, development of new tumours essentially ceased except for a number of small, rapidly involuting superficial keratoacanthomas.[11] It must be emphasized, however, that also less satisfactory observations on etretinate treatment of xeroderma pigmentosum have been published.[24]

Etretinate in Recessive Dystrophic Epidermolysis Bullosa

Both all-*trans*- and 13-*cis*-retinoic acid inhibit collagenase production in cultures of synovial cells[25] and of skin fibroblasts.[26] Since increased collagenase activity has been implied in the pathogenesis of recessive dystrophic epidermolysis bullosa, retinoids have been suggested as a rational approach to this barely tractable disorder. We used etretinate in one patient for 7 months (1.8mg/kg/day) but were unable to find any significant improvement in terms of frequency and intensity of blister formation and the ease to elicit the Nikolski sign. After withdrawal, no deterioration occurred. Absorption of the drug was clearly efficient for the presence of desquamative cheilitis.[12]

Etretinate in Sclerosing Disorders

Other than their profound effects in the epidermis, retinoids also induce important changes of the dermal connective tissue which have only recently met attention. In fibroblast cultures, all-*trans*-retinoic acid decreases cell proliferation as well as protein synthesis, particularly of collagen, and increases the production of glycoaminoglycans.[27-30] Based on these reports, we investigated the effects of etretinate in an open, uncontrolled study on eight patients with linear scleroderma and eight patients with lichen sclerosus. In both groups the majority of patients failed to show unequivocal responses to treatment. Clearing occurred both in two patients with scleroderma and two with lichen sclerosus; since occasional spontaneous clearing cannot be ruled out in both of these disorders, etretinate cannot be recommended as first choice treatment in either, pending new clinical data.

Conclusions

In our experience, etretinate has emerged as a powerful and safe drug which has revolutionized the treatment of a broad spectrum of dermatoses, some of which have hitherto not been amenable to any kind of therapy. Etretinate is the drug of choice in a number of ichthyoses and ichthyosiform disorders, Darier's disease and pityriasis rubra pilaris; caution is recommended in hyperkeratotic disorders which are characterized by associated features of inflammation and a propensity for erosions. Atopic patients should be excluded from etretinate therapy. Etretinate in monotherapy is only moderately effective in psoriasis but conditions the psoriatic plaques to become exquisitely sensitive to most types of conventional treatment. As an 'anti-neoplastic' agent, etretinate plays an insignificant role in the therapy of manifest skin epitheliomas with the possible exception of keratoacanthomas; as a prophylactic agent, it is capable, however, of retarding or preventing the development of neoplasms in xeroderma pigmentosum and similar states of genetically determined tumour propensity. Despite clear influence on fibroblast growth and metabolism *in vitro*, no unequivocal therapeutic effect of etretinate was observed in disorders of the dermal collagen, such as recessive dystrophic epidermolysis bullosa, linea scleroderma and lichen sclerosus.

References

1. Fritsch, P.O. (1979). Erythroderatodermia figurata variabilis Mendes da Costa: erfolgreiche Behandlung mit einem oralen aromatischen Retinoid (Ro 10-9359). *Hautarzt*, **30**, 161
2. Hönigsmann, H., Fritsch, P. and Jaschke, E. (1978). Hypertroph verhornende Variante des Morbus Darier. Erfolgreiche orale Behandlung mit einem aromatischen Retinoid (Ro 10-9359). *Hautarzt*, **29**, 601
3. Fritsch, P., Hönigsmann, H. and Jaschke, E. (1978). Epidermolytic hereditary palmoplantar keratoderma. Report of a family and treatment with an oral aromatic retinoid. *Br. J. Dermatol.*, **99**, 561
4. Fritsch, P., Hönigsmann, H., Jaschke, E. and Wolff, K. (1978). Augmentation of oral Methoxsalen-photochemotherapy with an oral retinoic acid derivative. *J. Invest. Dermatol.*, **70**, 178
5. Fritsch, P., Hönigsmann, H., Jaschke, E. and Wolff, K. (1979). Photochemotherapy bei Psoriasis: Steigerung der Wirksamkeit durch ein orales aromatisches Retinoid. *Dtsch. Med. Wochenschr.*, **103**, 1731
6. Elias, P.M., Fritsch, P.O., Lampe, M., Williams, M.L., Brown, B.E., Nemanic, M. and Grayson, S. (1981). Retinoid effects on epidermal structure differentiation and permeability. *Lab. Invest.*, **44**, 531
7. Fritsch, P.O., Pohlin, G., Längle, U. and Elias, P.M. (1981). Response of epidermal cell proliferation to orally administered aromatic retinoid. *J. Invest. Dermatol.*, **77**, 287
8. Fritsch, P. (1981). Oral retinoids in dermatology. *Dermatology*, **20**, 314
9. Wolff, K. and Fritsch, P.O. (1982). Retinoid – PUVA photochemotherapy. In Farber, E.M., Cox, A.J., Nall, L. and Jacobs, P.H. (eds.). *Psoriasis*. pp. 211–219. (New York: Grune & Stratton)
10. Nemanic, M.K., Fritsch, P.O. and Elias, P.M. (1983). Perturbations of membrane glycosylation in retinoid-treated epidermis. *J. Am. Acad. Dermatol.*, **6**, 801
11. Pichler, E. and Fritsch, P. (1983). Xeroderma pigmentosum: Tumorprophylaxe mit Etretinat. *Hautarzt*. (In press)
12. Fritsch, P., Klein, G., Auböck, J. and Hintner, J. (1982). Letter to the Editor, *J. Am. Acad. Dermatol.*, submitted
13. Ott, F. (1977). Behandlung der Psoriasis mit einem oral wirksamen aromatischen Retinoid. *Schweiz. Med. Wochenschr.*, **107**, 144
14. Orfanos, C.E. and Goerz, G. (1978). Orale Psoriasis-Therapie mit einem neuen aromatischen Retinoid (Ro 10-9359). *Dtsch. Med. Wochenschr.*, **103**, 195
15. Stollenwerk, R., Rischer-Hoinkes, H., Komenda, K. and Schilling, F. (1981). Clinical observations on oral retinoid therapy of psoriatic arthropathy (Ro 10-9359). In Orfanos, C.E., Braun-Falco, O., Farber, E.M., Grupper, Ch., Polano, M.K. and Schuppli, R. (eds.). *Retinoids: Advances in Basic Research and Therapy*. pp. 205-209. (Berlin, Heidelberg, New York: Springer-Verlag)

16. Rosenthal, M. (1979). Retinoid in der Behandlung von Psoriasis-Arthritis. *Schweiz. Med. Wochenschr.,* **109**, 1912

17. Fritsch, P., Rauschmeier, W. and Neuhofer, J. (1983). Response of psoriatic arthropathy to arotinoid (Ro 13-6298): a pilot study. (In press)

18. Milstone, L.M., McGuire, J. and Ablow, R.C. (1982). Premature epiphyseal closure in a child receiving oral 13-*cis*-retinoic acid. *J. Am. Acad. Dermatol.,* **7**, 663

19. Bollag, W. (1975). Prophylaxis of chemically induced epithelial tumors with an aromatic retinoid acid analogue (Ro 10-9359). *Eur. J. Cancer.,* **11**, 721

20. Sporn, M.B. and Newton, D.L. (1979). Chemoprevention of cancer with retinoids. *Fed. Proc.,* **38**, 2538

21. Haydey, R.P., Reed, M.L., Dzubow, L.M. and Shupack, J.L. (1980). Treatment of keratoacanthomas with oral 13-*cis*-retinoic acid. *N. Engl. J. Med.,* **303**, 506

22. Peck, G.L., Gross, E.G., Butkus, D. and DiGiovanna, J. (1982). Chemoprevention of basal cell carcinoma with isotretinoin. *J. Am. Acad. Dermatol.,* **6**, 815

23. Braun-Falco, O., Galosi, A., Dorn, M. and Plewig, G. (1982). Tumorprophylaxe bei Xeroderma pigmentosum mit aromatischem Retinoid (Ro 10-9359). *Hautarzt,* **33**, 445

24. Schnitzler, L. and Verret, J.L. (1981). Retinoid and skin cancer prevention. In Orfanos, C.E., Braun-Falco, O., Farber, E.M., Grupper, Ch., Polano, M.K. and Schuppli, R. (eds.). *Retinoids: Advances in Basic Research and Therapy.* pp. 385–388. (Berlin, Heidelberg, New York: Springer-Verlag)

25. Brinckerhoff, C.E., McMillan, R.M Dayer, J.-M. and Harris, E.D. (1980). Inhibition by retinoic acid of collagenase prodaction in rheumatoid synovial cells. *N. Engl. J. Med.,* **303**, 432

26. Bauer, E.A., Seltzer, J.L. and Eisen, A.M.(1982). Inhibition of collagen degradative enzyme by retinoic acid *in vitro. J. Am. Acad. Dermatol.,* **6**, 603

27. Nelson, D.L. and Balian, G. (1983). The influence of retinoic acid on collagen synthesis by skin fibroblasts. *J. Invest. Dermatol.,* **80**, 357 (A)

28. Hein, R., Krieg, T., Müller, P.K. and Braun-Falco, O. (1983). Einfluß von retinoiden auf die Regulation der Kollagensynthese mesenchymaler Zellen. *Arch. Derm. Res.* (In press)

29. Lacroix, A., Anderson, G.D.L. and Lippman, M.E. (1980). Retinoids and cultured human fibroblasts. Effects on cell growth and presence of cellular retinoic acid-binding protein. *Exp. Cell Res.,* **130**, 339

30. Jetten, A.M., Jetten, M.E.R., Shapiro, S.S. and Poon, J.P. (1979). Characterization of the action of retinoids on mouse fibroblast cell lines. *Exp. Cell Res.,* **119**, 289

6
PUVA-Etretinate Therapy in Chronic Plaque and Palmar Plantar Pustular Psoriasis

C.M. LAWRENCE, J. MARKS, S. PARKER, P.R. COBURN and
S. SHUSTER

Introduction

PUVA is an effective treatment for chronic plaque psoriasis[1] (CPP) and palmar plantar pustular psoriasis (PPPP).[2] However, large doses of UVA and many PUVA treatments may be required to achieve clearance. Etretinate has some effect of CPP[3] and PPPP[4] but does not usually clear the rash completely. Several open studies combining PUVA with etretinate (PUVA-etretinate) have shown that this combination is effective in CPP[5,6] and may be useful in PPPP.[7] We have compared PUVA etretinate and PUVA-placebo in two randomized, double-blind studies of CPP and PPPP.

Patients and Methods

Thirty patients of skin types II and III, one of whom had previously been PUVA resistant, with CPP involving 20–40 per cent of total body surface, and 20 patients, 17 of whom gave a history of pustule formation, with PPPP currently being treated in the Dermatology Department of the Royal Victoria Infirmary, Newcastle-upon-Tyne, were recruited. The nature of the study was explained to them and they agreed to take part. Patients with abnormal renal or hepatic function, those under 18 years of age and women of childbearing age (unless they agreed to use an effective method of contraception during and for 1 year after the study) were excluded from entry. Patients were randomly allocated, double-blind, to either PUVA-etretinate or PUVA-placebo.

Etretinate

Etretinate or placebo was started 14 days before PUVA therapy as identical capsules in a single daily dose according to body-weight (CPP approx. 0.75mg/kg, PPPP approx. 1mg/kg).

PUVA

8–methyoxypsoralen (0.6mg/kg) was given 2 hours before UVA therapy. The starting dose was based on skin type. (Type I 1.5J/cm^2; Type II 2.5J/cm^2; Type III 3.5J/cm^2; Type IV 4.5J/cm^2.) PUVA was given three times a week. Doses were increased by 1J/cm^2 every third treatment if the patient failed to improve; burning was an indication for decreasing the dose or missing treatments as described elsewhere.[1]

Other Treatment

Emulsifying ointment was the only topical treatment used during the trial. Topical therapy and other drugs were stopped 4 weeks before entering the trial in CPP and 1 week in PPPP.

Assessment of Response

The total UVA dose, number of treatments and time taken to clear were noted. Clearance was achieved when less than 2 per cent of the body surface area was covered by plaques in CPP and when all the pustules had disappeared and there was only mild or absent scaling and erythema in PPPP. Those patients who had not cleared within 10 weeks of starting PUVA for CPP or 18 weeks for PPPP were considered to be treatment failures and PUVA-etretinate or PUVA-placebo was stopped.

In the patients with PPPP, erythema and scaling were scored from 0–3, and the total number of fresh pustules were counted before the trial and at weeks 10 and 20 or on clearing.

Investigations

In patients with CPP weekly full blood count, serum bilirubin, alkaline phosphatase, aspartate transaminase, and γ-glutamyl transferase were measured and pre- and post-treatment urea and electrolytes, thyroid function tests, fasting serum lipids and HDL cholesterol, and a hand X-ray with step wedge for densitometry were performed.[8]

In the patients with PPPP a full blood count, liver function screen, fasting lipids and cholesterol were measured before and at the end of the trial.

Results

28 of the 30 CPP patients and 19 of the 20 patients with PPPP completed

the trial. Two were withdrawn because of an unrelated intercurrent illness and another because of failure to attend.

Response to Treatment

Chronic Plaque Psoriasis (Table 1)

Table 1. Clearance data on 28 patients with chronic plaque psoriasis who completed the trial.

	Number of patients treated	Number of patients who cleared	Total UVA dose (J/cm²) to clear Mean ± SE	Number of exposures to clear Mean ± SE	Duration of treatment to clear (days)* Mean ± SE
Etretinate	15	14	62.1 ± 8.9	17.1 ± 1.7	40.3 ± 4.3
Placebo	13	9	77.3 ± 15.8	18.2 ± 2.1	49.4 ±6.7
			NS ($p>0.05$)	NS ($p>0.05$) NS ($p>0.05$)	NS ($p>0.05$)

*Excludes 14-day pre-PUVA period.

One patient failed to clear after 10 weeks PUVA therapy in the PUVA-etretinate group and four failed in the PUVA-placebo group ($p>0.05$ Fisher's exact test). The time, total cumulative UVA dose and number of treatments required to achieve clearance were all lower in the PUVA-etretinate group (Table 1) but the differences were not significant ($p>0.05$). The greater time to clear in the PUVA-placebo group as compared to the PUVA-etretinate group despite a similar number of PUVA exposures is due to temporary withdrawal of treatment due to burning and missed treatments due to holidays.

Palmar Plantar Pustular Psoriasis (Table 2)

All patients in the PUVA-etretinate group cleared compared with four treatment failures, after 18 weeks PUVA treatment, in the PUVA-placebo group ($p=0.03$ Fisher's exact test). There was a significant ($p<0.05$ Wilcoxon rank-sum test) reduction of the duration of treatment and the number of PUVA treatments required to clear in the PUVA-etretinate group compared with the PUVA-placebo group. The mean cumulative and final PUVA dose required to clear the rash was considerably reduced in the PUVA-etretinate group, but this did not achieve significance ($p<0.05$).

Pustule count fell to zero in all five patients in the PUVA-etretinate group who had pustules at the start of the trial. In the PUVA-placebo group, where six patients had pustules, counts fell to zero in three but three others still had numerous pustules at the end of the trial. Erythema and scale scores fell in nine of the ten PUVA-etretinate patients and six of the nine PUVA-placebo group ($p>0.05$ Fisher's exact test).

Table 2. Clearance data on 19 patients with hand and foot psoriasis who completed the trial.

	Number of patients treated	Number of patients who cleared	Total UVA dose (J/cm^2) to clear (Mean ± SE)	Final UVA dose (J/cm^2) to clear (Mean ± SE)	Number of treatments to clear (Mean ± SE)	Duration of PUVA treatment to clear (days) (Mean ± SE)
PUVA-etretinate	10	10	53.9 ±18.5	4.5 ± 0.7	13.1 ±2.9	30.3 ±7.1
PUVA-placebo	9	5	113.1 ± 33.4	6.1 ± 0.8	23.2 ± 4.2	59.2 ± 11.5
		$p=0.03$†	$p>0.05$* NS	$p>0.05$* NS	$p<0.05$*	$p<0.05$*

*Wilcoxon rank-sum test †Fisher's exact test

Side-Effects

Clinical

Table 3. Clinical side-effects in 28 patients with chronic plaque psoriasis who completed the study.

	Etretinate ($n = 15$)	Placebo ($n = 13$)
Dry cracked sore lips	13	7
Nausea	2	6
Dry mouth	5	6
Headaches	2	4
Hair loss	3	0
Itching	6	6
Palmo-plantar desquamation	3	1
Nose bleeds	0	0
Sore eyes	2	2
Loss of appetite	1	1
Thirst	0	2
Paronychia	0	1
Sweating	3	3
Drowsiness	2	3

The patients with CPP (Table 3) were asked to report on specific side-effects according to a check list handed to them at the end of the trial. This produced a much greater number of reported side-effects both in the etretinate and placebo group than those found in the PPPP patients who were asked about side-effects at each visit and at the end of the trial, without being prompted by a check list. Dryness and cracking of the lips occurred much more commonly in the etretinate group (Table 4), so that it seriously interfered with the double-blind nature of the trial. Hair

Table 4. Clinical side-effects in 19 patients with hand and foot psoriasis who completed the trial.

	PUVA-etretinate (n = 10)	PUVA-placebo (n = 9)
Cheilitis	6	0
Hair loss	4	0
Peeling skin	2	0
Itching	1	0
Dryness of nasal mucosa and nose bleeds	1	0
Nail softening	1	0
Nausea	0	1

loss occurred in seven of the 25 patients who received etretinate and was severe in three, two of whom first noticed hair loss after stopping etretinate. In no case did side-effects necessitate stopping treatment.

Haematological, Biological and Bone Density Measurements

Liver function tests, full blood count, bone density urea and electrolytes were unchanged. There was significant increase in fasting triglyceride levels in patients with PPPP treated with PUVA-etretinate.

Discussion

In CPP there was no significant benefit of adding etretinate to a PUVA regime; more patients cleared and the cumulative UVA dose, number of treatments and time to clear were less in the PUVA-etretinate group but none of these differences achieved statistical significance. This contrasts with the findings of other workers[5-7] who have shown a significant benefit of PUVA-etretinate over PUVA alone. These studies differed from ours in several respects: their patients were not randomly allocated;[6,7] in two studies[6,7] the patients were probably more severe than ours with more than 30–40 per cent surface involvement; PUVA was given four times a week instead of our three and the starting dose of UVA was different[5-7] which was partially due to the inclusion of patients of all skin types; the etretinate dose (1mg/kg) was higher[6,7] and it was started 4 days[7] or 4 weeks[5] before PUVA therapy. It is possible that we were using an unnecessary high dose of UVA with the etretinate although this was not apparent from the day-to-day erythemal response. A second possibility is that we used an insufficient dose of etretinate; this seems unlikely as other workers[5] have demonstrated a significant reduction of PUVA required to clear CPP with a similar dose. Lastly, it is still possible that the small differences noted would achieve significance if the trial was extended.

In PPPP our findings show that the inclusion of etretinate to a standard PUVA regime for PPPP significantly decreases the number of treatment failures and the time and number of treatments required to clear. The cumulative UVA dose was also less in the PUVA-etretinate group, although this was not statistically significant ($p>0.05$). These findings are similar to those of Fritsch et al.[7] although his patients required fewer treatments to clear (mean = 7 compared with 13 in our patients).

Side-effects due to etretinate were relatively common but did not necessitate withdrawal from the trial in any patient. Their characteristic features enabled the observer to identify those receiving etretinate and although patients could be allocated double-blind to either placebo or etretinate the trial could not be conducted in this way. The high rate of side-effects reported by the CPP PUVA-placebo group was probably due to the method of assessing them by questionnaire and it seems likely that the side-effects described by the patients with PPPP more accurately reflect the true incidence of side-effects due to etretinate. Hair loss was almost certainly due to etretinate and occurred in seven of the 25 patients treated. Although temporary, it was severe in three and upset the patients considerably.

In summary, unlike some other studies, we could not demonstrate a significant advantage of PUVA-etretinate over PUVA alone in CPP. In contrast, in PPPP we demonstrated a significant benefit of PUVA-etretinate over PUVA alone, more patients responding in a significantly faster time with less PUVA.

Acknowledgements

We should like to thank Dr A.J. Miller of Roche Products Ltd. for his assistance with the trial. Dr Parker was supported by the Newcastle Health Authority Research Committee.

References

1. Rogers, S., Marks, J., Shuster, S., Vella Briffa, D., Warin, A. and Greaves, N. (1979). Comparison of photochemotherapy and dithranol in the treatment of chronic plaque psoriasis. *Lancet*, **1**, 455
2. Murray, D., Corbett, M.F. and Warin, A.P. (1980). A controlled trial of photochemotherapy for persistent palmoplantar pustulosis. *Br. J. Dermatol.*, **102**, 659
3. Lassus, A. (1980). Systemic treatment of psoriasis with an oral retinoic acid derivative (Ro 10-9359). *Br. J. Dermatol.*, **102**, 195
4. Reymann, F. (1982). Two years experience with Tigason treatment of pustulosis palmo-plantaris and eczema keratoticum manum. *Dermatologica*, **164**, 209
5. Lauharanta, J., Juvakoski, T. and Lassus, A. (1981). A clinical evaluation of the effects of an aromatic retinoid and PUVA, and PUVA alone in severe psoriasis. *Br. J. Dermatol.*, **104**, 325
6. Grupper, C. and Berretti, B. (1981). Treatment of psoriasis by oral PUVA therapy combined with aromatic retinoid (Ro 10-9359; Tigason). *Dermatologica*, **162**, 404
7. Fritsch, P.O., Honigsmann, H., Jaschke, E. and Wolff, K. (1978). Augmentation of oral methoxsalen-photochemotherapy with an oral retinoic acid derivative. *J. Invest. Dermatol.*, **70**, 178
8. Anderson, J.B., Shimmins, J. and Smith, D.A. (1966). A new technique for the measurement of metacarpal density. *Br. J. Radio.*, **39**, 443

7
The Use of Tigason (Etretinate) in Darier's Disease

S. M. BURGE and J. D. WILKINSON

Introduction

This study was designed to establish the use of Tigason by a group of patients with Darier's disease. Eighteen patients with Darier's disease were treated with Tigason in 1980, in a study to establish the efficacy of the drug.[1] Seventeen out of 18 patients improved. A questionnaire was sent to this group to document their subsequent course, use of the drug and drug-related side-effects.

Results

The questionnaire was sent to 17 patients. One patient had died in 1980 after completing the initial study and one patient did not reply.

Of the remaining 15 patients, five patients were still taking Tigason regularly. One with severe disease took 50mg per day and two with severe disease took 25mg per day. Two with moderate disease took 25mg on alternate days. Several patients had raised triglycerides, but no other serious side-effects.

Three patients with either moderate or mild disease took prophylactic Tigason before a stimulus they knew would provoke their disease (e.g. sun exposure).

The remaining seven patients were not using Tigason because it "did not help"(2); the disease was so mild(3), or the side-effects were worse than the disease(2). These patients used emollients, weak steriods and sun-screens.

In summary, five out of 14 patients were still taking Tigason regularly; three out of 14 used the drug intermittently, and six no longer used the drug. The patients who were using the drug were all on a low dose (maximum 50mg per day) and did not find the side-effects a major problem.

In our original study, we stated that long-term therapy was likely to be necessary for most patients, but intermittent therapy may be appropriate for some patients. We recommended a dose of 50mg per day for most patients to reduce the incidence of side-effects. We do not know the effect of persistently elevated triglycerides, but none of the patients in this study had serious medical problems.

This long-term follow-up study supports the conclusions made in our initial paper and also demonstrates once more that patients with mild disease are unlikely to tolerate this treatment.

Reference

1. Burge, S.M., Wilkinson, J.D., Miller, A.J. and Ryan, T.J. (1981). The efficacy of an aromatic retinoid, Tigason (etretinate), in the treatment of Darier's disease. *Br. J. Dermatol.*, **104**, 675

8
Etretinate in the Ichthyosiform Erythrodermas

D.J. ATHERTON and R.S. WELLS

Introduction

The treatment of the more severe types of congenital ichthyosis represents a major problem in paediatric dermatology. Of these disorders the greatest difficulties are presented by bullous ichthyosiform erythroderma (syn. epidermolytic hyperkeratosis) and by non-bullous ichthyosiform eyrthroderma (syn. lamellar ichthyosis). Intensive topical therapy with emollients and keratolytics provides only limited and short-lived relief in the worst affected cases, and though high dosage oral vitamin A and later oral retinoic acid were definitely beneficial, this effect was nullified by the considerable toxicity of both agents. When etretinate became available, it was hoped that a superior therapeutic index would be achieved, and early reports[1,2] of its value in these ichthyoses were encouraging. As far as we are aware, all trials of etretinate in the ichthyoses have so far been conducted on an open basis, at least partly because the epithelial effects of the drug make it difficult to maintain strictly double-blind conditions. Another problem in trial design is the need for careful tailoring of the dose for the individual patient. We nevertheless believed that the benefits of etretinate in the ichthyoses did require confirmation in a properly controlled study, and employed a novel trial design in an attempt to overcome these problems.

Patients and Methods

Eleven children with bullous ichthyosiform erythroderma (BIE) were treated (age range 3–14 years; mean 9.9 years; seven boys, four girls), and nine children with non-bullous ichthyosiform erythroderma (NBIE) (age range 1–10 years; mean 6.2 years; five boys, four girls).

The trial was divided into two parts, (1) an initial dose-finding study conducted on an open basis, and (2) a placebo-controlled double-blind trial of maintenance therapy.

Initial Open Study

The children were seen at 6-weekly intervals for 24 weeks, and assessed clinically at each visit. Renal and hepatic function were checked at the first and final visits.

Clinical assessments were made by selecting those areas of the patient's skin showing the most severe degrees of erythema and scaling at the outset, and scoring each of these on a 5 point scale (0–4) at each visit. The degree of palmo-plantar keratoderma was similarly scored on a 5 point scale (0–4). The proportion of the skin surface affected was estimated as a percentage of the total body surface area. At each visit a global comparison was made both by the parents and by the clinician of the change in the child's skin relative to its initial condition, i.e. much worse, slightly worse, unchanged, slightly improved, much improved. Parents were also asked at each visit to record any possible adverse effects.

Initial dosage of etretinate was 0.5mg/kg, given as a single daily dose. Dosage was increased by increments of 0.5mg/kg daily at each visit (up to a maximum of 2mg/kg/daily) until clearance or the onset of dose-limiting side-effects. In several cases, the dose was reduced to obtain relief of such side-effects.

Double-Blind Trial of Maintenance Therapy

Parents who wished their children to continue treatment at the conclusion of the initial open study were invited to take part in a 24-week controlled trial of maintenance treatment. Those agreeing to enter this study were randomly allocated by the pharmacist to take either etretinate capsules (10mg/capsule) or identical placebo capsules, containing lactose filler only. The dose selected was the maintenance dose determined for that patient during the initial open study.

The children were seen at the start of the controlled study, and twice more at 8-weekly intervals. Assessments were made by parents and clinician as in the initial study, but the parents were given the opportunity to contact the clinician at any time to request withdrawal from the study in the event of significant deterioration in the child's skin condition. The final assessment was then brought forward, and the child withdrawn.

Informed consent was obtained from parents before both studies. Exemption from the need for a clinical trial certificate was obtained from the Licensing Authority of the DHSS, and approval for the trial was obtained from the Hospital's Ethical Committee.

Results

Open Study

Non-Bullous Ichthyosiform Erythroderma

Of the nine children with this disorder who initially entered the study, six completed it. The other three children were withdrawn because of a rapid deleterious effect of treatment on their skin. In each case, within 3–4 days of starting treatment at the initial dose of 0.5mg/kg/day, the skin started to peel away in extensive sheets leaving raw red areas beneath. Two of the patients tried again on at least one occasion, but had the same experience each time.

Table 1. Open study; global assessments

	Non-bullous ichthyosiform erythroderma (n=9)		Bullous ichthyosiform erythroderma (n=11)	
	Parents	Clinician	Parents	Clinician
Much improved	4	4	6	6
Slightly improved	1	1	5	5
No change	–	1	–	–
Slightly worse	1	–	–	–
Much worse	3	3	–	–

Global Assessments (Table 1) – Both the parents and clinician considered that the skin condition had been much improved in four of the nine children, with slight improvement in one other. Three were regarded as having been made much worse by etretinate, as described above, and these children were withdrawn from the study. One other child was considered by the parents to have become slightly worse on treatment, though no change could be discerned by the clinician. This child's parents elected to discontinue treatment at the end of the study, the parents of the five patients who had improved electing to continue.

Clinical Scores (Table 2) – In the six children completing the study, there was a 40 per cent mean improvement in scores for erythema (range 0–100

Table 2. Open study: clinical scores (means).

	Non-bullous ichthyosiform erythroderma (n = 9)			Bullous ichthyosiform erythroderma (n = 11)		
	Initial	Final	Δ	Initial	Final	Δ
Erythema (0–4)	1.67	1.00	− 0.67 (− 40%)	2.18	1.36	− 0.92 (− 38%)
Scaling (0–4)	2.67	1.33	− 1.33 (− 50%)	3.73	1.36	− 2.37 (− 63%)
Palmo-plantar keratoderma (0–4)	2.17	1.17	− 1.00 (− 40%)	2.36	1.00	− 1.36 (− 58%)
Area (0–100%)	100	83.3	− 16.7 (− 16.7)	76.82	72.27	− 4.55 (− 6)

per cent), a 50 per cent mean improvement in scores for scaling (range 50–67 per cent), a 40 per cent mean improvement in scores for palmo-plantar keratoderma (range 0–100 per cent) and a 17 per cent mean decrease in area affected (range 0–50 per cent).

Optimal Dosage – The mean final dose in the six patients completing 6 months treatment was 1.5mg/kg/day (range 0.5–2.1).

Side-Effects – The development by three patients of an early idiosyncratic exfoliative reaction has been described above. Two further children complained of a mild degree of pruritus, which in both cases resolved without a change in dosage. One other child's skin was described by the parents as having become fragile, so that scratching or accidental trauma caused painful raw erosions; this was the child who elected to discontinue treatment at the end of the open study, though this decision was largely based on lack of effect. Three children experienced no side-effects whatsoever, and all five children who elected to continue treatment were free of any side-effects at the end of the 6-month study period.

Bullous Ichthyosiform Erythroderma

All 11 children entering the study completed the 6 months period of treatment.

Global Assessments (Table 1) – The skin condition of all 11 children was regarded as being improved by treatment both by the parents and clinician, half of them much improved, the other half slightly improved. All 11 elected to continue treatment.

Clinical Scores (Table 2) – There was a 38 per cent mean improvement in erythema during the course of the study (range 0–100 per cent), a 63 per cent mean improvement in scaling (range 50–75 per cent), a 58 per cent mean improvement in palmo-plantar keratoderma (range 25–100 per cent) and a 6 per cent decrease in area affected (range 0–35 per cent).

Optimal Dosage – The mean final dose in the 11 patients was 1.2mg/kg/day (range 0.6–1.8).

Side-Effects – Three children experienced no side-effects whatsoever. Three children reported minor dryness of the lips. Six children reported mild pruritus, which in every case was associated with increased fragility of the skin, so that scratching, or rubbing from clothing, or accidental knocks would produce erosions with a raw red base. All these side-effects were relieved by small reductions in dosage, and none of the patients had any side-effects to record at the end of the study.

Controlled Trial

Thirteen children agreed to enter this phase of the study. Three other

Table 3. Controlled trial: global assessments.

	Active		Placebo	
	Parents	Clinician	Parents	Clinician
Non-bullous ichthyosiform erythroderma				
	n = 2		n = 2	
Much improved	–	–	–	–
Slightly improved	–	–	–	–
No change	2	2	–	–
Slightly worse	–	–	–	–
Much worse	–	–	2	2
Bullous ichthyosiform erythroderma				
	n = 2		n = 7	
Much improved	–	–	–	–
Slightly improved	–	–	–	–
No change	2	2	–	–
Slightly worse	–	–	1	3
Much worse	–	–	6	4

children, while not wishing to enter the double-blind trial, did elect to continue therapy at the end of the open study.

Unfortunately, due to a misunderstanding in our pharmacy, allocation to active or placebo therapy was not well balanced in the children with bullous ichthyosiform erythroderma, seven out of the nine cases being allocated to placebo.

Global Assessments (Table 3) – Both parents and clinician recorded no change in those children with either disorder who were maintained on active therapy. On the other hand, the parents of seven of the nine children allocated to placebo asked to withdraw early from the study because of rapid deterioration, in most cases within 4 weeks of entry. All children receiving placebo were recorded by both parents and clinician to have deteriorated either at the time of early voluntary withdrawal, or at the end of the full 6 month study period.

Table 4. Controlled trial: clinical scores (means).

	Initial	Active Final	Δ	Initial	Placebo Final	Δ
Non-bullous ichthyosiform erythroderma						
		n = 2			n = 2	
Erythema (0–4)	1.00	1.00	0	0.50	1.00	+0.5 (+5%)
Scaling (0–4)	1.50	1.00	−0.50 (−33%)	1.00	2.50	+1.50 (+150%)
Palmo-plantar keratoderma (0–4)	1.00	1.00	0	1.00	2.00	+1.00 (+100%)
Area (0–100%)	95	95	0	90	97.5	+7.5 (+8%)
Bullous ichthyosiform erythroderma						
		n = 2			n = 7	
Erythema (0–4)	2.50	2.50	0	1.29	1.86	+0.57 (+44%)
Scaling (0–4)	2.00	2.00	0	1.57	3.14	+1.57 (+100%)
Palmo-plantar keratoderma (0–4)	2.00	2.00	0	1.00	1.86	+0.86 (+86%)
Area (0–100%)	100	100	0	70.71	73.57	+2.86 (+4%)

Clinical Scores (Table 4) – Three of the four children with either condition who continued active treatment showed no change in any score. One child with non-bullous ichthyosiform erythroderma showed a small further improvement in scaling. On the other hand, quite marked deterioration in all scores was recorded for the patients who were transferred from active to placebo treatment.

Side-Effects – None of the children reported any side-effects during the controlled trial.

Discussion

These results confirm the findings of others,[1-3] that oral etretinate is an effective therapy for many children with ichthyosiform erythroderma.

What we currently recognize and classify as non-bullous ichthyosiform erythroderma probably includes a heterogeneous group of disorders. It appeared subjectively that those children with the more lamellar pattern of large polygonal scales and lesser degrees of erythroderma showed a better therapeutic response to etretinate than those children with more branny scaling and a greater degree of erythroderma. It was patients in this latter category who demonstrated the idiosyncratic exfoliative response during initial treatment, which required cessation of etretinate therapy, and it was a girl with this type of disease whose parents discontinued treatment at the end of the open study, because of both a lack of effect and increased skin fragility. Those children with non-bullous ichthyosiform erythroderma who benefited from treatment showed wide variability in their response. Several of the children showed a definite decrease in eythema, though the greatest and most reliable effects were those on scaling and palmo-plantar keratoderma. Most of the children had universal involvement, and this largely remained the case on treatment, though severity was diminished. In one of the five children benefiting from treatment, the skin became virtually normal.

The response in the children with bullous ichthyosiform erythroderma was also variable, only six of the 11 children demonstrating clinically really significant improvement. Two of these six showed virtually complete clearance of disease. Subjectively, it appeared that those children with the most severe disease, particularly those with persistent blistering, were the least likely to benefit, in contrast to those with more stable, predominantly hyperkeratotic disease. Once again, there was a definite improvement in erythema in many cases, but the most impressive benefits were reduced hyperkeratosis and palmo-plantar keratoderma. It was noticeable that the reduction in hyperkeratosis was most marked on the dorsa of the hands and feet, important areas from the patients' viewpoint. Once again, any diminution in area affected was small.

When considering the results of the controlled trial, it has to be borne in mind that only patients who had benefited from oral etretinate were invited to enter. Clearly the results reflect the bias inherent in this method of patient selection. Nevertheless, it was impressive that seven of the nine placebo-treated patients showed such rapid and marked deterioration, that their parents pressed for an early break of code, and subsequent re-establishment of active treatment. Every child was who switched to placebo deteriorated, whereas no change (other than a slight continued improvement in one case) was recorded in any of the children who were treated with etretinate throughout. Although the degree of benefit is variable in both disorders, the parents of all nine children who were allocated to placebo wished to restart active treatment at the end of the study, providing strong evidence that the benefit is both real and worthwhile.

The dosage level providing maximum therapeutic effect with minimal side-effects varied widely in our patients, from 0.5–2.1mg/kg/day, the mean daily dose being 1.3mg/kg. This level is perhaps relatively high, but reflects our own experience that children tolerate a higher dose per unit weight than adults. Whether they actually require a higher dose per unit weight to achieve the same therapeutic effect is not clear, but is certainly appears that children experience less problems with side-effects at equivalent doses per unit weight. None of our patients reported or manifested any noticeable degree of hair loss at any time, and although some of the children reported cheilosis during early treatment, this was always mild and none were experiencing this problem by the end of the open study. The principal dose-limiting adverse effect seen in our patients was increased skin fragility[4] and this was a particular problem in the children with bullous ichthyosiform erythroderma. The exfoliative reaction experienced by three of the patients with non-bullous ichthyosiform erythroderma appeared to be idiosyncratic, in so far as it could be induced even by single 10mg doses. It may nevertheless simply reflect a very exaggerated degree of the same type of increased fragility.

Acknowledgements

We are very grateful to Mrs M. Hurst and Dr A.J. Miller of Roche Products Ltd., for their assistance with these studies.

References

1. Pehamberger, H., Neumann, H. and Holubar, K. (1978). Oral treatment of ichthyosis with an aromatic retinoid. *Br. J. Dermatol.*, **99**, 319
2. Tameyo, L. and Ruiz-Maldonado, R. (1980). Oral retinoid (Ro 10-9359) in children with lamellar ichthyosis epidermolytic hyperkeratosis and symmetrical progressive erythrokeratoderma. *Dermatologica*, **161**, 305

3. Marks, R., Finlay, A.Y. and Holt, P.J.A. (1981). Severe disorders or keratinization: effects of treatment with Tigason (etretinate). *Br. J. Dermatol.*, **104**, 667
4. Williams, M.L. and Elias, P.M. (1981). Nature of skin fragility in patients receiving retinoids for systemic effect. *Arch. Dermatol.*, **117**, 611

9
Lupus Erythematosus and Etretinate

Ch. GRUPPER and B. BERRETTI

Over the last 6 years, numerous authors have reported on the efficacy of etretinate (Tigason) in the treatment of disturbances in keratinization (dermatosis in association with hyper-, para-or dyskeratosis), but also for various other dermatoses, from lichen planus to mycosis fungoides. These results were confirmed at the October 1980 meeting on retinoids.[1]

Etretinate has a wide therapeutic spectrum. Laboratory studies demonstrate a possible effect upon the mechanisms of inflammation and the parameters of the immune response.[2–4,7,9] Hyperkeratotic forms of chronic discoid lupus erythematosus (CDLE) are frequent. We therefore considered that CDLE might constitute an interesting indication for this drug and we have treated patients with CDLE resistant to the usual forms of treatment.

A first report concerning out initial, highly favourable results in the treatment of seven patients was delivered at the Berlin Symposium. Currently, this study has been extended to a total of 25 patients and etretinate has proven efficacious in many of these. Nevertheless, in light of some less favourable results and due to considerable difficulties in therapeutic management of some patients, our initially enthusiastic appraisal must be somewhat modified.

Patients

The protocol of this trial required the following tests before patient-inclusion: clinical examination, standard histology and lupus band test from cutaneous lesions and covered healthy skin, laboratory tests (blood count, sedimentation rate, urea, creatinine, transaminases, alkaline phosphatase, serum protein, cholesterol, triglycerides and urinalysis) and immunological tests for antinuclear antibodies. Twenty-five patients entered into our study, 15 males and ten females with a mean age of 49 years and extremes at 15 and 85. All of these patients had CDLE evolving over more than 2 years and were refractory to conventional agents (antimalarials, corticosteroids, thalidomide). In addition, some patients presented retinopathy, a formal contra-indication to the use of anti-malarials. From the clinical standpoint, nine patients had a hyperkeratotic form (Figures 1 and 2) and 15 others a more inflammatory type (Figure 3) (lupus tumidus (Figure 4), cicatrical lupus with active borders). In these 24 patients, all clinical, laboratory and immunological parameters were normal.

The last patient was a 43-year-old female presenting a highly poly-morphous cutaneous eruption, papular and nodular, relapsing and chronic (Figures 5 and 6). Histology from cutaneous eruption lesions showed lympho-cytic vasculitis and the lupus band test was negative, as were results of visceral examination. Laboratory tests showed an inflammatory syndrome with high ESR (60/120), hyper α_2- and hyper γ-globulins. Standard antinuclear antibodies were negative but anticytoplasmic Ro antibodies were present.

Therapeutic Management

Our initial schedule involved administration of etretinate at a daily dosage of 1mg/kg. Nevertheless, numerous and severe unexpected side-effects in patients presenting the inflammatory form required certain changes in the standard treatment protocol.

Clearing Treatment

Etretinate was used alone in 13 patients. The initial daily dosage of 1mg/kg could be maintained only in the hyperkeratotic form shown by five patients, clinical results and incidence of side-effects here being excellent. In the remaining patients with inflammatory forms, daily etretinate dosage was quickly reduced to 0.50 and to 0.25mg/kg or less. Furthermore, in some patients etretinate had to be withdrawn owing to poor tolerance. Etretinate was used in conjunction with antimalarials in 12 patients, either initially or after failure of etretinate monotherapy. Daily dosage was of 0.50 or 0.25mg/kg or less, depending upon side-effects and clinical results. The duration of the clearing phase was 4–6 weeks.

Maintenance Treatment and Follow-up

All cleared patients continued to receive maintenance treatment.

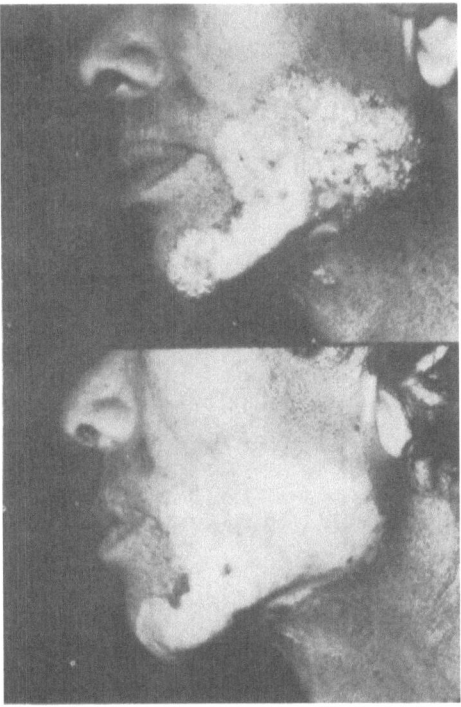

Figure 1. Upper: hyperkeratotic discoid lupus erythematosus before therapy; lower: after 2 months therapy with etretinate.

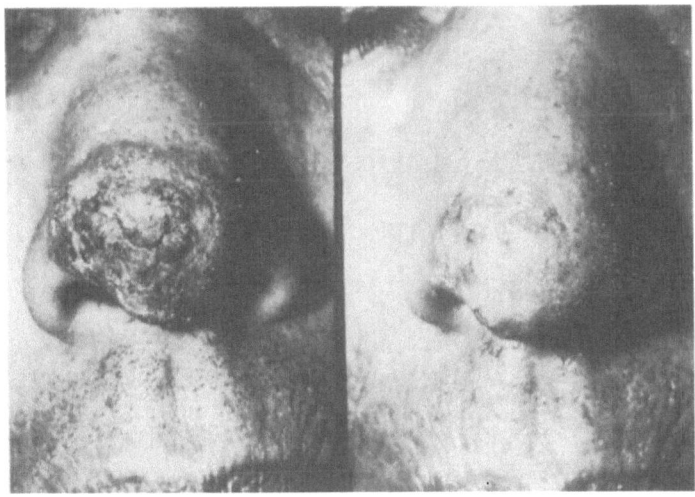

Figure 2. Left: hyperkeratotic discoid lupus erythematosus before therapy; right: after 2 months therapy with etretinate.

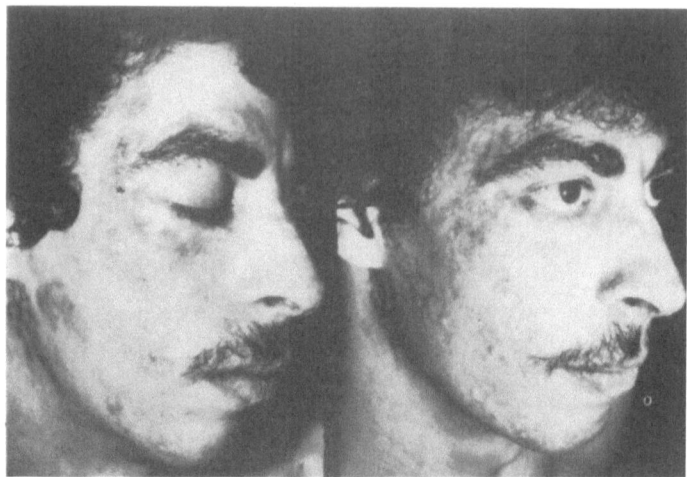

Figure 3. Left: psoriasiform type of discoid lupus erythematosus; right: after 1 month combination therapy with etretinate and antimalarials.

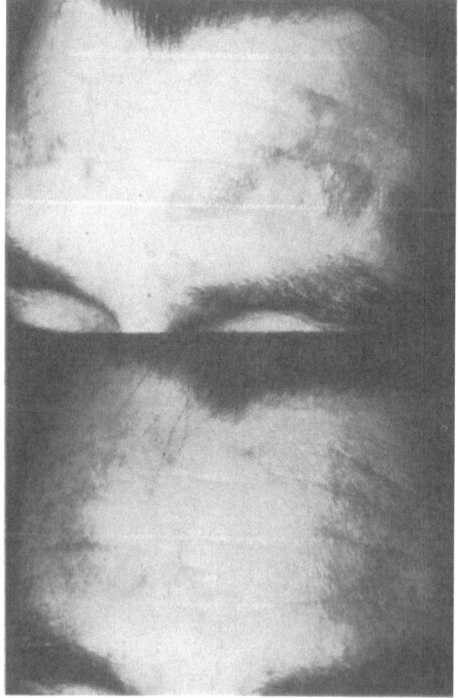

Figure 4. Upper: tumid type of discoid lupus erythematosus; lower: after 1 month combination therapy with etretinate and antimalarials.

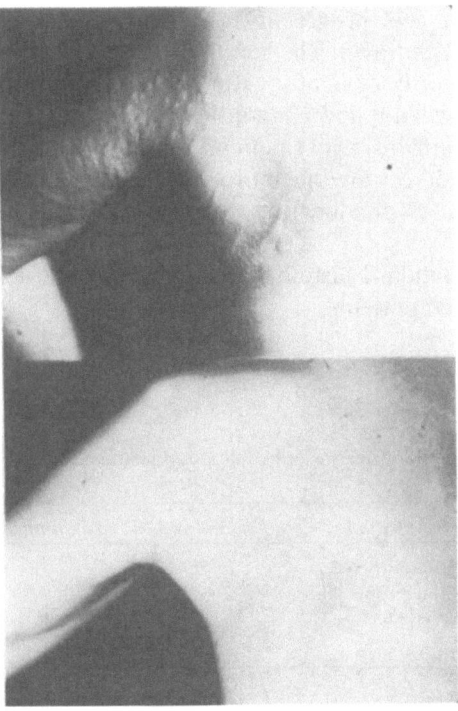

Figure 5. Upper: subacute lupus erythematosus with plaque of non-pruriginous urticaria before therapy; lower: after 2 months therapy with etretinate.

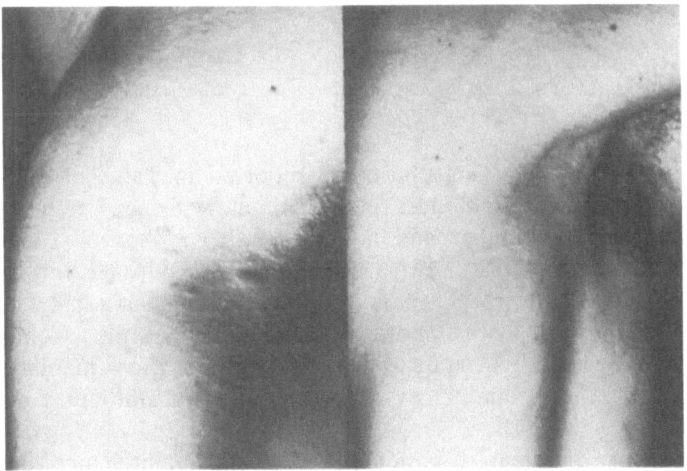

Figure 6. Upper: papular type of discoid lupus erythematosus, lower: after 2 months therapy with etretinate.

Etretinate dosage was progressively reduced over 3–6 months, and the drug was finally withdrawn. The length of remission as well as chronology, incidence and severity of relapses were noted. Duration of this follow-up study ranged between 9 and 12 months.

During the treatment, every patient was subject to standard laboratory tests in order to detect any haemotological, hepatic, renal or lipoprotein toxicity. Women of childbearing age received adequate contraceptive methods.

Comparative standard histological and lupus band tests were obtained from seven cleared patients.

Results

Table 1. Clearing schedule for hyperkeratotic CDLE. ($n = 9$).

Methods	Good results	Good tolerance
Etretinate ($n = 5$)	4/5	5/5
Etretinate plus anti-malarials ($n = 4$)	4/4	4/4
Total	8/9	9/9

Table 2. Clearing schedule for inflammatory CDLE. ($n = 16$).

Methods	Good results	Good tolerance
Etretinate ($n = 8$)	2/8	2/8
Etretinate plus anti-malarials ($n = 8$)	5/8	7/8
Total	7/16	9/16

The results of the clearing phase are reported in Tables 1 and 2. We classed the last patient amongst the inflammatory forms: cutaneous polymorphic eruption, papular and nodular, with lymphocytic vasculitis, a negative lupus band test, severe inflammatory syndrome and anticytoplasmic Ro antibodies. In this patient, etretinate alone at a daily dosage of 1mg/kg cleared all cutaneous lesions after 2 months. Comparative histology showed the disappearance of all pathological manifestations. Nevertheless, the inflammatory syndrome and Ro antibodies were still present.

All of the 15 cleared patients underwent maintenance treatment (etretinate alone or in conjunction with antimalarials). During this period, no patient relapsed.

Table 3. Follow-up study.

Duration = 3–6 months after etretinate cessation
Patient population: 15 cleared patients
  1 death (cause other than CDLE)
  2 dropouts
  4 persistent remissions (without treatment)
  4 persistent remissions under antimalarials, minimal
    doses
  4 relapses: positive reponse to etretinate reintroduction.

Our follow-up study is reported in Table 3. In the patient with Ro anti-bodies, cessation of etretinate was rapidly followed by a relapse. A new course of etretinate at a daily dosage of 1mg/kg again cleared cutaneous lesions. This patient currently remains cleared under maintenance treatment with etretinate at a daily dosage of 0.25mg/kg. Results of comparative histological and immunological studies are shown in Table 4.

Table 4. Pathology and immunopathology. Seven comparative cutaneous samples before and after clinical clearing.

		Before	*After*
5 {	Pathology	+	+
	BMZ	+	+
2 {	Pathology	+	−
	BMZ	+	−

Discussion

Etretinate proved effective in hyperkeratotic forms of CDLE. A good response was obtained after 4–8 weeks of etretinate, alone or in conjunction with antimalarials, in eight of nine patients. Clinical side-effects were moderate (cheilitis and palmoplantar desquamation). In more inflammatory forms of CDLE, results were less spectacular. A good response was obtained after 4–8 weeks of etretinate treatment in only seven of 16 patients. Clinical intolerance explains this partial efficacy of etretinate. Indeed, seven of ten failures withdrew from the trial due to severe intolerance after only 1–3 weeks of treatment. Numerous and severe unexpected side-effects were noted: severe cheilitis, massive palmoplantar ragged desquamation, severe and diffuse pruritus, intense and diffuse erythematosquamous or erosive paronychia, and diffuse papular dermatosis. All of these patients had inflammatory forms of CDLE: six patients had been treated with etretinate alone and one with etretinate in conjunction with antimalarials.

Considering these results, we can offer the following suggestions:

(1) Clinical results are a function of CDLE clinical form: virtually all hyperkeratotic forms cleared (eight of nine patients) whereas in inflammatory forms of CDLE, only half of the patients showed improvement (seven of 16).

(2) Good results are contingent upon good clinical tolerance: seven of ten failures were attributable to voluntary dropout owing to severe side-effects.

(3) Treatment schedules should be appropriate to the clinical form. Etretinate alone should probably be reserved for hyperkeratotic forms, where a dose of 1mg/kg/day is adequate. It seems that, where possible, the combination of etretinate with antimalarials could be recommended as a standard approach to treatment of CDLE, both of the hyperkeratotic and the inflammatory forms. This combination appears more efficacious than etretinate alone and clinical tolerance is much better.

Our follow-up study is still too limited to enable us to draw definitive conclusions. Nevertheless, maintenance treatment with small daily doses of etretinate/antimalarials seemed to provide the longest remissions. The decision of whether or not to institute maintenance treatment must be made individually, carefully weighing the risk–benefit ratio in each case.

Results of the comparative histological study were concordant with clinical results in only two of seven cases. In the remaining five, standard histology and lupus band tests showed persistence of modifications.

It is very difficult to explain the action of etretinate in a mesenchymatous disease such as CDLE. Even hypotheses are hazardous. Indeed, the immunology and physiopathology of CDLE has been subject to less study than has systemic lupus erythematosus. Biesecker[10] reported the presence of immune complexes in CDLE cutaneous lesions and suggested that these complexes could activate complement, inducing lytic processes and membranous lesions. Gilliam[11] suggested that dermal T cells could secrete lymphokinins in response to altered DNA of epidermal origin, and that these lymphokinins might be responsible for lesions seen in lupus. Bauer[2] found that etretinate inhibits *in vitro* lymphocytic response to PHA-M and PWM mitogens. According to Gilliam's hypotheses, *in vivo*, etretinate could inhibit dermal T-cell stimulation by altered epidermal DNA.

Conclusions

Considering the results of this study, we can offer the following conclusions:

(1) Etretinate appears to be of use in the treatment of forms of CDLE

resistant to the usual agents, as well as in patients where antimalarials are formally contra-indicated.

(2) Etretinate apparently potentiates previously ineffective antimalarial therapy; combination of etretinate with antimalarials is to be preferred to etretinate alone.

(3) Management of inflammatory forms is difficult. Etretinate dosage should be carefully adapted on a case-by-case basis. Small doses (0.2mg/kg or less) are frequently effective.

(4) Hyperkeratotic forms respond better than do the more inflammatory forms and clinical safety is better here.

Thus, etretinate may constitute a novel and efficacious approach to the treatment of refractory CDLE. Nevertheless, its use in this dermatosis remains delicate, with indications being limited to certain specific cases.

References

1. Orfanos, C.E. *et al.* (1981). *Retinoids: Advances in Basic Research and Therapy.* (Berlin, Heidelberg, New York: Springer-Verlag)
2. Bauer, R. and Orfanos, C.E. (1981). Influence of retinoid of human blood cells *in vitro.* TMMP retinoids inhibits the mitogenic properties of lectins and modulates lymphocytic response. In Orfanos, C.E. *et al.* (eds.). *Retinoids: Advances in Basic Research and Therapy.* pp. 153–160. (Berlin, Heidelberg, New York: Springer-Verlag)
3. Bialasiewicz, A.A., Lubach, D. and Marghescu, S. (1981). Immunological features of psoriasis: effects of Ro 10-9359, Concavalin A, pokeweed mitogen and methotrexate on cultivated lymphocytes. In Orfanos, C.E. *et al.* (eds.). *Retinoids: Advances in Basic Research and Therapy.* pp. 335–338. (Berlin, Heidelberg, New York: Springer-Verlag)
4. Hercend, T.H., Bruley-Rosset, M., Florentin, I. and Mathe, G. (1981). *In vivo* immunostimulating properties of two retinoids Ro 10-9359 and Ro 13-6297. In Orfanos, C.E. *et al.* (eds.). *Retinoids: Advances in Basis Research and Therapy.* pp. 21–29. (Berlin, Heidelberg, New York: Springer-Verlag)
5. Orfanos, C.E. (1980) Oral retinoids – present status. *Br. J. Dermatol.,* **103**, 473–481
6. Peck, G.L. (1980). Retinoids in dermatology. An interim report editorial. *Arch. Dermatol.,* **116**, 283
7. Rhodes, J. and Oliver, S. (1980) Retinoids as regulators of macrophage functions. *Immunology,* **40**, 467
8. Sopp, A.M., Soppi, E. and Jansen, C.T. (1981). Effect of systemic Ro 10-9359 treatment on immunological parameters in Darier's disease. In Orfanos, C.E. *et al.* (eds.). *Retinoids: Advances in Basic Research and Therapy.* pp. 321–324. (Berlin, Heidelberg, New York: Springer-Verlag)
9. Plewig, G. and Wagner, M. (1981). Anti-inflammatory effects of 13-cis retinoic acid. *Arch. Dermatol. Res.,* **270**, 89
10. Biesecker, G., Lavin, L., Ziskind, M. and Kofler, D. (1982). Cutaneous localisation of the membrane attack complex in discoid and systemic lupus erythematosus. *N. Engl. J. Med.,* **306**, 264
11. Gilliam, J.N. (1981). Immunopathology and pathogenesis of cutaneous lupus erythematosus. In Safai, B.B. and Good, R.A. (eds.). *Comprehensive Immunology.* Vol. 7. *Immunodermatology.* pp. 323–332. (New York: Plenum Medical)

10
Etretinate Treatment in Erosive Lichen Planus of the Oral Mucosa

N. HAMMERSLEY, M.M. FERGUSON and N.B. SIMPSON

Introduction

Lichen planus of the oral mucosa may present in various forms. White striae and plaques are symptomless but atrophic areas with erosions and desquamative gingivitis cause considerable discomfort. Unlike the cutaneous form, involvement of the oral mucosa tends to be prolonged, lasting for many years. Whereas some patients have concurrent lesions on the skin and oral mucosa, the majority appear to be restricted to one or other of these sites.

The diagnosis of lichen planus in the oral mucosa can sometimes present difficulty as both the clinical lesion and the histopathological appearance of a biopsy may be relatively non-specific.

The aetiology of lichen planus remains unknown. Treatment is therefore empirical and in the erosive and desquamative gingivitis form this usually consists of topical corticosteroids. Success has been reported recently with systemic etretinate.[1-7] In these studies the side-effects have been prominent and hence it is impractical to conduct blind parallel or cross-over studies. The side-effects commonly reported with etretinate therapy include cheilitis, dryness of the mucous membranes, exfoliation of the feet and hands, hair loss, paronychia and pruritus.

Methods

(a) Patients

Ten patients (seven female, three male) with severe erosive lichen planus were entered into the trial. Their median age was 54 years (range 39 years to 67 years), and the duration of their oral disorder ranged from 6 months to 6 years (mean 2.3 years). In each case the clinical diagnosis was confirmed by mucosal biopsy.

(b) Trial Design

The clinical trial was conducted over a 14-week period, with each patient attending at 2-weekly intervals. The selection of patients was confined to adult females, who were either sterilized or beyond child-bearing age, and to adult males. Informed consent was obtained routinely and the study was conducted with local Ethical Committee approval.

Placebo capsules were given for the first 2 weeks after which etretinate was to be given orally for 8 weeks at a dose of one 25mg capsule, thrice daily. In most cases it was necessary to decrease the dose after the first 2 weeks of treatment due to the severity of side-effects. A final assessment was made 4 weeks after completing the etretinate therapy.

(c) Assessment

After initial examination and biopsy, all patients were assessed by one clinician and the area of ulcerated mucosa drawn on a standard diagram of the oral cavity. The areas of ulceration before and after treatment were measured planimetrically.

The maximal parotid salivary flow rates were measured bilaterally using a Teflon modified Carlson–Crittenden cup and flooding 10 per cent citric acid solution onto the dorsum of the tongue every 10 seconds. Measurements were performed at the start of the trial, 8 weeks after etretinate therapy and 4 weeks after stopping treatment.

The following haematological and biochemical investigations were performed on entry and after 8 weeks: full blood count, fasting triglycerides and cholesterol, serum electrolytes, urea, uric acid, creatinine, albumin alkaline phosphatase, bilirubin, γ-GT, SGOT, SGPT, calcium and phosphate.

The patients were asked to score on a 10cm visual analogue scale with respect to oral discomfort at each attendance without reference to previous scores.

Statistical analysis of the data was by the Wilcoxon ranked-pair test.

Results

Two of the 10 patients were withdrawn from the trial after 4 weeks of

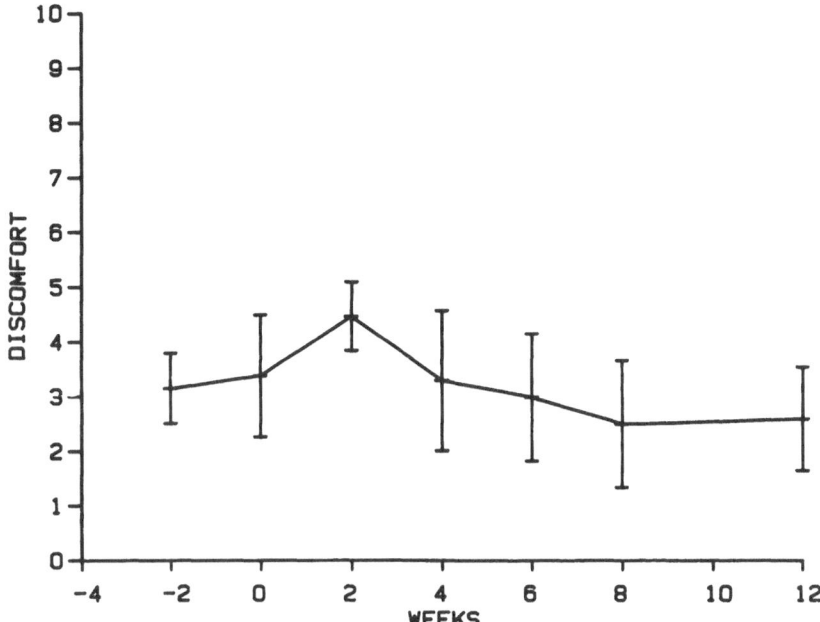

Figure 1. Visual analogue scale of oral discomfort, ranging from 0cm (no pain at all) to 10cm (severe, intolerable pain). Mean values ± SEM at 2-weekly intervals during placebo and etretinate therapy.

etretinate therapy due to intolerable discomfort from cheilitis and generalized pruritus. Only one patient tolerated the full dose of 75mg daily for the entire 8-week period, although three others were able to resume this dose after reducing the dose to 1 or 2 capsules daily during the third and fourth weeks of active treatment. The remaining four patients were maintained at the lower dose.

The size of ulcerated areas was reduced significantly from a mean initial value of 2.73cm² to 1.39cm² ($p < 0.05$). This was not reflected in the patients' objective discomfort score by visual analogue scale (Figure 1) which was unchanged during the placebo phase of the trial but showed a consistent increase after 2 weeks of full dosage etretinate therapy. The scoring from this point on is difficult to assess as dosage schedules differed from patient to patient. However, there was a mean reduction in discomfort recorded after 8 weeks of treatment compared with initial values. Although white striae and plaques were not accurately charted, it was apparent that there was a decrease in these.

The clinical side-effects encountered are listed in Table 1. It should be emphasized that although there was often oral discomfort, no patient complained of dryness affecting the mouth or any other mucosal surface. Neither was there any clinical evidence of xerostomia.

Table 1. Side-effects encountered with etretinate therapy in
10 patients with erosive lichen planus.

Rash and pruritus	7
Cheilitis	6
Desquamation of hands and feet	6
Paronychia	4
Onychomadesis	2
Hair loss (temporary)	1
Dry mouth	0

The rash consisted of an intensely itchy, generalized symmetrical maculo-papular eruption, particularly marked over the limbs. A biopsy of this rash from one patient revealed a non-specific acute dermatitis reaction. Although the rash was most suggestive of an allergic reaction, it tended to fade with time despite the continuation of etretinate albeit at a reduced dosage.

The maximal stimulated parotid flow rates were all well within accepted normal values at the start of the trial (mean 2.4ml/min) and there was no significant change at either 8 weeks (mean 2.2ml/min) or 4 weeks after stopping treatment (mean 2.3ml/min).

No alterations were seen overall in any of the haematological or biochemical investigations performed. However, two individuals who were initially normal, showed elevations in the serum γ-GT, SGOT and SGPT concentrations. These had returned to normal values 4 weeks later in one of these patients and was improving by that time in the other.

Discussion

Despite the widespread use of topical corticosteroids, erosive lichen planus of the oral mucosa and the desquamative gingivitis form are often resistant to therapy, even in high dosage, and several alternative approaches have been examined.

Earlier reports of retinoic acid used topically in oral lichen planus suggested that this was effective in some forms.[8-10] Subsequent studies with systemic etretinate described some success in lichen planus, although side-effects were sufficiently common to cause patients to stop treatment.[5-7] Reticulate and plaque forms of lichen planus are asymptomatic and consequently the use of etretinate is inappropriate. Despite this, Hersle et al.[5] reported on its success in these forms of lichen planus and similar improvements were observed in coexisting striae in the present series.

In this study of ten patients, there were no dramatic improvements in their erosions during the 8 weeks of active treatment and none of the patients elected to resume further therapy at the completion of the investigation. On the other hand, there was a marginal decrease in the visual analogue discomfort scale and the areas of ulceration were reduced significantly.

Side-effects were prominent and several patients developed cheilitis with vertical fissuring. Despite the previous reporting of dry mouth this was not a feature in the group and it is feasible that the term 'dry mouth' has been used loosely to describe a burning or scalded sensation, which accompanies the cheilitis. Similar features occur intra-orally in excessive vitamin A dosage.[11]

Whereas salivary gland changes with xerostomia and metaplasia of the ductal epithelium can develop in vitamin A deficiency,[12,13] no salivary abnormalities have been identified in hypervitaminosis A. The maximum stimulated parotid flow rates are used as a standard assessment of salivary gland function[14] and the present data indicate that there is no functional change in the salivary glands during etretinate therapy.

Changes in serum triglyceride levels[15] and liver function tests[16] are recognised consequences of etretinate ingestion. In the present limited group of patients there was no general trend in these parameters but two patients did develop abnormalities of γ-GT, SGOT and SGPT.

The conclusion of this clinical trial is that etretinate was of minimal value in the management of erosive lichen planus of the oral mucosa when used in doses of 25–75mg daily for 8 weeks. Side-effects were common and troublesome and none of the patients considered any possible improvement in their condition to outweigh the discomfort of the various other effects. Possibly alternatives dosage schedules for etretinate should be investigated.

Acknowledgement

We are grateful to Dr A.J. Miller of Roche Products Limited for the supply of etretinate (Tigason) and placebo capsules.

References

1. Scheiber, W. and Plewig, G. (1978). Behandlung des Lichen ruber mucosae mit Vitamin-A-Saure-Derivaten. *Dermatologica*, **157**, 171
2. Schuppli, R. (1978). The efficacy of a new retinoid (Ro 10-9359) in lichen planus. *Dermatologica*, **157**, (Suppl 1) 60
3. Maidhof, R. (1979). Zur systemischen Behandlung des oralen Lichen planus mit einem aromatischen Retinoid (Ro 10-9359). *Z. Hautkr.*, **54**, 873
4. Ehrl, P.A. (1980). Klinische Untersuchung eines aromatischen Retinoids (Ro 10-9359) zur Behandlung oralen Hyperkeratosen. *Dtsch. Zahnraerzh. Z.*, **35**, 554
5. Hersle, K., Mobacken, H., Sloberg, K., and Thilander, H. (1982). Severe oral lichen planus: treatment with an aromatic retinoid (etretinate). *Br. J. Dermatol.*, **106**, 77

6. Mahrle,G., Meyer-Hamme, S. and Ippen, H. (1982). Oral treatment of Keratinizing disorders of Skin and Mucous Membranes with Etretinate. *Arch. Dermatol.*, **118**, 97

7. Schell, H., Hornstein, O.P., Deinlein, E. and Bauer, G. (1983) Epithelial Cell Proliferation of Oral Lichen Planus in Patients Treated with an Aromatic Retinoid. *Acta Derm-Venereol. (Stockholm)*, **63**, 66

8. Ebner, H., Mischer, P. and Raff, M. (1973). Lokal Behandlung des Lichen Ruber Planus der Mundehlermhaut mit Vitamin-A-Säure. *Z. Haukr.*, **48**, 735

9. Günther, S. (1973). Vitamin A acid in treatment of oral lichen planus. *Arch. Dermatol.* 107

10. Günther, S. (1973). The therapeutic value of retinoic acid (vitamin A acid) in lichen planus of the oral mucous membrane. *Dermatologica*, **147**, 130

11. Smith, J.H. (1964). Hypervitaminosis A: report of a case. *Oral Surg.*, **17**, 305–307

12. Salley, J.J. (1959). The effect of chronic vitamin A deficiency on dental caries in the Syrian hamster. *J. Dent. Res.*, **38**, 1038

13. Hayes, K.C., McComb, H.L. and Faherty, T.P. (1970). The fine structures of vitamin A deficiency. I Parotid duct metaplasia. *Lab. Invest.* **22**, 81

14. Wiesenfeld, D. and Ferguson, M.M. (1983) Salivary inflammatory exocrinopathy : diagnosis and treatment. *Aust. Dent. J.*, **28**, 87

15. Ellis, C.H., Swanson, N.A., Greikin, R.C., Goldstein, N.G. Bassett, D.R., Anderson, T.F. and Voorhees, J.J. (1982). Etretinate therapy causes increased in lipid levels in patients with psoriasis. *Arch. Dermatol.*, **118**, 559

16. Schmidt, H. and Foged, E. (1981). Some hepatotoxic side effects observed in patients treated with an aromatic retinoid (Ro 10-9359). In Orfanos, C.E. *et al.* (eds.). *Retinoids. Advances in Basic Research and Therapy.* pp. 359–362. (Berlin, Heidelberg and New York: Springer-Verlag)

Section 2

Etretinate – Mechanism of Action

11
Overview of Mode of Action of Retinoids

R. MARKS, A.D. PEARSE, T. HASHIMOTO and S. BARTON

It is astonishing that even in the highly sophisticated and scientific time in which we live the bulk of useful drugs derive from serendipity rather than inductive reasoning. Because of this it is not infrequent that we are presented with compounds that are therapeutically effective but whose mode of action remains mysterious. It is worthwhile bearing in mind that it is only in the past 20 or 30 years that we have understood how digitalis and morphine work despite the fact that they were in use for between one and a half to two centuries previously. We are still not clear how the corticosteroids exert their anti-inflammatory effect even with the extensive research on the subject in the 30 odd years since their development. It is especially difficult to determine which biological result of their use is the main one when the drugs in question have multiple actions and therapeutic benefits (as with the corticosteroids). This is certainly the case with the retinoids. Here are drugs that are active in psoriasis (plaque type, erythrodermic, pustular and arthropathic), the disorders of keratinization (including the ichthyotic disorders, erythrokeratoderma variabilis and Darier's disease), acne and cutaneous malignancies. To make matters even more difficult they possess a variety of immunomodulating effects and act as immune adjuvants as well as having a prophylactic effect on various tumours. Is it possible that all these actions can be explained by one major biochemical mechanism?

As the synthetic retinoids all derive from vitamin A (retinol) it does not seem unreasonable to ask whether they are not merely replacing a deficiency when they are successfully used in patients. That this is not the case is probably the most certain information that we possess. In the first place the clinical manifestations of the diseases for which they are given do not remotely resemble experimental vitamin A deficiency. Secondly, patients with the various disorders treated with the retinoids are not vitamin A deficient biochemically. Lastly, the retinoids do not replace vitamin A as far as its functions in reproduction, growth and visual physiology and do not possess all the toxic effects of vitamin A, especially the neurotoxic and hepatotoxic side-effects. It seems, then, that they act in a truly pharmacological sense rather than via a physiological mechanism.

As stated previously, one major problem with sorting out the underlying mechanisms of action with potent drugs is the fact that they are so active. It may be almost impossible to determine whether an observed effect is due to the fundamental action of the drug or is merely an epiphenomenon and due to some biochemical effect much further back in metabolism. In addition, several of the tissue responses observed after administration of the retinoid drugs appear biphasic or at least time dependent. Without making observations over the complete course of the reaction it is impossible to work out the overall effect on the tissues, let alone how the effect is mediated.

Studies of the effect of retinoids on epidermal cell proliferation provide examples of both type of difficulty. In most *in vitro* studies of epidermal cells grown in the presence of retinoids there is a reduction in cell proliferation. However, this is not always very pronounced as a recent study in our laboratory clearly shows (Table 1). The topical administration of retinoic acid causes an increase in the rate of epidermal cell production in small mammals and man. Fritsch et al.[1] found that systemic etretinate increased epidermal cell production in mice. But administration of etretinate causes little change in thymidine autoradiographic epidermal labelling index measurement in normal skin after 4 weeks (Table 2). However, in psoriasis treated with etretinate there is at first no change in parameters of epidermal cell production and later, as the disease improves, there is a decrease. Verma and Boutwell's work[2] showed that there is a decrease in ornithine decarboxylase (ODC) activity in the tumours of animals treated with retinoids, and Lowe et al.[3] have also demonstrated reduction of ODC activity in retinoid-treated psoriasis.

It may also be that cell proliferation is influenced secondarily by alterations in epidermal cell membranes caused by changes in glycosyl and mannosyl radical transfer. Certainly there is now a considerable body of evidence that there are marked changes in glycoprotein synthesis after retinoid administration. De Luca[4] has found that vitamin A enhances glycoprotein synthesis in rat liver and that specifically it is the cell membrane fraction that is affected. Wolf et al.[5] have found that retinol participates in the transfer of residues via a retinol-linked sugar (mannosyl retinyl phosphate). King and Tabiowo[6] found that retinoic acid stimulates incorpo-

Table 1. Effect of vitamin A and retinoids on human epidermal cell growth in cell culture.

Treatments	Number of experiments	Number of colonies /cm²±SD	Number of cells /cm²±SD	Cells/colonies ± SD
UVC treated*				
FCS	10	95.3±60.8	88.6±66.9	84.8±25.3
Control	13	100	100	100
Vitamin A (1×10⁻⁷mol/l)	13	99.7±28.8	102.2±40.0	97.7±18.3
Vitamin A (1×10⁻⁶mol/l)	13	89.2±53.9	95.2±76.8	91.0±35.4
Vitamin A (1×10⁻⁵mol/l)	11	45.6±38.4	40.5±42.5	67.0±34.4
All trans-				
Vitamin A acid (1×10⁻⁷mol/l)	8	83.0±30.5	103.0±61.7	100.0±21.5
All trans-				
Vitamin A acid (1×10⁻⁶mol/l)	8	40.5±29.6	40.0±37.3	77.5±44.0
All trans-				
Vitamin A acid (1×10⁻⁵mol/l)	8	29.5±33.7	26.4±32.6	56.0±42.9
Etretinate (1×10⁻⁷mol/l)	13	101.3±55.6	104.6±79.6	95.6±18.7
Etretinate (1×10⁻⁶mol/l)	13	97.7±56.7	79.8±43.6	87.2±30.0
Etretinate (1×10⁻⁵mol/l)	11	78.5±36.4	81.9±57.7	94.5±36.3

The data indicate the mean of the percentages against the control in each experiment.

Epidermal cells obtained from human foreskin were cultured in Ca²⁺ free media supplemented with 5 per cent FCS with or without various concentrations of vitamin A or retinoids in the presence of 3T3 cell feeder layers for 7 days. All cultures contain 0.05–0.1 per cent ethanol.

*Vitamin A depleted FCS by irradiation with ultra violet of short wavelength (UVC) was added instead of untreated FCS.

ration of glucosamine into glycosaminoglycans and glycoproteins of pig ear slices. Alteration in the lectin binding properties of mouse epidermis after retinoid treatment was reported by Nemanic et al.[7] and provided morphological evidence of the changes in the cell membrane caused by retinoids.

Table 2. Labelling index expressed as a percentage of the number of labelled basal cells to the total number of basal cells in normal subjects.

Volunteer subject	0 days	28 days
1	4.6	7.5
2	6.9	12.9
3	4.5	7.9
4	3.7	2.5
5	4.9	3.3
Mean ± SD	4.9±1.2	6.8±4.2

The difference between the two labelling indices is not significant.

There are also changes in proteoglycan and glycolipid synthesis after retinoid administration. In view of the high concentration of ceramide in the stratum corneum and its possible importance in the process of desquamation, the action on glycolipids might have particular importance for the treatment of scaling dermatoses. Because of the effects on glycosaminoglycan and proteoglycan synthesis and the high concentrations of these substances in the dermis as well as the influence the dermis has for the epidermis, we thought it relevant to monitor dermal structure after treatment. Histologically and histochemically no marked changes were found in a group of normal subjects given etretinate for 4 weeks. Dermal thickness measurements made with the ultrasound dermal depth detector device also did not show any marked change after a period of treatment (Table 3).

In view of the apparent involvement of sugar residue transfer in the mediation of the retinoid effect it seemed important to investigate the activity of enzymes of the Krebs cycle and the pentose shunt pathway in the epidermis. For this reason we have studied the changes in the cytochemical profile of succinic dehydrogenase (SDH) and glucose-6-phosphate dehydrogenase activities in the epidermis of normal human volunteer subjects and of patients with ichthyotic disorders before and after 4 weeks treatment with etretinate.[8] We used an automated image analysis system (Quantimet 720 image analysis computer) to measure the formazan reaction product deposited through the thickness of the epidermis. Different results were obtained for epidermis from patients with disorders of keratinization as compared to epidermis from healthy skin. The pentose shunt enzyme glucose-6-phosphate dehydrogenase (G6PDH) showed enhanced activity in the pretreatment epidermis of patients, which was reduced by the retinoid treatment (Figure 1).

Table 3. Skin thickness as determined by ultrasound measurements (mm) in normal subjects, before, during and after 28 days etretinate treatment.

Volunteer subject	0 days	14 days	28 days	Difference
1	0.61	0.61	0.61	0
2	0.76	0.76	0.76	0
3	0.61	0.61	0.61	0
4	0.61	0.61	0.61	0
5	0.76	0.76	0.76	0
6	0.61	0.53	0.53	−0.08
7	0.76	0.61	0.61	−0.15
8	0.76	0.76	0.76	0
9	0.61	0.61	0.61	0
10	0.46	0.46	0.46	0

There is no difference in dermal thickness during the period of etretinate administration.

Interestingly, etretinate administration increased the activity of this same G6PDH activity in normal epidermis. As far as SDH is concerned, etretinate treatment enhanced enzyme activity in normal subjects and decreased the abnormally high activity levels found in the epidermis from patients with disorders of keratinization. From these studies it can be concluded that etretinate certainly does alter the pattern of epidermal enzyme activity but that it does so differently in normal and abnormal skin, and that in the disease studied there is a 'normalizing effect'.

One observation that has to be fitted into the framework of any hypothesis to explain the mode of action of retinoids concerns the utrastructural appearances of skin of individuals treated by retinoids. Several investigators have noted the presence of a finely granular material between epidermal cells (e.g. Kanerva et al.[9]). Although some reports suggest that the material stains with substances identifying glycoprotein and glycosaminoglycan, this reaction is inconstant. Furthermore, sometimes similar material is seen in untreated skin, although not in great quantities. There certainly is much more present following retinoid treatment, and the material, although predominantly finely granular, is also coarsely granular after retinoid administration (Figure 2).[10] We believe that this appearance may be the result of yet another action of the retinoids (sometimes termed a 'non-specific effect') – the labilization of lysosomal membranes. Release of lysosomal hydrolases and proteases can result in cell death and could account for some of the effects on keratinization (Figure 3). Certainly lysomal membrane release appears to have a role in normal keratinization. As an extension to the cytochemical studies mentioned above, non-specific esterase activity (measuring the indoxyl acetate splitting activity) was measured in the epidermis before and after etretinate administration in patients and

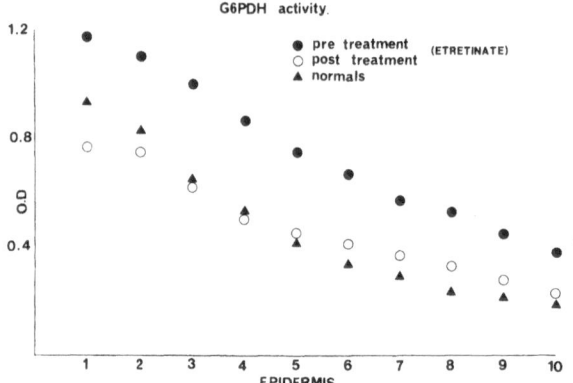

Figure 1. Glucose-6-phosphate dehydrogenase (G6PDH) activity as assessed by optical density of patients before and after treatment with etretinate and normal subjects across the epidermis.

normal subjects. Increase in enzyme activity was found in the normal epidermis subsequent to treatment and a decrease in the abnormally high levels of patients' epidermis. We have noted that patients with epidermolytic hyperkeratosis sometimes develop more blisters subsequent to treatment. Is this perhaps due to protease release after retinoid treatment? Clearly lysosomal membranes of all cells do not lyse to allow liberation of enzymes after retinoid treatment. Perhaps it is only those membranes at a particular stage of differentiation or which have been perturbed in some other way that react in this way after retinoid administration.

We have only made passing reference to the effects of retinoids on the inflammatory reaction and, although this is not the place to cover this topic in any depth, it is pertinent to say that this aspect of their action may be of great importance to their clinical effects. They enhance delayed hypersensitivity responses and tumoricidal action of peritoneal macrophages,[11] and have an adjuvant effect on immediate hypersensitivity.[12] They also inhibit the release of neutrophil enzymes and superoxide anion production.[13] These effects may well be relevant to the action of etretinate and 13-*cis*-retinoic acid in the inflammatory dermatoses psoriasis and acne.

Finally, we want briefly to consider which of the various retinoid effects operate in two apparently very different diseases – psoriasis and acne. In psoriasis the effects on epidermal cell proliferation, epidermal differentiation and on the inflammatory process may all be important. As the retinoids are so efficacious in pustular psoriasis it may be surmised that the effects on neutrophils may be most important and that effects on epidermal differentiation are a 'bonus', so to speak. However, there is little hard evidence

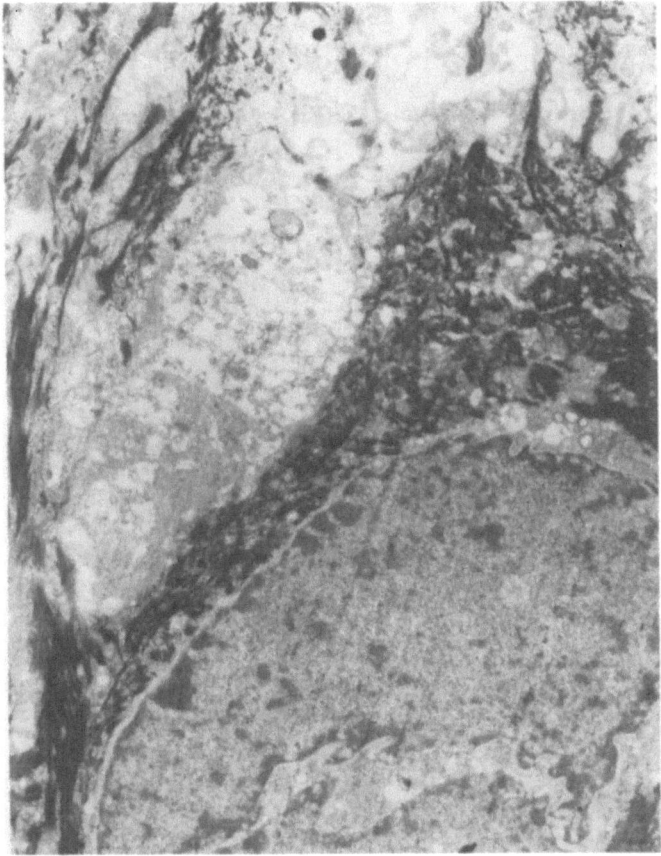

Figure 2. Evidence of cell breakdown in the upper Malpighian layer of a solar keratosis lesion from a patient treated with arotinoid. A mixture of find and coarse granular material and small membrane bound vesicles are present between two cells. (× 4900)

to back this view and more work in this area is required.

As far as acne is concerned, the most striking effect, apart from the resolution of the disease, is the marked diminution of the rate of sebum secretion.[14,15] The reasons for the inhibition of sebaceous gland secretion are not understood. Suppression of sebocyte proliferation, alteration of sebocyte differentiation and inhibition of lipogenesis are possibilities but more work is required to decide which one (or more) is most important. Reduction of sebum secretion takes place before the clinical response but returns to pretreatment values some weeks after stopping treatment. It is interesting that the sebum secretion is restored to normal but the acne rarely returns. Under these circumstances it is reasonable to ask whether some other action of retinoids is producing the clinical effect. There are at least two other possibilities that merit serious consideration. The first rela-

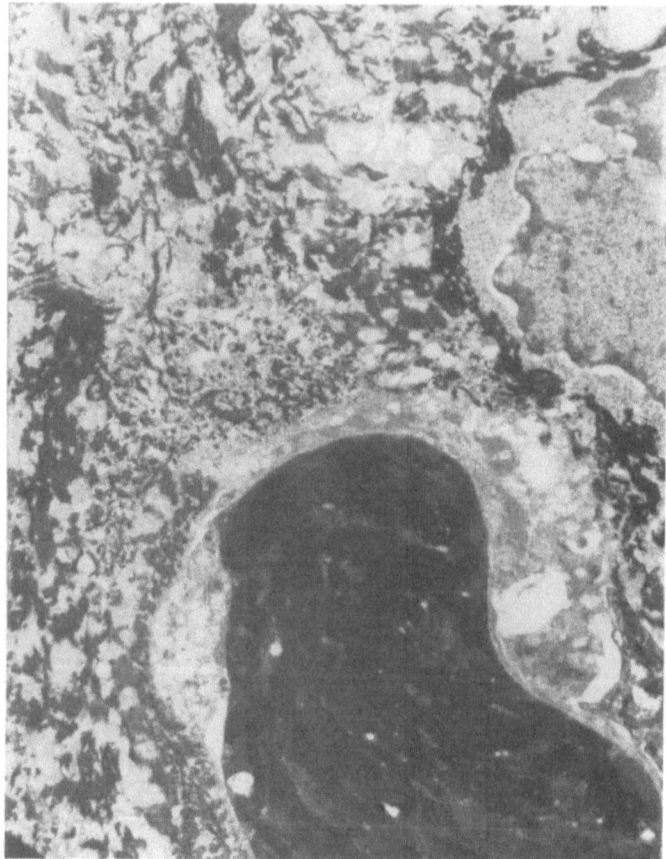

Figure 3. Large dense apoptotic body in the stratum granulosum of a solar keratosis lesion after arotinoid treatment. (× 4900)

tes to the abnormal follicular keratinization in acne. Topical retinoic acid certainly causes a shedding of comedones and it seems likely that systemic retinoids have a similar action. In addition to this comedolytic or keratolytic action, the anti-inflammatory actions of 13-*cis*-retinoic acid must be considered as candidate modes of action. It has been demonstrated that pustulation is much less easy to induce during treatment and presumably inhibition of neutrophil aggregation could contribute to the therapeutic effect.[16] Modulation of lymphocyte reactivity may also be relevant to the treatment of acne but there is very little evidence to guide us on this issue.

The development of the retinoids is a most important milestone in the slow march along the therapeutic trail. But even more impressive than the benefit that these drugs confer on patients is their potential for future development. Clearly, if we could gain clearer insight into their mode of action, it would be much easier to design and choose more active and less toxic compounds.

References

1. Fritsch, P.O., Pohlin, G., Langle, U. and Elias, P.M. (1981). Response of epidermal cell proliferation to orally administered aromatic retinoid. *J. Invest. Dermatol.*, **77**, 287
2. Verma, A.K. and Boutwell, R.K. (1977). Vitamin A acid (retinoic acid) a potent inhibitor of 12-*O*-tetradecanoylphorbol-13-acetate induced ornithine decarboxylase activity in mouse epidermis. *Cancer Res.*, **37**, 2196
3. Lowe, N.J., Kaplan, R. and Breeding, J. (1982). Etretinate treatment for psoriasis inhibits epidermal ornithine decarboxylase. *J. Am. Acad. Dermatol.*, **6**, 697
4. De Luca, L.M. (1977). The direct involvement of vitamin A in glycosyl transfer reactions of mammalian membranes. *Vit. Hormones*, **35**, 1
5. Wolf, G., Kiorpes, T.C., Masushig, S., Schreiber, J.B., Smith, M.J. and Anderson, R.S. (1979). Recent evidence for the participation of vitamin A in glycoprotein synthesis. *Fed. Proc.*, **38**, 2540
6. King, I.A. and Tabiowo, A. (1981). The effect of all-*trans*-retinoic acid on the synthesis of epidermal cell surface associated carbohydrates. *Biochem. J.*, **194**, 341
7. Nemanic, M.K., Fritsch, P.O. and Elias, P.M. (1982). Perturbations of membrane glycolysation in retinoid treated epidermis. *J. Am. Acad. Dermatol.*, **6**, 801
8. Pearse, A.D., Gaskell, S.A. and Marks, R. (1983). Effects of aromatic retinoid Ro 10-9359 on epidermal cell production and metabolism in normals. Society for Investigative Dermatology and European Society for Dermatological Research Joint Meeting April/May 1983. Abstract. *J. Invest. Dermatol. (Suppl.)*, **80**, 357
9. Kanerva. L., Niemi, K.M., Lauharanta, J., Juvakoski, T. and Lassus, A. (1981). Electron microscopic characterization of the mucus-like material of the epidermis before and after retinoid and retinoid-PUVA (rePUVA) treatment of psoriasis. In Orfanos, C.E. *et al.* (eds.). *Advances in Basic Research and Therapy.* pp. 467–472. (Berlin, Heidelberg, New York: Springer-Verlag)
10. Barton, S. and Marks, R. (1983). (In preparation)
11. Hercend, Th., Bruley-Rosset, M., Forentin, I. and Mathé, G. (1982). *In vivo* immuno-stimulating properties of two retinoids: Ro 10-9359 and Ro 13-6298. In Orfanos, C.E. *et al.* (eds.). *Retinoids: Advances in Basic Research and Therapy.* pp. 21–30. (Berlin, Heidelberg, New York: Springer-Verlag)
12. Jurin, M. and Tannock, I.F. (1972). Influence of vitamin A on immunological response. *Immunology*, **23**, 283
13. Camisa, C., Eisenstat, B., Ragaz, A. and Weissmann, G. (1982). The effects of retinoids on neutrophil function *in vitro*. *J. Am. Acad. Dermatol.*, **6**, 620
14. Strauss, J.S., Peck, G.L., Olsen, T.G., Downing, D.T. and Windhorst, D.B. (1978). Alteration of skin lipid composition by oral 13-*cis*-retinoid acid: comparison of treatment and pre-treatment value. *J. Invest. Dermatol.*, **70**, 223
15. Strauss, J.S., Thomsen, R.J., Farrell, L.N. and Stranieri, A.M. (1981). Oral retinoids: effects on human sebaceous glands and nodulocystic acne. In Orfanos, C.E. *et al.* (eds.). *Retinoids: Advances in Basic Research and Therapy.* pp. 237-244. (Berlin, Heidelberg, New York: Springer-Verlag)
16. Plewig, G., Wagner, A., Nikolowiski, J. and Landthaler, M. (1981). Effects of two retinoids in animal experiments and after clinical application in acne patients: 13-*cis*-retinoic acid Ro 4-3780 and aromatic retinoid Ro 10-9359. In Orfanos, C.E. *et al.* (eds.). *Retinoids: Advances in Basic Research and Therapy.* pp. 219–236. (Berlin, Heidelberg, New York: Springer-Verlag)

12
Effects of Synthetic Retinoids on Human Peripheral Blood Lymphocytes and Polymorphonuclears *in Vitro*

R. BAUER and C.E. ORFANOS

Introduction

Synthetic retinoids are obviously effective in the treatment of psoriasis, Darier's disease, lichen planus, ichthyoses, keratoderma palmoplantare, pityriasis rubra pilaris, etc. In these conditions, the site of action of retinoids seems to focus on the pathologically keratinizing epidermis. A large number of disorders of keratinization (DOK) of the skin showing ortho- or para-keratosis appear to respond to oral retinoids.

Interestingly enough, the pustular variant of psoriasis also responds extremely well to the aromatic retinoid Ro 10-9359 (Tigason). In contrast to the relatively slow clinical progression in the disorders of keratinization mentioned above, the pustules in psoriasis recede in a remarkable short period of time. As a rule, a beneficial effect is seen in both the localized palmoplantar form and the generalized Zumbusch type of the disease in a few days, or 1–2 weeks. Severe pustular psoriasis currently represents a main indication for oral retinoid treatment.

On the basis of these clinical observations, several experiments were carried out by our group during the last 4–5 years in order to answer the question as to whether synthetic retinoids may also influence the function of peripheral blood cells, in addition to their effect on epidermal keratinocytes. Our investigations have clearly demonstrated that indeed both human polymorphonuclear granulocytes (PMNs) and peripheral blood lymphocytes must be regarded as target cells for retinoids. The individual retinoid compounds may differ considerably in their affinity to blood cells as well as in their effect on this particular target. In the present paper we review our findings on retinoid-induced effects on human peripheral blood cells using different models.

Techniques

During these studies the following retinoid compounds* were investigated: (a) the aromatic retinoid Ro 10-9359 (etretinate, Tigason), (b) its main metabolite Ro 10-1670 (aromatic retinoic acid, TMMP-RA), (c) the 13-*cis*-retinoic acid (isotretinoin, Roaccutane), and (d) the new potent retinoid, the arotinoid Ro 13-6298.

Visual Analysis of Vital PMN Locomotion and Migration in Vitro

For investigating the functional state of PMNs before and under oral retinoid therapy a simple *in vitro* model designed by Engel[1-3] was used in patients under oral retinoid treatment. Addition of retinoid *in vitro* was found inappropriate.

A drop of venous blood is taken from the finger tip with a cover glass on a slide free of fat and dust. The drop must be so small that it just spreads uniformly to the edges of the cover glass, using slight pressure. Then all blood cells lie separately side by side, the specimen being about 3μm thick. 21 × 26mm cover glasses and pure white, alkali-free slides were used for this experiment. In order to prevent the specimens from drying, they were sealed on all sides with warmed paraffin using a fine brush and were then examined by light microscopy at room temperature over 48 hours. Selected areas of some specimens were documented by microcinematography over the entire period of the experiment. Technical data: Zeiss Standard WL light microscope condenser; V/Z (1,4); objective: Apo Ph 100/1.32; ocular: 6.3×; filter: interference green and heat protection filter; light source: low-voltage lamp and Zeiss Ukatron 60 W; camera: Contax; film material: Kodak Panatomic X; image scale: 1,800:1 or 1,000:1.

Oxalate-Induced Radial Segmentation Test

This technique has been designed by Norberg[4,5] and his collaborators as a screening test for metaphase blocking agents. It was applied here in order to elucidate the effect of synthetic retinoids on the microtubular cell system.

Heparinized venous blood (10IU/ml) was obtained from three healthy individuals and was diluted with an oxalate solution containing 0.97 per cent (w/v) potassium oxalate and 0.85 per cent ammonium oxalate.

*The retinoids were kindly supplied by Hoffman-La Roche, Grenzach-Basel

0.2ml of this oxalate solution was added to 0.8ml blood. After incubation for 6 hours at room temperature, mononuclear blood cells were isolated with a ficoll–hypaque gradient as described above. The cells were smeared, were stained with Pappenheim's stain, and the percentage of cells with radially segmented mononuclear cell nuclei was determined by counting 500 cells. In order to investigate the influence of retinoids the compounds were dissolved in $10\mu l$ DMSO and were added $(0.025-\mu/\text{ml})$ to the heparinized blood before addition of the oxalate solution. The further procedure was identical to control preparations without retinoid. Five experiments were performed per concentration level.

Isolation and Cultivation of Lymphocytes

Several investigations were performed on normal cultured lymphocytes under addition of various synthetic retinoids. Lymphocytes were isolated from heparinized blood (100IU/ml) with a ficoll–hypaque gradient. The heparinized blood was diluted 1:1 with 0.9 per cent NaCl solution and was layered via single-stage ficoll–hypaque gradient at a ratio of 3:1 (blood to gradient). After centrifugation for 30 minutes at $400g$, the lymphocytes were drawn off above the gradient layer with a pasteur pipette and were washed 2–3 times for 10 minutes at $400g$ in RPMI 1640. After the last washing procedure, the samples were adjusted to 5×10^5 cells/ml. 5×10^5/ml lymphocytes were then cultured in RPMI 1640 with 20mmol/l hepes, 200mmol/l L-glutamine, 10 per cent calf serum, $10\mu g$/ml neomycin and 0.5U/ml bacitracin at a total volume of 0.5ml in plastic tubes. $25\mu l$ of phytohaemagglutinin M (PHA-M), phytohaemagglutinin P (PHA-P), concanavalin A (ConA) and pokeweed mitogen (PWM) were added for mitogenic stimulation; their concentration was adjusted to maximal stimulation values. After 48 hours incubation, $3\mu Ci$ ^{3}H-thymidine (New England Nuclear; specific activity 6.7Ci/mmole) per sample was added for radioactive labelling over 18 hours. Labelled lymphocytes were then treated with 0.5ml 10 per cent trichloracetic acid (TCA). After having been separated by centrifugation, the precipitates were washed 3 times with 1ml 5 per cent TCA and before the last washing procedure were extracted once with 95 per cent methanol. The sediment was taken up in $100\mu l$ 1N KOH, was transferred to an aquasol/H_2O scintillator and the radioactivity was measured in a Tricarb (Packard).

Density Gradient Centrifugation of Homogenated Lymphocytes with ^{3}H-Labelled 13-cis-retinoic acid

10^7 human peripheral blood lymphocytes were homogenized in 0.05M of

Tris–HCl buffer pH 7.8. The homogenate was centrifuged at 15,000 rpm in a Sorvall centrifuge for 30 minutes. The supernatant was then incubated at 0°C for 18 hours with 1μM ^{3}H-13-*cis*-retinoic acid (specific activity 1.78 Ci/mmole), was subsequently dialysed against 0.05M of tris–HCl pH 7.8 and the dialysate was layered in 200μl portions on a continuous saccharose density gradient of 5–20 per cent (w/v).The gradient volume amounted to 5ml. The gradient was produced in 0.05M of tris–HCl buffer at pH 7.8. Centrifugation was performed at 50,000 rev./min for 18 hours in a Beckmann centrifuge with the swing-out-rotor SW 50. Control preparations contained, in addition to the radioactive retinoid, an excess of non-labelled retinoid (200μM). After centrifugation, the gradient was fractionated and the radioactivities of test and control samples were measured.

Results and Discussion

In Vitro *Observations on Vital PMNs Before and After Oral Retinoid Therapy*

Peripheral blood PMNs of several healthy persons and from 12 patients with extensive plaque-like psoriasis were examined before and after 2–3 weeks of oral retinoid administration. In the *in vitro* model used here PMNs develop their migratory activity in three consecutive stages with smooth transition from one stage to the other (stage of resting and adaptation, stage of movement, stage of migration). Before treatment, the *resting stage* was characterized by vigorous and rapid intracellular granular kinetics, lasting for about 15 minutes. The cell granula were moving centripetally towards the cytocentrum. The *movement stage* began with the formation of multiple cytoplasmic protrusions at the cell surface of varying size and shape. The cells started to move forth and back within a small area for 15 additional minutes, leading to a continuously changing and bizarre cell picture. A constant pseudopod was then formed on the plasma cell membrane, the cells became elongated, the cytoplasmic organelles arranged themselves orderly around the cytocentrum and the cells moved into the *migration stage*, which lasted for up to 30 hours. A rectilinear directional cell migration was then measurable with a maximum of *ca.* 20μm/minute, 2–3 hours after the preparation of the specimen. The survival time of the PMNs in *vitro* was approximately 48 hours under these conditions.

Influence of Etretinate (Ro 10-9359)

After 2–3 weeks of oral treatment (1mg/kg/day) venous blood was obtained from the same 12 patients and the *in vitro* activity of PMNs was investigated under the same conditions as described above. Visual analysis *in vitro* showed a reduced granula kinetics in all PMNs during the resting stage. In some cells granula movement was only recognizable by time-lapse microcinematography, indicating some functional disorders of the centrosphere. The resting and adaptation stage was considerably prolonged under Ro 10-9359, in some cells up to 7 hours. With great delay most PMNs entered into a slow and uncoordinated cell movement stage. Some pseudopods were formed and migration forms were also seen, nevertheless, the inner order of the cell organelles was not achieved in most cases. Measurable migration did not occur. The *in vitro* survival time of PMNs was clearly reduced by 50 per cent under retinoid treatment, thus amounting to approximately 24 hours.

Cell degeneration was also different under oral aromatic retinoid compared to cells from non-treated persons or before·treatment: non-treated PMNs developed multiple, long, beaded cytoplasmic branches with granula and degenerated; whereas, after oral retinoid administration only a few short and crude protrusions were developed, which finally disappeared again.

Influence of 13-*cis*-Retinoic Acid (Ro 4-3780)

Vital PMNs from four patients with severe acne conglobata and from two patients with psoriasis vulgaris were examined before and after oral treatment (4 weeks) with 13-*cis*-retinoic acid (1mg/kg/day). In contrast to the changes seen under oral aromatic retinoid (Ro 10-9359), the behaviour of peripheral blood PMNs *in vitro* was only slightly altered under treatment with 13-*cis*-retinoic acid (Ro 4-3780). Though there was a 2–3 fold prolongation of the resting and adaptation stage, all cells passed via the movement stage into the stage of migration and moved in straight lines for hours. Their survival time amounted to 36–40 hours and was thus only insignificantly shorter than before treatment.

Influence of Arotinoid (Ro 13-6298)

The *in vitro* activity of peripheral blood PMNs of nine patients with the new potent retinoid compound arotinoid (Ro 13-6298) was also examined. The patients were suffering from severe psoriasis vulgaris ($n = 3$), Darier's disease ($n = 1$), ichthyosis congenita ($n = 1$) keratosis palmoplantaris ($n = 3$) and multiple superficial basal cell carcinomas ($n = 1$). The daily dose of arotinoid varied between 0.05 and 0.1mg per day. The investigations were carried out 2 and 4 weeks after onset of treatment. Alterations could be recognized after 2 weeks and became even more pronounced after 4 weeks of oral arotinoid therapy. The resting and adaptation phase was prolonged to about 5 hours. The transition to the movement phase was hesitant and slow and was clearly prolonged to *ca.* 1–2h. However, the movements of the cells under arotinoid did not differ from those in control specimens. Transition from the movement stage into the migration stage was achieved by all cells observed, showing rectilinear migration. Also, the values of measurable migration and of the survival time of the cells remained unchanged.

Discussion

These observations suggest that oral retinoids may influence and alter the functional behaviour of polymorphonuclear granulocytes *in vitro*.[6,7] The aromatic retinoid etretinate (Tigason) had the strongest effect on vital PMNs, whereas the influence of arotinoid and of 13-*cis*-retinoic acid was less developed.

The *in vitro* migration of polymorphonuclear leukocytes is a complex process. Söderström *et al.*[8] distinguished between (a) *non-stimulated chance movement,* (b) *stimulated chance-movement,* (c) *antitubulin-resistant chemotaxis* and (d) *antitubulin-sensitive chemotaxis.* Under standardized conditions PMNs pass through characteristic time-dependent

Table 1. Behaviour of vital PMNs *in vitro* under oral therapy with various retinoids.

	Before therapy	*Tigason*	*Therapy with Roaccutane*	*Arotinoid Ro 13-6298*
Diagnosis	Psoriasis, acne, healthy volunteers	Psoriasis (n=12)	Acne congl. (n=4) Psoriasis (n = 2)	Psoriasis (n=3) DOK (n=5) MBCC (n=1)
Duration of treatment	0	2–3 weeks	4 weeks	2–4 weeks
Dose	0	75mg/day	1mg/kg/day	0.05–0.1mg/day
Stages (1) Resting & adaptation	15 min	→ 7h	30–45 min	→ 5h
(2) Movement in loco	15 min	→ 15h	30–45 min	→ 2h
(3) Migration	30h	0	24–30h	24h
Migration Maximum	20μm/min after 1–2h	0	10–20μm/min after 3–5h	20μm/min after 6–7h
Survival time *in vitro*	48h	24h	36–40h	48

DOK = Disorders of keratinization
(Darier's disease, ichthyosis congenita, palmo-plantar keratosis).

MBCC = Multiple superficial basal cell carcinomas.

stages which finally lead to a directional, rectilinear cell migration. As a rule, subantimitotic concentrations of colchicine and podophyllin can inhibit the antitubulin-sensitive chemotaxis of PMNs *in vitro* without influencing the basic mechanisms of cellular movement.[9] Amoeboid motility of peritoneal macrophages and PMNs may still occur under colchicine and vinblastine.[10,11] In other words, one may assume that antitubulins have little or no influence on the locomotor system of the cell and that cytoplasmic microtubuli are probably not involved in non-stimulated or stimulated chance movements. Functional activity of microtubuli seems necessary only for directional rectilinear migration on a concentration gradient.[12,13] The functional alterations of vital PMNs *in vitro* under oral retinoid therapy indicate clear parallels to the mode of action of antitubulins: amoeboid cell motility still exists, however, a rectilinear cell migration is distinctly reduced or fails to appear. For this reason we suggest that oral treatment with etretinate may interfere with the cytoplasmic microtubular system of the PMNs and therefore reduce or inhibit their rectilinear migration.

Recent investigations suggest that microtubule organizing centres are localized in the cytocentrum associated with the centrosome.[14] They represent an accumulation of cytoplasmic microtubuli and control their number, length, alignment, functional activity etc. Thus, the cytocentrum is considered to be of great importance for the formation of axial microtubuli which enable the cell to alter its cytoplasmic architecture and its shape and enter into the migratory stage.[15]

Inhibition of Oxalate-Induced Radial Segmentation of Mononuclear Cell Nuclei by Aromatic Retinoic Acid (Ro 10-1670) In Vitro

In order to obtain more information on the influence of retinoids on the functional state of the microtubuli, we performed further experiments using the *in vitro* oxalate-induced segmentation test. The addition of oxalate solutions to a cell system *in vitro* leads to the appearance of regular and deep indentations of the mononuclear cell nuclei, obviously by inducing instability or disassembly of the cytoplasmic microtubuli. The cell nuclei then appear segmented. Substances which interfere with the function of the microtubuli were shown to inhibit or reduce the segmentation of the nuclei.[4,5] Oxalate-induced radial segmentation has been proposed as a screening test for antitubulins, especially metaphase-blocking agents.

With the technique described on p.102 we tested the main metabolite of aromatic retinoid, the free acid Ro 10-1670 (TMMP-RA), for its ability to inhibit oxalate-induced radial segmentation. A statistically significant reduced number of segmented nuclei was measured if $2.5\mu g/ml$ retinoid

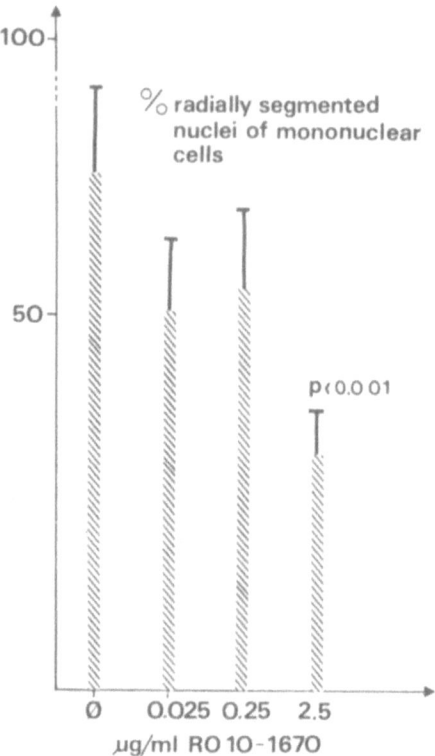

Figure 1. Influence of the free aromatic acid (Ro 10-1670) on the oxalate-induced radial segmentation of mononuclear cell nuclei. Reduction to 46.3 per cent of the pretreatment value ($p < 0.001$)

were added to the cell system (Figure 1). Concentration levels between 0.025 and 0.25μg/ml TMMP-RA also led to some reduction of the number of radially segmented nuclei compared to control preparations without TMMP-RA. These findings support the opinion that etretinate especially its main metabolite Ro 10-1670 may act similar to antitubulins on peripheral blood cells.

Influence of Retinoids on Lymphocyte Cultures

Binding of Retinoids to Protein

Previous experiments had shown that aromatic retinoic acid (TMMP-RA, Ro 10-1670) is practically insoluble in aqueous solutions. The same grade or water solubility showed for 13-*cis*-retinoic acid. For using these retinoids in cultures of lumphocytes we incubated each compound in the complete medium RPMI 1640 (with calf serum) for 1h at 37°C. Photometric analysis of the incubated solutions showed a clear maximum at 340nm indicating that both retinoids were bound to the protein. The unbound insoluble surplus was removed by centrifugation for 15min at 3,000 rev./min. The culture medium thus loaded with retinoid was used for subsequent experiments. Arotinoid is more soluble in water than TMMP-RA and 13-*cis*-retinoic acid. In the present series of experiments, however, it was used bound on protein, like the other compounds, for comparison.

Influence of Aromatic Retinoid (Ro 10-1670) on Cultured Lymphocytes

No effect of ^{3}H-thymidine uptake in non-stimulated cultured lymphocytes could be detected *in vitro* after addition of 5ng to 50µg TMMP-RA per ml culture medium. The rate of ^{3}H-thymidine incorporation amounted to 846 ± 427 counts/min per 2.5×10^5 lymphocytes in all concentrations used. Control preparations stimulated by PHA showed an incorporation rate of 48, 621 ± 6482 counts/min per culture. Addition of TMMP-RA (0.025–25µg/ml) in the medium followed by addition of mitogens led to a dose dependent inhibition of DNA-synthesis in mitogen-stimulated lymphocytes (Figure 2). Here the stimulation with T-cell mitogens (PHA, ConA) was more clearly inhibited than stimulation with PWM as a

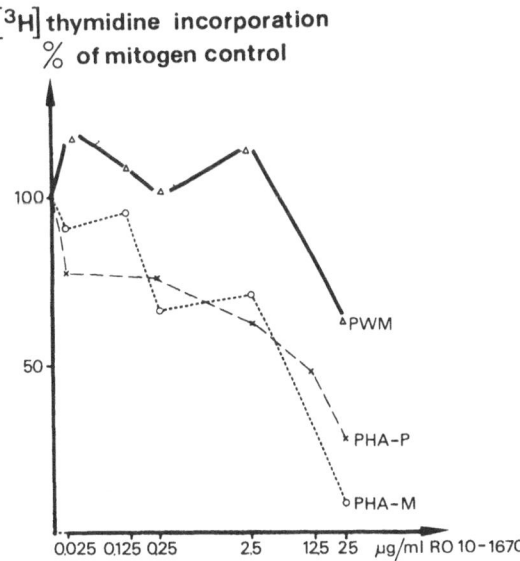

Figure 2. Influence of the free aromatic acid (Ro 10-1670) on the ^{3}H-thymidine uptake of cultured lymphocytes stimulated by lectins.

B-cell mitogen. Trypan blue exclusion tests showed no changes indicative for TMMP-RA-induced alterations whatsoever.

Influence of 13-*cis*-Retinoic Acid (Ro 4-3780)

After addition of 0.1–10μg/ml Ro 4-3780 into the cultures ^{3}H-thymidine incorporation showed no increase of ^{3}H-thymidine uptake in non-stimulated lymphocytes. Under 13-*cis*-retinoic acid and stimulation with mitogens, a mitogen-dependent and dose-dependent modulation of DNA synthesis occured. A low dose of 13-*cis*-retinoid (0.1μg/ml) increased ConA-stimulated DNA-synthesis, whereas, higher doses (5–10μg/ml) significantly reduced cell proliferation down to 25 per cent of the initial values (Figure 3). Similar findings were registered under stimulation with PHA. In the presence of 13-*cis*-retinoic acid and PWM in a wide range of doses (0.1–5μg/ml) DNA synthesis remained unaltered. Only if 10μg or

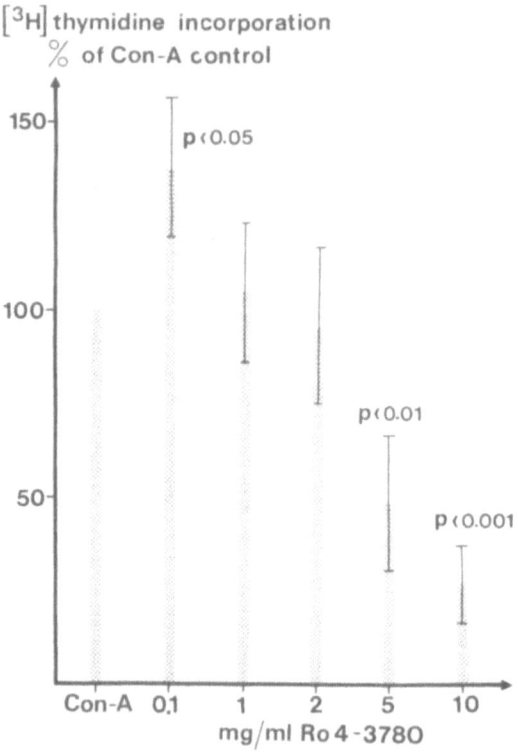

Figure 3. Dose dependent modulation of ConA-stimulation by 13-*cis*-retinoic acid *in vitro*. The inhibition of ^{3}H-thymidine uptake under higher doses (5–10μg/ml) is clearly significant ($p < 0.01$).

110

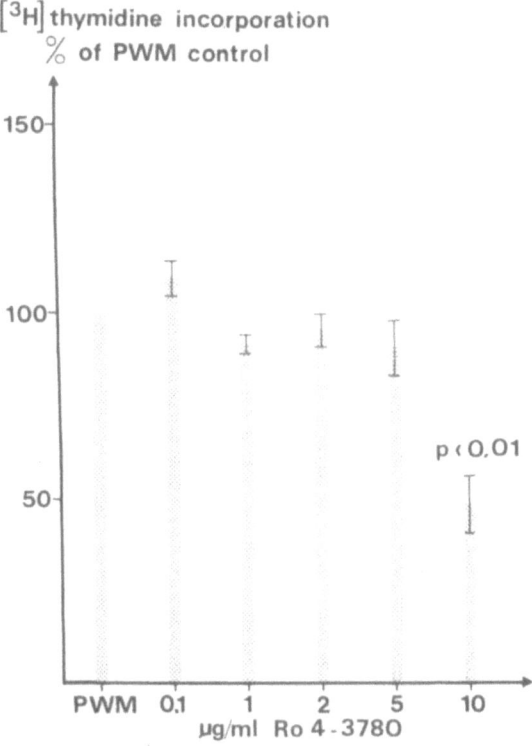

Figure 4. ³H-thymidine uptake in cultured lymphocytes stimulated with PWM in presence of of 13-*cis*-retinoic acid.

more per ml culture were added, the stimulus of PWM was inhibited (Figure 4). Trypan blue exclusion tests revealed no alterations in cell vitality due to 13-*cis*-retinoic acid in doses 0.1–5μg/ml. At 10μg/ml culture medium, however, increased amounts of stainable lymphocytes were seen (*ca.* 12 per cent) indicating some cytotoxicity.

Influence of Arotinoid (Ro 13-6298)

Doses of arotinoid between 0.1ng and 10μg/ml culture had no influence on DNA synthesis of non-stimulated cultured lymphocytes. Also after addition of PWM no changes were seen in this wide range of dose (Figure 5). In contrast, arotinoid altered the lymphocytic response to ConA at dose levels between 1 and 10ng/ml culture and led to a distinct increase of the ³H-thymidine uptake at these doses, as compared to controls (Figure 6). Higher doses had no influence. The trypan blue exclusion test showed no cell alterations due to arotinoid (0.1ng/ml–10μg/ml).

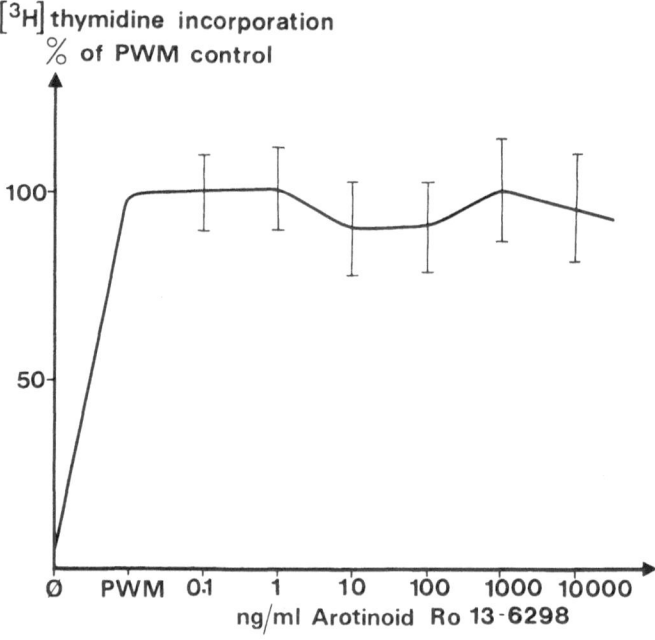

Figure 5. ³H-thymidine uptake in cultured lymphocytes stimulated with PWM in the presence of arotinoid Ro 13-6298.

Discussion

The findings presented here confirmed and extended our previous results on the influence of retinoids on cultured lymphocytes.[16-19] After some years of continuing experience we can state that human peripheral blood lymphocytes may be regarded as target cells for synthetic retinoids *in vitro*. The influence of retinoids, however, may vary according to (a) the type of mitogen, (b) the particular retinoid compound used and (c) the level of the given retinoid dose:

(*a*). In general, a difference is apparent concerning the type of mitogen: PHA and ConA which most likely correspond to T-cell stimulating agents are clearly influenced by the addition of retinoids in culture; whereas, stimulation of lymphocytes with PWM, which is largely regarded as a B-cell mitogen, remains unaltered under retinoids *in vitro*. Only doses of retinoids close to cytotoxic levels, as shown in the trypan blue exclusion test, may also inhibit PWM-stimulation.

(*b*). The influence of retinoids on the T-cell mitogens PHA and ConA may differ according to the type of retinoid used. The free aromatic acid TMMP-RA (Ro 10-1670) clearly inhibits PHA and ConA-induced stimulation. 13-*cis*-retinoic acid (Ro 4-3780) seems to stimulate in low and

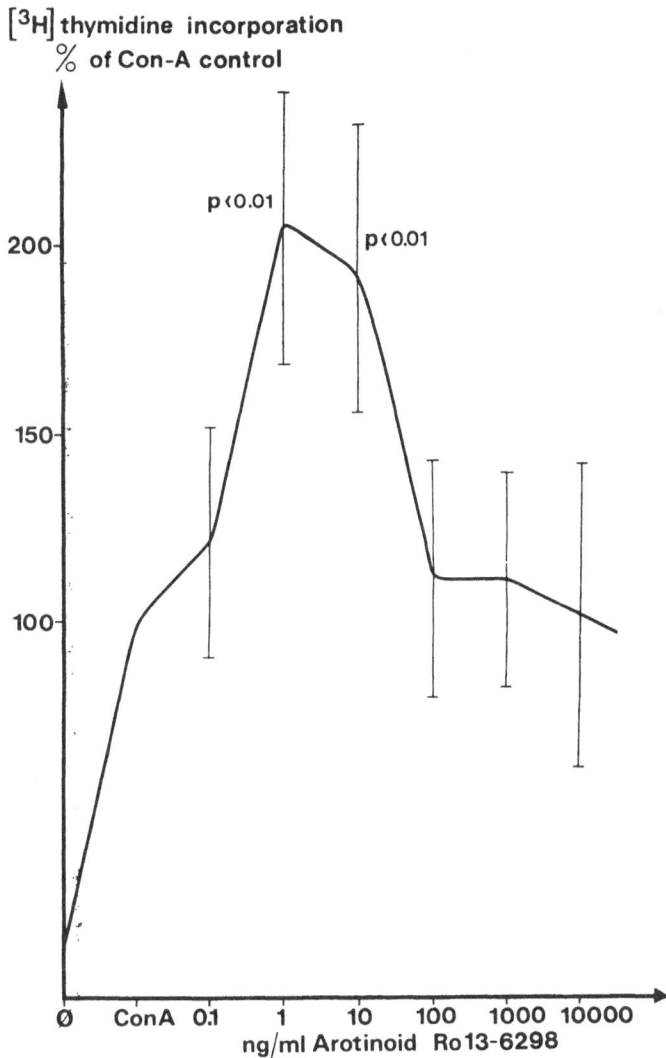

Figure 6. Influence of arotinoid Ro 13-6298 on ^{3}H-thymidine uptake of cultured lymphocytes stimulated with ConA.

to inhibit in higher, non-cytotoxic doses. The new arotinoid (Ro 13-6298)
enhances ConA-induced stimulation in lowest doses and has no influence
whatsoever at higher doses.

(c). The levels of dose being effective *in vitro* differ considerably among
the various retinoids: the free aromatic acid acts in a dose level of
2–12.5μg/ml to inhibit T-cell stimulation; 13-*cis*-retinoic acid acts in a range

of dose of 0.1–5µg/ml culture, leading to enhancement or inhibition of T-cell stimulation; 10µg/ml are obviously cytotoxic. Arotinoid acts at dose levels 1,000× or even lower (1–10g/ml) than the free aromatic acid and enhances T-cell stimulation with ConA.

These results strongly suggest an immunomodulatory effect of retinoids on peripheral blood cells *in vitro*. Interestingly, the modulatory effect becomes evident only in the presence of lectins. We were not able to observe any direct influence of the three retinoid compounds tested on the ³H-thymidine uptake of cultured lymphocytes. At doses close to therapeutic blood levels 13-*cis*-retinoic acid and arotinoid acted as co-mitogens; whereas, the free acid of the aromatic retinoid inhibited DNA synthesis induced by PHA and ConA. It is clearly shown, therefore, that in cell systems *in vitro* changes of the retinoid molecule undoubtedly lead to different or even the opposite pharmacological effects.

Abb and Deinhardt[20] investigated the effect of all-*trans*-retinoic acid and reported results similar to the effect of 13-*cis*-retinoic acid reported here. Low concentrations of all-*trans*-retinoic acid increased PHA-induced lymphocyte proliferation, whereas high doses inhibited the cell response. Soppi *et al.*[21] reported that the response of peripheral blood lymphocytes of patients with Darier's disease treated with aromatic retinoid was clearly lower than that of non-treated patients. In another publication, the same group of authors stated that they had not observed any change of ³H-thymidine uptake after addition of Ro 10-9359 *in vitro*.[22] Bialasiewicz *et al.*[23] on the other hand, found an inhibitory effect with Ro 10-9359 on IgG-synthesis in an *in vitro* system.

In conclusion, we feel that synthetic retinoids exert distinct modulatory effects on the lymphocytic response *in vitro*, particularly on the mitogen-induced T-cell stimulation.

Binding of Retinoids to Various Proteins. A 2S-Intracytoplasmic Isotretinoin-Binding Protein in Human Lymphocytes

In additional experiments the possible interaction between mitogens and TMMP-RA was examined more carefully. 50mg of the drug were given to 2ml physiological saline and the following proteins were added in different solutions: 12mg calf serum protein, 1.5mg ConA, 0.6mg PWM, 2.4mg PHA-M and 320mg polyvalent immunoglobulin. All solutions were incubated for 30 min at room temperature and were then centrifuged for 30 min at 10,000 rev./min to separate unbound amounts of retinoid. Photo-metric analysis of the above solutions at 340nm compared to physiological saline containing the proteins alone or retinoid alone provided evidence that well-defined amounts of TMMP-RA were bound to lectins and, to a

Table 2. Binding capacity of various proteins (lectins) for TMMP-RA (Ro 10-1670).

	E_{340}/mg protein
Calf serum protein	0.05
Con-A	0.9
PWM	1.4
PHA-M	0.44
Immunoglobulin	0.016
Saline	0.00

lesser extent, to calf serum protein and to immunoglobulin (Table 2).

In a further experiment density gradient centrifugation of homogenized lymphocytes incubated with ³H-labelled 13-*cis*-retinoic acid was performed, as described on p.103. The findings revealed evidence for a 2S-protein, binding 13-*cis*-retinoic acid in the homogenate of lymphocytes. Displacement of the ³H-labelled compound by an excess of unlabelled 13-*cis*-retinoic acid was in favour of a specific binding protein in the cell homogenate (Figure 7).

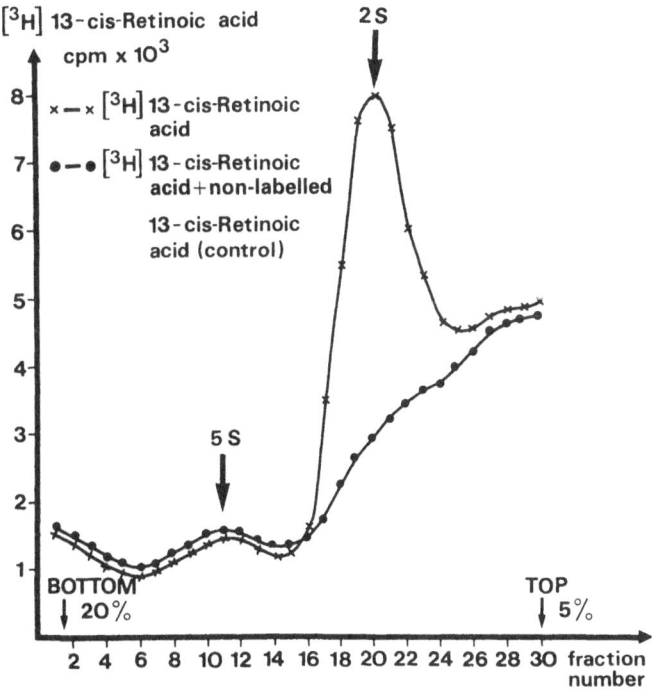

Figure 7. Density gradient centrifugation analysis of homogenized lymphocytes with ³H-labelled 13-*cis*-retinoic acid.

Discussion

The extremely poor solubility of vitamin A derivatives in water must be overcome *in vivo* and also *in vitro* by binding of retinoids to proteins.[24,25] In the experiments described above it became evident that lectins possess a rather high binding capacity for the retinoids tested. For example, their relative binding capacity for TMMP-RA was found to be 10–30-fold higher than that of calf serum. In culture, therefore, a transfer of the retinoid from serum protein to the lectin must take place, which may alter the interaction between lectin and lumphocytes. Interestingly, a region of non-polar, hydrophobic side-chains of amino-acid residues occurs in the ConA-molecule near the carbohydrate-binding site. This region may be bound by aromatic aglycones and alter the functional activity of the lectin.[26,27] One may suspect, that the same region interacts with aromatic retinoid molecules. In other words, aromatic retinoids may exert their particular effects by interacting with polypeptide chains and influencing the functional groups of regulating proteins.

In a previous report we provided evidence that also the plasma cell membrane of lymphocytes binds aromatic retinoid,[15] possibly on the basis of the same mechanism. This interaction undoubtedly contributes to the altered response of cultured lymphocytes to lectins. The affinity of TMMP-RA to cell membranes is in agreement with other reports indicating an altered viscosity of the plasma cell membrane under the influence of all-*trans*-retinoic acid.

A third possible site of retinoid-binding was shown in this study: density gradient centrifugation of ^{3}H-labelled 13-*cis*-retinoic acid evidenced the presence of a specific 2S-binding-protein in homogenized lymphocytes. It is conceivable, therefore, that this binding-protein may provide intra-cytoplasmic transfer of 13-*cis*-retinoic acid to the cell nucleus and influence DNA-synthesis in cultured lymphocytes under certain conditions, similar to all-*trans*-retinoic acid.[28–30] Retinoid–protein complexes may be of major significance as regulatory compounds with controlling properties. From this point of view retinoids may act as hormone-like substances.

Conclusions and Summary

Peripheral blood PMNs are likely to represent target cells for synthetic oral retinoids. Drug influence on the function of these cells, however, may vary depending on the particular retinoid derivative used: Etretinate (Ro 10-9359) had a distinct effect on PMNs from patients with psoriasis (n = 12). Their migration was clearly inhibited *in vitro* after 2–3 weeks oral treatment with Tigason. Visual analysis including microcinematography suggested a disturbance of the microtubular function. In addition, the reduction of radially segmented mononuclear cell nuclei, induced by oxalate as an *in vitro* screening test, supported this suggestion for the main metabolite of etretinate, the free aromatic acid Ro 10-1670. Oral therapy with other retinoids, such as 13-*cis*-retinoic acid (Ro 4-3780) and arotinoid (Ro 13-6298), seemed to slow down PMN activity but failed to show a major influence on the *in vitro* migration of PMNs of patients with psoriasis ($n = 5$), severe acne conglobata ($n = 4$), palmo-plantar keratosis ($n = 3$), Darier's disease ($n = 1$), ichthyosis congenita ($n = 1$) and multiple basal cell carcinomas ($n = 1$).

The response of normal cultured lymphocytes to mitogens was also influenced by retinoids. In particular, T-cell stimulation induced *in vitro* by PHA and ConA was clearly modulated by all retinoids tested. Thus, the aromatic retinoid TMMP-RA inhibited ^{3}H-thymidine uptake of normal cultured lymphocytes stimulated with ConA and PHA, at concentration levels close to those expected under therapeutic doses of Tigason. 13-*cis*-retinoic acid, on the other hand, increased the response of normal cultured lymphocytes to ConA and PHA in low doses and showed some inhibition only in higher doses, which were suspected to be cytotoxic. The arotinoid Ro 13-6298 stimulated the T-cell response to ConA in doses 1,000–1,200× lower than that of the other two retinoids. Higher doses of arotinoid had no influence.

Further experiments confirmed the finding, that retinoids obviously interact with lectins *in vitro*. The binding capacity of lectins for TMMP-RA is 10–30× stronger than that of serum protein. In addition, density gradient centrifugation evidenced a 2S-specific carrier protein in homogenates of normal lymphocytes. These and other results of other authors support the view that retinoids act mainly in their protein-bound form and can be regarded as hormone-like regulatory compounds.

References

1. Engel, H.J., Schütz, R. and Zerbst, E. (1974). Die Blutzellen im Vitalpräparat. *Publ. Wiss. Film. Sekt. Med.*, **2**, 227
2. Engel, H.J. (1963). Neutrophile Granulozyten – Homo sapiens. *Publ. Wiss. Film. Sekt. Med.*, **2**, 245
3. Engel, H.J. (1968). Untersuchungen zur LE-Zellgenese im Supravitalpräparat. *Blut*, **17**, 93
4. Norberg, B. (1969). Neutrophil segmentation and radial segmentation. *Scand. J. Haematol.*, **6**, 274
5. Norberg, B. and Uddman, R. (1973). The oxalate-induced radial segmentation of the nuclei of lymphocytes and monocytes from peripheral blood. *Blut*, **26**, 261
6. Bauer, R., Schütz, R. and Orfanos, C.E. (1982). Granulozyten-Migration in vitro bei Psoriasis-Patienten unter aromatischem Retinoid. *Z. Hautkr.*, **57**, 1247
7. Dubertret, L., Lebreton, C. and Touraine, R. (1982). Inhibition of neutrophil migration by etretinate and its main metabolite. *Br. J. Dermatol.*, **107**, 681
8. Söderström, U.B., Simmingsköld, G., Norberg, B., Bäck, O. and Rydgren, L. (1979). Analysis of polymorphonuclear leukocyte (PMN) migration by the leading front technique. *Exp. Cell. Res.*, **121**, 325
9. Allan, R.B. and Wilkinson, P.C. (1978). A visual analysis of chemotactic and chemo-kinetic locomotion of human neutrophil leucocytes. *Exp. Cell Res.*, **111**, 191

10. Bhisey, A.N. and Freed, J.J. (1971). Ameboid movement induced in cultured macrophages by colchicine or vinblastine. *Exp. Cell Res.*, **64**, 419
11. Ramsey, W.S. and Harris, A. (1973). Leukocyte locomotion and its inhibition by antimitotic drugs. *Exp. Cell. Res.*, **82**, 262
12. Bandmann, U., Rydgren, L. and Norberg, B. (1974). The difference between random movement and chemotaxis. *Exp. Cell Res.*, **88**, 63
13. Bäck, O., Bandmann, U., Norberg, B. and Söderström, U.B. (1978). Direct chemotaxis and leucocyte-induced chemotaxis of poly-morphonuclear leucocytes. *Scand. J. Haematol.*, **20**, 108
14. Solomon, F. (1980). Organizing microtubules in the cytoplasm. *Cell*, **22**, 331
15. Rydgren. L., Simmingsköld, G. Bandmann, U. and Norberg, B. (1976). The role of cytoplasmic microtubules in polymorphonuclear leukocyte chemotaxis. *Exp. Cell Res.*, **99**, 207
16. Bauer, R. and Orfanos, C.E. (1981). Influence of retinoid on human blood cells in vitro. TMMP-retinoid inhibits the mitogenic properties of lectins and modulates the lymphocytic response. In Orfanos, C.E. *et al.* (eds.). *Retinoids. Advances in Basic Research and Therapy.* pp. 153–160. (Berlin, Heidelberg, New York: Springer-Verlag)
17. Bauer, R. and Orfanos, C.E. (1981). Trimethylmethoxyphenyl retinoid acid (Ro 10-1670) inhibits mitogen-induced DNA-synthesis in peripheral blood lymphocytes in vitro. *Br. J. Dermatol.*, **105**, 19
18. Bauer, R., Stadler, R., Gollnick, H., Brand, G. and Orfanos, C.E. (1983). Modulation of mitogen-induced lumphocytic response in vitro by a new synthetic retinoid, the arotinoid Ro 13-6298. *Arch. Dermatol. Res.* (In press)
19. Bauer, R., Gollnick, H., Brand. G. and Orfanos, C.E. (1983). Proliferation of stimulated lumphocytes under 13-cis retinoic acid. Abstract. *Arch Dermatol. Res.* (In press)
20. Abb, J., Abb, H. and Deinhardt, F. (1982). Retinoic acid suppression of human leukocyte interferon production. *Immunopharmacology*, **4**, 303
21. Soppi, A.M., Soppi, E. and Jansen, C.T. (1981). Effect of systemic retinoid Ro 10-9359 treatment on immunological parameters in Darier's disease. In Orfanos C.E. *et al.* (eds.). *Retinoids. Advances in Basic Research and Therapy.* pp. 321-322. (Berlin, Heidelberg, New York: Springer-Verlag)
22. Soppi, E., Tertti, R., Soppi, A.M., Toivanen, A. and Jansen, C.T. (1982). Differential in vitro effects of etretinate and retinoic acid on the PHA and ConA induced lymphocyte transformation, suppressor cell induction and leukocyte migration inhibitory factor (LMIF) production. *Int. J. Immunopharmac.*, **4**, 437
23. Bialasiewicz, A.A., Lubach, D. and Marghescu, S. (1981). Immunological features in psoriasis: Effects of Ro 10-9359, Concanavalin A (ConA), pokeweed mitogen (PVM) and methotrexate (MTX) on cultivated lymphocytes. In Orfanos, C.E. *et al.* (eds.). *Retinoids. Advances in Basic Research and Therapy.* pp. 335–338. (Berlin, Heidelberg, New York: Springer-Verlag)
24. Chytil, F. and Ong, D.E. (1979). Cellular retinol- and retinoic acid-binding proteins in vitamin A action. *Fed. Proc.*, **38**, 2510
25. Smith, J.E. and Goodman, D.S. (1979). Retinol-binding protein and the regulation of vitamin A transport. *Fed. Proc.*, **38**, 2504
26. Edelman, G.M., Cunningham, B.A., Reeke, G.N., Becker, J.W., Waxdal, M.J. and Wang, J.L. (1972). The covalent and three dimensional structure of Concanavalin A. *Proc. Natl. Acad. Sci. USA*, **69**, 2580
27. Poretz, R.D. and Goldstein, I.J. (1971). Protein-carbohydrate interaction on the mode of binding of aromatic moieties to ConA, PHA and the jack bean. *Biochem. Pharmacol.*, **20**, 2727
28. Ong, D.E. and Chytil, F. (1976). Presence of cellular retinol and retinoic acid binding proteins in experimental tumors. *Cancer Lett.*, **2**, 25
29. Sani, B.P. and Corbett, T.H. (1977). Retinoic acid-binding protein in normal tissues and experimental tumors. *Cancer Res.*, **37**, 209
30. Ong, D.E., Page, D.L. and Chytil, F. (1975). Retinoic acid binding protein: Occurrence in human tumors. *Science*, **190**, 60

13
Effects of Retinoids on Chondrogenesis and Epidermogenesis *In Vitro*

D. TSAMBAOS, B. ZIMMERMANN and C.E. ORFANOS

Introduction

In the last few years, the mouse limb bud culture has been successfully used as a test system for studies in developmental biology and prenatal toxicology.[1-5] In this highly reproducible system, which was originally developed by Kochhar[6] and Aydelotte and Kochhar,[7] the chondrogenesis and epidermogenesis *in vitro* proceed in a well-organized fashion simulating the corresponding processes of morphogenetic differentiation *in vivo*.[8,9] In this paper we review our recent work on the effects of various retinoids on chondrogenesis and epidermogenesis *in vitro*, using the mouse limb bud culture as an experimental model.[10-13]

Material and Methods

Forelimb buds were dissected from 11-day-old NMRI mouse embryos (day 0 = day of conception) and were grown for 3 or 6 days in an organ culture,[14] as modified by Aydelotte and Kochhar.[7] Detailed descriptions of this technique have been published elsewhere.[1,5] The growth medium consisted of BGJ-medium (Gibco-Biocult) supplemented with 20 per cent fetal calf serum (Boehringer, Mannheim) and $75 \mu g/ml$ ascorbic acid. The following synthetic retinoids* were used: Ro 4-3780 (13-*cis* retinoic acid), Ro 10-1670 (trimethylmethoxyphenyl analogue of retinoic acid),

---

*All retinoids used in our studies were kindly supplied by Dr W. Bollag, Hoffmann-La Roche, Switzerland and Dr R. Hennes, Hoffmann-La Roche, Germany.

Ro 11-1430 (trimethylmethoxyphenyl analogue of retinoic acid ethyl amide) and Ro 13-6298 (arotinoid ethyl ester). Considering the biological activity of these compounds, as found by Bollag[15] in the antipapilloma test and based on the results of a pilot study performed in our laboratory, we added the retinoids (dissolved in DMSO) to the medium to give final concentrations of 0.1, 0.5, 1.0, 5.0, 10.0 and 15.0 μg/ml (Ro 4-3780, Ro 10-1670, Ro 11-1430) and 0.1, 0.5, 1.0, 5.0, 10.0 and 15.0 ng/ml (Ro 13-6298). Equivalent amounts of 0.1 per cent DMSO were added to the medium of the control cultures. The limb buds were exposed to retinoids from day 1 to day 3. A part of the limb buds was then processed for electron microscopy. The other part was transferred to and cultivated in the control medium for 3 additional days. The limb buds were fixed in 2 per cent glutaraldehyde and 1 per cent tannic acid in 0.1 mol/l phosphate buffer (pH 7.2) and postfixed in 1 per cent OsO_4. Then the specimens were dehydrated in ethanol and embedded in Epon. Ultrathin sections stained with lead citrate and uranyl acetate were examined with a Zeiss Em 10 C or a Siemens EM 101 electron microscope.

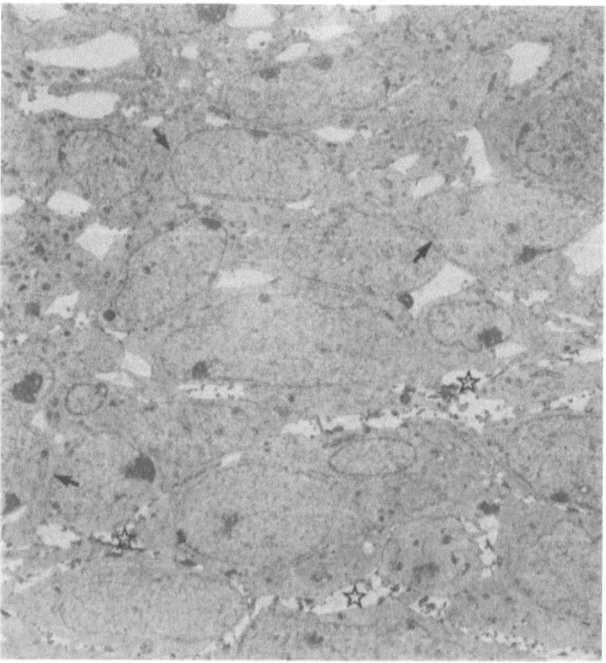

Figure 1. Blastema cells after 3 days of cultivation in the control medium. The densely packed cells reveal considerable numbers of close contacts, particularly of the gap junction type (arrows) and begin to produce tannin-positive matrix (stars) ($\times$ 3,200).

Results

Chondrogenesis[10,11]

Control Cultures

After a 3-day-cultivation in the control medium the densely packed blastema cells were round or oval in shape, possessed a large nucleus and

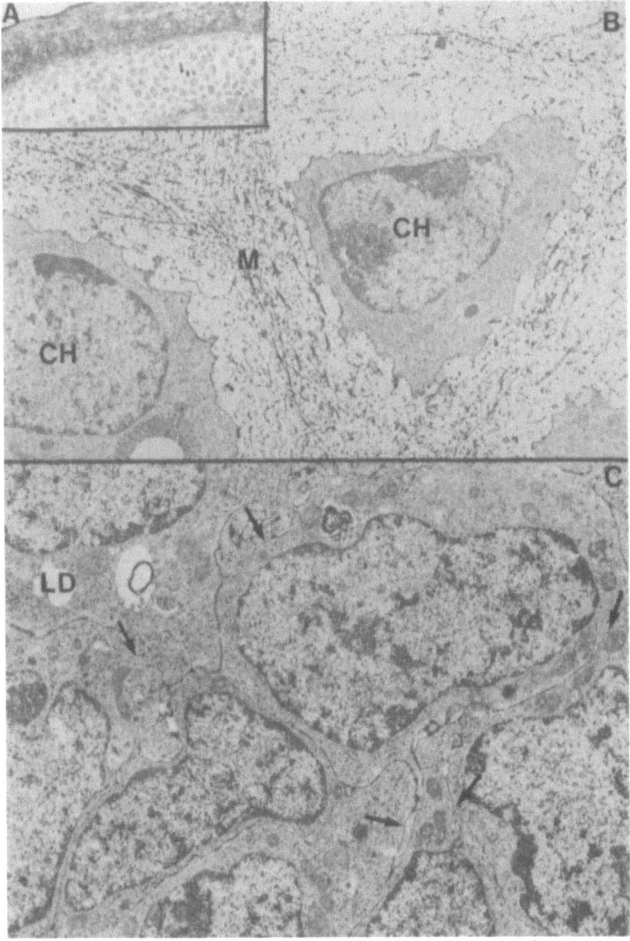

Figure 2. (A) Cartilaginous differentiation of the digits in control limb buds after 6 days in culture (× 360). (B) Differentiated chondrocytes (CH) with well-developed rough endoplasmic reticulum, separated from each other by wide areas containing cartilage specific matrix (M); (control medium; days 1 to 6) (× 6,600). (C) Subsequent to treatment with 10.0μg/ml Ro 4-3780 (days 1 to 3). Extensive formation of gap junctions (arrows) between the treated cells, which maintain their mesenchymal characteristics and produce no matrix (LD=lipid droplets) (× 8,400).

small amounts of cytoplasm with several mitochondria and some rare profiles of endoplasmic reticulum (Figure 1). Blastema cells exhibited considerable numbers of specific contacts of the gap junction type. In some intercellular spaces small amounts of tannin-positive matrix could be already seen.

After 6 days of cultivation in the control medium a cartilaginous differentiation was evident in the distal parts of the limb buds (Figure 2(a)). Chondrocytes were round or oval in shape and at most places showed a decrease in the nuclear to cytoplasmic ratio, as compared to blastema cells. They exhibited prominent nucleoli, a well-developed rough endoplasmic reticulum and several mitochondria. They were separated from each other by wide intercellular spaces, which were occupied by the components of the cartilage matrix (Figure 2 (b)). At higher magnification,

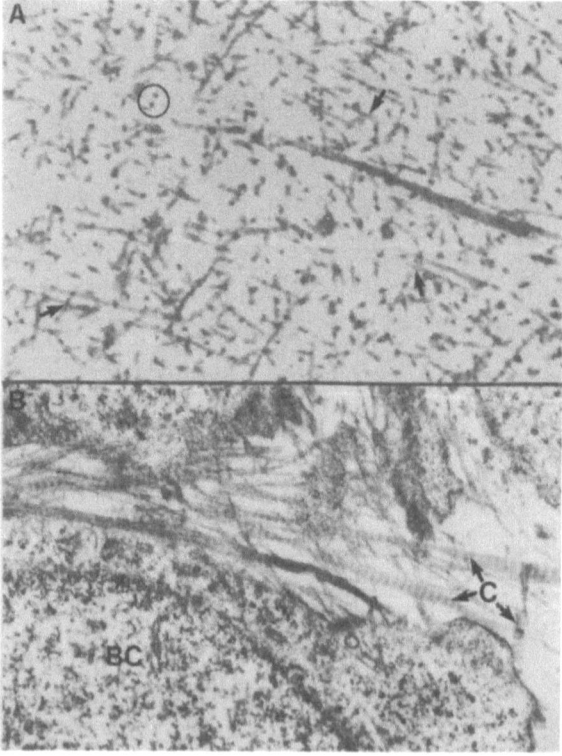

Figure 3. (A) Cartilage specific matrix in control limb buds after 6 days in culture, consisting of proteoglycan matrix granules (circle) and collagen fibrils (arrows) (× 33,000). (B) Blastema cells (BC) treated with 10.0μg/ml Ro 4-3780 (days 1 to 3) do not differentiate to chondrocytes even after transfer to and cultivation in the control medium for 3 additional days. Proteoglycan matrix granules are lacking. Cells predominantly produce thick and banded collagen fibrils (C) (× 20,000).

the latter consisted of mostly unbanded and thin collagen fibrils (10–20nm) and proteoglycan matrix granules (Figure 3 (a)).

Retinoid-Treated Cultures

All retinoids were capable of inducing a dose-dependent inhibition of the differentiation of limb buds from the blastema stage (day 11 of gestation) to the cartilaginous anlagen of skeleton. A detailed analysis of the dosage–effect relationship for each retinoid will be published elsewhere. It should be noted, however, that the first signs of inhibition of chondrogenic differentiation appeared when Ro 4-3780 and Ro 10-1670 were added to the medium in concentrations 0.5–1.0μg/ml, compared to 10.0μg/ml and 0.5ng/ml for Ro 11-1430 and Ro 13-6298 repectively Since in ultrastructural terms, the effects of the tested retinoids on the blastema cells were very similar, they will be described here together.

After a 3-day-cultivation with retinoids the condensation of blastema cells was more pronounced, as compared to the controls. In the large and lobulated nuclei of the treated cells irregular chromatin clumps were seen. The cytoplasm contained increased numbers of coiled membrane figures and phagolysosomes, as compared to the controls. There was a marked increase in the formation of gap junctions. After subsequent cultivation of the limb buds in the control medium for 3 additional days, the blastema cells retained the ultrastructural features seen after the 3-day-treatment with retinoids (Figure 2 (c)). Extremely close apposition of plasma membranes (4–8nm) often occurred at the contact zones of the cells, whereas the formation of gap junctions was extensive. In the narrow intercellular spaces varying amounts of collagen fibrils were seen. Most of them were banded (65nm periodicity) and revealed a diameter ranging between 38 and 55nm, while others were unbanded and much thinner (7–10nm) (Figure 3 (b)). The proteoglycan matrix granules were markcdly reduced or completely absent.

Epidermogenesis[10,12,13]

Control Cultures

After 3 days of cultivation in the control medium, the embryonic epithelium (apart from the region of the apical ectodermal ridge) consisted of three clearly defined strata (Figure 4). The cuboidal cells of the stratum basale revealed round or oval nuclei and contained several mitochondria, small amounts of glycogen and a few cisternae of rough endoplasmic

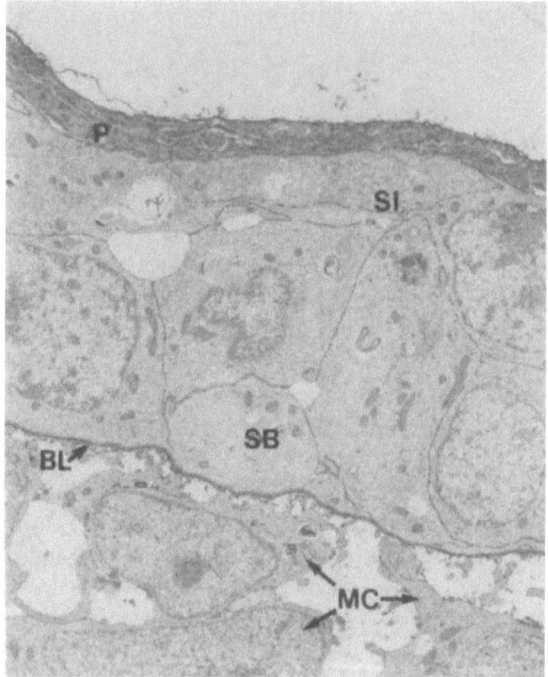

Figure 4. Embryonic epithelium of control limb buds after 3 days in culture. Epithelial cells reveal a very low level of differentiation and are arranged in three strata:stratum basale (SB, stratum intermedium (SI) and periderm (P) (BL=basal lamina; MC=mesenchymal cell) (× 5,500)..

reticulum. Desmosomes and hemidesmosomes were relatively rare and poorly developed; free tonofilaments could not be detected. The intercellular spaces were of variable width. The cells of the stratum intermedium were polygonal or slightly flattened with their long axis parallel to the surface of the epidermis, and contained increased amounts of immature desmosomes, as compared to the basal cells. At some places short and thin bundles of tonofilaments could be seen. The cells of the stratum intermedium were covered by extremely flattened, electron-dense peridermal cells, which contained spindle-shaped nuclei and considerable numbers of membrane-bound vesicles.

After a 6-day-cultivation in the control medium the embryonic mouse epidermis revealed the morphological features of a normally keratinizing, squamous epithelium and consisted of four strata. The cells of the stratum basale were cuboidal or cylindrical in shape and their nuclei were oriented with the long axis perpendicular to the continuous basal lamina (Figure 5C)), which revealed frequent hemidesmosomes. A few mitochondria, small amounts of glycogen and some profiles of rough endoplasmic

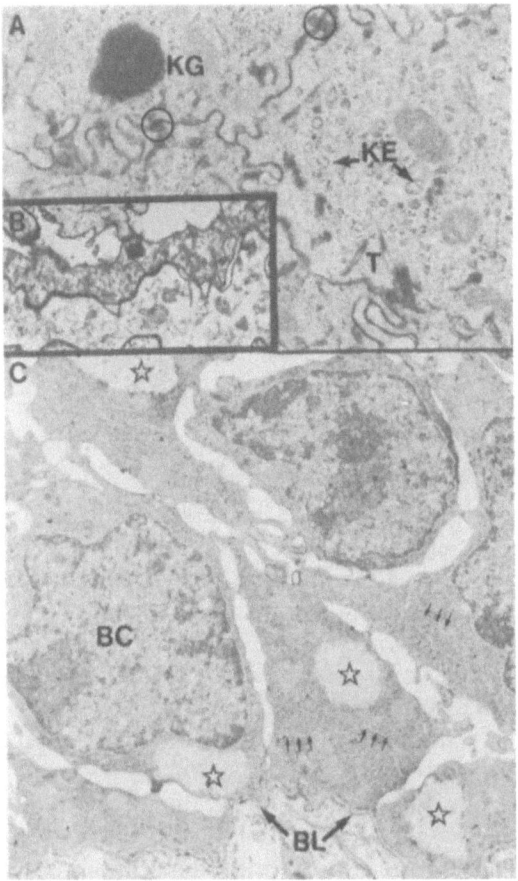

Figure 5. Embryonic epithelium of control limb buds after 6 days in culture. (A) In the stratum spinosum, epithelial cells reveal an advanced stage of differentiation containing tonofilaments (T), desmosomes (circles), keratohyalin granules (KG) and keratinosomes (KE). The intercellular spaces are very thin (× 21,000). (B) The stratum corneum consists of flattened corneocytes with thickened plasma membranes and rather uniformly dense filaments closely resembling a normal keratin pattern (× 9,000). (C) The stratum basale consists of cuboidal or cylindrical cells (BC) with small numbers of free tonofilaments and desmosomes and considerable amounts of glycogen (stars). Arrows point to profiles of rough endoplasmic reticulum. The intercellular spaces are mostly wide (BL=basal lamina) (× 8,600).

reticulum were visible. Small numbers of desmosomes and free tonofilaments were regularly seen; the intercellular spaces were wide. In the lower stratum spinosum the epithelial cells were polygonal in shape, whereas in the upper stratum spinosum they became flattened. In contrast to the basal cells, they revealed an advanced stage of differentiation containing considerable amounts of free tonofilaments, keratinosomes and several keratohyalin granules (Figure 5 (A)). In the narrow intercellular spaces interdigitating cell processes could be observed, held together by desmosomes. The number of the latter was higher, as compared to the stratum basale. Occasionally, gap junctions were seen. The cells of the stratum spinosum were remarkedly flattened; their long axes oriented parallel to the surface of the epidermis. They contained numerous free tonofilaments, keratinosomes, and keratohyalin granules. The intercellular spaces were narrow. Large numbers of desmosomes were seen, connecting neighbouring cells. The stratum corneum consisted of four to six flattended corneocytes, which showed thickened plasma membranes and rather uniformly dense filaments closely resembling a normal keratin pattern (Figure 5 (B)).

Retinoid-Treated Cultures

All retinoids were capable of inducing a dose-dependent and persistent inhibition of the differentiation of mouse embryonic epithelium *in vitro*. However, they exerted their inhibitory effects starting at different levels of concentration. Thus, Ro 4-3780 was active in concentrations $\geq 5.0 \mu g/ml$, Ro 10-1670 in $\geq 1.0 \mu g/ml$, Ro 11-1430 in $\geq 10.0 \mu g/ml$, whereas Ro 13-6298 was active in concentrations $\geq 1.0 ng/ml$. A detailed analysis of the dosage–effect relationship for each retinoid will be published elsewhere. Since in ultrastructural terms the effects.of the tested compounds on the epithelial cells were very similar, they will be described here together.

After a 3-day-cultivation with retinoids, the thickness of the embryonic epithelium was increased, as compared to the control cultures. The basal lamina revealed at some places gaps and reduplications (Figures 6(A)) and 6(B)). Through the former, cytoplasmic projections of mesenchymal cells were occasionally contacting the epithelial cells of the stratum basale. In all epidermal layers, cells often revealed prominent nucleoli; in their cytoplasm increased numbers of profiles of rough endoplasmatic reticulum, Golgi membranes and ribosomes were visible. Hemidesmosomes could not be detected and immature desmosomes were very rare or absent. Epithelial cells were densely packed and revealed high numbers of gap junctions. At some places the plasma membranes were flabby and fused. In the vicinity of the cellular surface and in the intercellular spaces coiled membrane figures could be seen. The cells of periderm were sometimes lacking; when present they revealed no alterations.

In limb buds, which were treated with retinoids for 3 days and were then transferred to and cultivated in the control medium for 3 additional days, the thickness of the embryonic epidermis was increased, as compared to the controls (Figure 7(A)). The basal lamina revealed alterations almost identical to those seen after 3 days of cultivation in the presence of

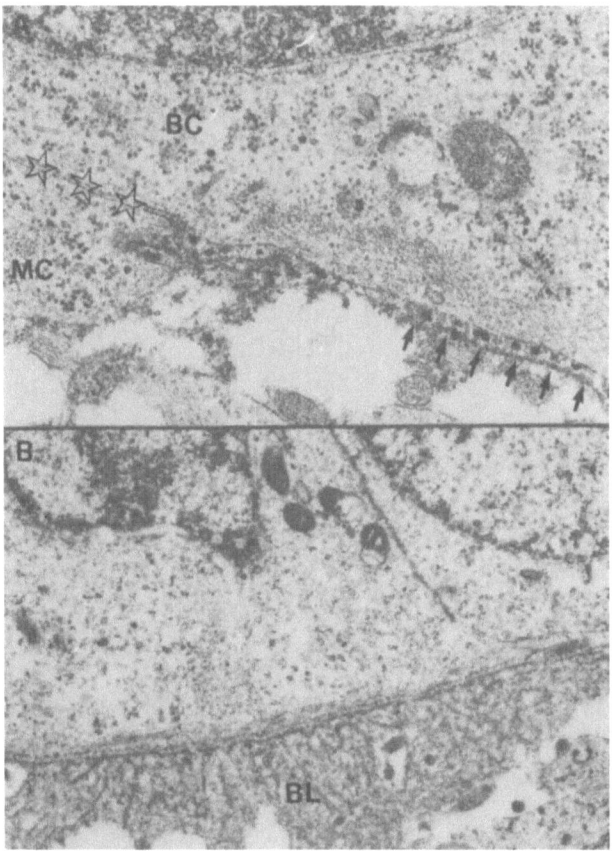

Figure 6. (A) Dermo-epidermal junction of limb buds treated with 1.0ng/ml Ro 13-6298 (days 1 to 3), after 6 days in culture. Through the gaps of the basal lamina (stars), cytoplasmic projections of mesenchymal cells (MC) are contacting the basal cells (BC). Arrows point to areas with intact basal lamina (× 39,000). (B) Dermo-epidermal junction of limb buds treated with 10.0μg/ml Ro 10-1670 (days 1 to 3) after 6 days in culture. Note the marked reduplications of the basal lamina (BL) (×16,000).

retinoids. The densely packed epithelial cells revealed no or or very low levels of differentiation. Their ultrastructural features resembled those of the underlying mesenchymal cells. Tonofilaments and desmosomes were very rare or absent (Figure 7(B)). Keratinosomes and keratohyalin granules were very rare or completely lacking. The fusion of plasma membranes of adjacent cells was prominent and the formation of gap junctions was extensive (Figures 8(B) and 8(C)). Particularly in the upper epithelial layers, large number of coiled membrane figures were present (Figure 8(A)). The horny layer was poorly developed or absent.

127

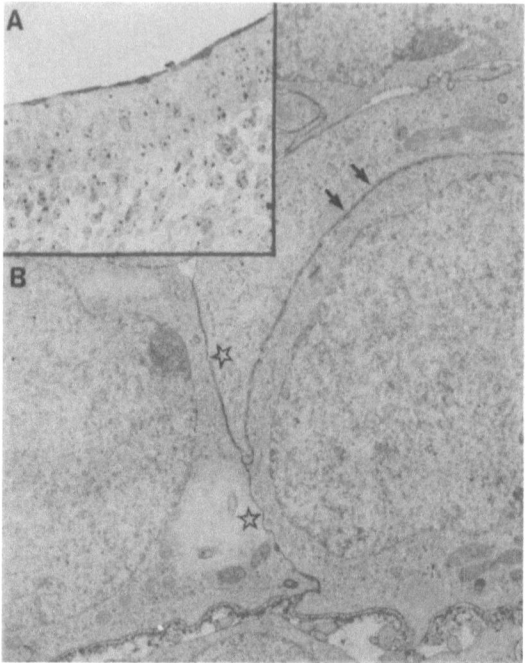

Figure 7. Epithelium of limb buds treated with 10.0ng/ml Ro 13-6298 (days 1 to 3) after 6 days in culture. (A) The densely packed epithelial cells reveal prominent nucleoli; keratohyalin granules are not visible. Peridermal cells are still present here (× 380). (B) Tonofilaments and desmosomes are absent in the basal cells, whose features resemble those of the underlying mesenchymal cells. Arrows point to areas with membrane fusion and stars point to gap junctions (× 10,000).

Discussion

Chondrogenesis

The results of our studies showed that a 3-day-cultivation of limb buds (from 11-day-old mouse embryos) in the presence of retinoids results in a dose-dependent and persistent inhibition of chondrogenesis. Marked quantitative differences were found between the tested retinoids with regard to the expression of their inhibitory effects, even between compounds with very similar molecular structure, such as Ro 10-1670 and Ro 11-1430. In ultrastructural terms, however, the treated blastema cells uniformly responded to all retinoids, provided that the latter were applied in sufficient amounts. The early stages of chondrogenesis in limb buds grown in a retinoid-free medium are characterized by a condensation of mesenchymal cells, which gives rise to the blastema.[16] As their close contacts are progressively disrupted, the blastema cells differentiate to

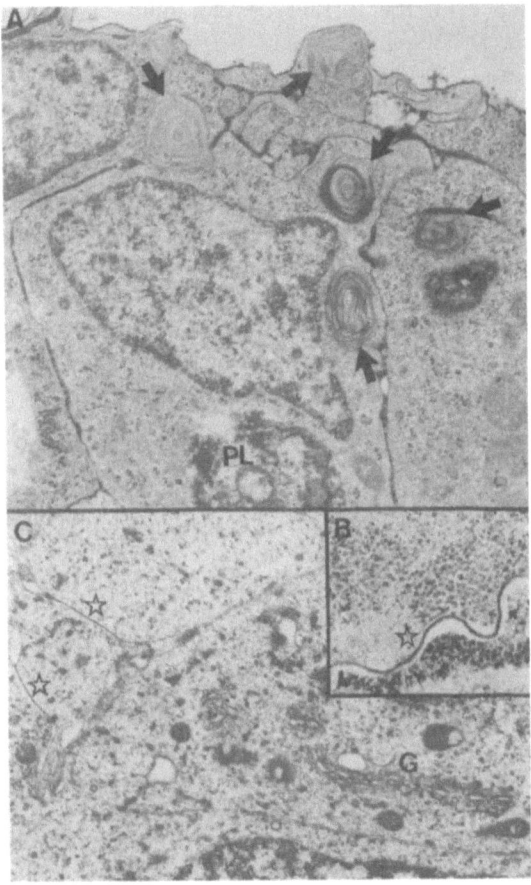

Figure 8. (A) Epithelium of limb buds treated with 10.0ng/ml Ro 13-6298 (days 1 to 3) after 6 days in culture. In the upper epithelial layers large number of coiled membrane figures (arrows) can be seen. Keratohyalin granules and keratinosomes are lacking. There is no evidence of cornification (PL=phagolysosome) (× 20,000). (B), (C) Epithelium of limb buds treated with 10.0μg/ml Ro 10-1670 (days 1 to 3) after 6 days in culture. Extensive formation of gap junctions (stars) and well-developed Golgi membranes (G) ((B)× 32,000; (C)× 17,000).

chondrocytes and produce the cartilage specific matrix.[17] Under treatment with retinoids, as shown in our studies, the disruption of the condensation process does not take place and the development of close contacts, particularly that of gap junctions is further enhanced. The blastema cells maintain their mesenchymal morphological characteristics and produce – instead of matrix – mostly thick and banded collagen fibrils with minimal amounts of or no proteoglycan granules.

The mechanisms by which retinoids exert their inhibitory effects on the mouse limb bud chondrogenesis *in vitro* are unknown. Considering the maintenance and even the further development of extensive and close membrane contacts between the cells, it is reasonable to suggest that the retinoids may induce modifications in their surface. The resulting changes in the cell communication, together with a possible interaction with nuclear components may be implicated in the mechanisms of antichondrogenic action of retinoids. This hypothesis is strongly supported by the findings of Hassell et al.[18] and Lewis et al.[19] These authors found that, in high density cultures of mesenchymal cells derived from chick or mouse embryos, the chondrogenesis is inhibited by retinoic acid and that the treated cells reveal surface features different from those seen in the control cultures. The retinoic acid-treated cells retain the 220,000 dalton surface glycoprotein (fibronectin) of the prechondrogenic phase, which is lost with normal differentiation and contain smaller amounts of the 80,000 dalton surface protein, as compared to the controls. Finally, in other cell lines[20] vitamin A, which also inhibits the chondrogenesis in vitro, induces an increase in the gangliosides of the cellular surface.

Epidermogenesis

In our studies the epidermis of 11-day-old mouse embryos showed a dose-dependent inhibition of differentiation after a 3-day-treatment with retinoids, which persisted even after transfer of the limb buds to and further cultivation in the control medium for 3 additional days. Ultra-structural evidence for mucous production by or in the epithelial cells could not be found even in those specimens which were treated with excessive doses of these compounds. However, since in our experiments only 11-day-old mouse embryos were used, we cannot exclude the possibility that mucous production may appear in the limb bud epithelium if it is exposed to the retinoids at an earlier or later stage of its development. Evidence in favour of this possibility comes from New,[21] who could demonstrate mucous production in rat tongue under vitamin A in 16-day-old embryos but not in 20-day-old embryos, which responded only with an inhibition of keratinization.

Occurrence of gaps in the basal lamina has been previously reported in organ cultures of embryonic mouse and chick skin treated with vitamin A and retinoic acid.[22–24] Since these alterations preceded all other changes in the embryonic epithelium, Hardy et al.[24] suggested that the basal lamina may be primarily affected by the retinoids. The defects of the basal lamina could be casually related to the mucous metaplasia of the epithelium, since they may have allowed 'inappropriate' dermal signals to reach the epidermal cells and modulate their differentiation. This hypothesis was supported by the results of another study of Hardy et al.,[25] which had revealed that areas of hair follicle walls with intact basal lamina maintain their normal structure in organ culture of mouse skin in the presence of excess vitamin A; on the contrary, areas with a vitamin A-induced breakdown of the basal lamina showed metaplastic changes of the epithelial cells. In our studies the gaps of the basal lamina did not precede the morphological changes of the embryonic epithelium under the retinoids tested here and they were not as extensive as reported under vitamin A. Furthermore, we could detect no differences in the expression of retinoid effects in the embryonic mouse epithelium between areas with basal lamina breakdown and those with intact basal lamina. Since inhibition of keratinization can be also seen in isolated embryonic epidermis subsequent to treatment with retinoids,[13] it seems likely to us that epithelial-mesenchymal interactions are not of primary importance for the retinoid action on the embryonic epithelium. On the other hand, since the basal lamina is thought to be produced by the basal epithelial cells,[26] its breakdown under retinoids may represent a consequence rather than the cause of the alterations in the epithelial cells.

In our studies the increase of gap junctions, the fusion of adjacent plasma membranes and the occurrence of numerous coiled membrane figures were prominent changes of the embryonic mouse epithelium in response to retinoids. These alterations possibly reflect distinct effects of retinoids on the structure and turnover of cell membranes. Increase of gap junctions was also found in human or animal skin after topical and oral application of retinoic acid and etretinate respectively.[27-29] It seems, therefore, that both embryonic and adult epidermis respond to the influence of retinoids with an increased formation of gap junctions. Since the latter are considered to play an important role in the communication, growth and differentiation of epithelial cells,[30] their increase under retinoids may be implicated in the mechanisms of the pharmacological action of these compounds.

In conclusion, the results of our studies indicate that all retinoids tested here are capable of exerting a dose-dependent and persistent inhibition of chondrogenesis and epidermogenesis *in vitro*. Marked quantitative but no qualitative differences were found between these compounds with regard to the expression of their effects at the ultrastructural level. Ro 13-6298 was the most potent retinoid and Ro 11-1430 the compound with the weakest effects. The mouse limb bud culture seems to be a useful *in vitro* test system for the comparative evaluation of the antichondrogenic and antikeratinizing effects of various synthetic retinoids.

References

1. Neubert, D., Merker, H.J. and Tapken, S. (1974). Comparative studies on the prenatal development of mouse extremities *in vivo* and in organ culture. *Naunyn-Schmiedeberg's Arch. Pharmacol.*, **286**, 251

2. Merker H.J. (1975). Significance of the limb bud cultures system for investigations of teratogenic mechanisms. In Neubert, D. and Merker, H.J. (eds.). *New Approaches to the Evaluation of Abnormal Embryonic Development*. pp. 161–199. (Stuttgart: Georg Thieme Publishers)

3. Zimmermann, B., Neubert, D., Bachmann, D. and Merker, H.J. (1975). Induction of skeletal malformations in organ cultures of mouse limb buds. *Experientia*, **31**, 227

4. Merker, H.J. (1977). Considerations on the problem of critical period during the development of limb skeleton. In Bergsma, D. and Lenz, W. (eds.). *Birth Defects*. pp. 179–202. (New York: Alan R. Liss)

5. Zimmerman, B. (1978). The development of alkaline phosphatase activity in limb buds of mouse embryos *in vitro* and its relation to chondrogenesis. *Anat. Embryol.*, **153**, 95

6. Kochhar, D.M. (1970). Effects of azetidine-2-carboxylic acid, a proline analog on chondrogenesis in cultured limb buds. In Bass, R., Beck, F., Merker, H.J., Neubert, D. and Randhahn, R. (eds.). *Metabolic Pathways in Mammalian Embryos during Organogenesis and its Modification by Drugs*. pp. 475–482. (Berlin: Free University of Berlin)

7. Aydelotte M.B. and Kochhar, D.M. (1972). Development of mouse limb buds in organ culture:chondrogenesis in the presence of a proline analog, L-azetidine-2-carboxylic acid. *Dev. Biol.*, **28**, 191

8. Schultz-Ehrenburg, U. (1975). Differentiation of the epidermis in the limb bud culture. In Neubert, D. and Merker, H.J. (eds.). *New Approaches to the Evaluation of Abnormal Embryonic Development*. pp. 213–225. (Stuttgart: Georg Thieme)

9. Merker, H.J., Zimmerman, B., Barrach, H.J., Grundmann, K. and Ebel, H. (1981). Simulation of steps of limb skeletogenesis *in vitro*. In Merker, H.J., Nau, H. and Neubert, D. (eds.). *Teratology of the Limbs*. pp. 137–151. (Berlin, New York: Walter de Gruyter & Co.)

10. Zimmermann, B. and Tsambaos, D. (1982). Effects of different retinoids on ectoderm and mesoderm of embryonic limb buds *in vitro*. *Arch. Dermatol. Res.*, **273**, 165

11. Zimmermann, B. and Tsambaos, D. (1983). Retinoid-induced persistence of mesenchymal cell condensation and inhibition of chondrogenic differentiation *in vitro*. In press

12. Tsambaos, D. and Zimmerman, B. (1983). Effects of arotinoid Ro 13-6298 on the differentiation of embryonic mouse epidermis *in vitro*. In press

13. Tsambaos, D. and Zimmermann, B. (1983). Retinoid-induced inhibition of differentiation in isolated embryonic epidermis. In preparation

14. Trowell, O.A. (1959). The culture of mature organs in a synthetic medium. *Exp. Cell Res.*, **16**, 118

15. Bollag, W. (1982). Chemistry and pharmacology of retinoids. In Farber, E.M., Cox, A.J., Nall, L. and Jacobs, P.H. (eds.). *Psoriasis. Proceedings of the Third International Symposium, Stanford* (July 3–17 1981). pp. 175–183. (New York, London: Grune and Stratton)

16. Thorogood, P.V. and Hinchcliffe, J.R. (1975). An analysis of condensation process during chondrogenesis in the embryonic chick hind limb. *J. Embryol. Exp. Morphol.*, **33**, 581

17. Grüneberg, H. and Lee, A.J. (1973). The anatomy and development of brachypodism in the mouse. *J. Embryol. Exp. Morphol.*, **30**, 119

18. Hassell, J.R., Pennypacker, J.P., Yamada, K.M. and Pratt, R.M. (1978). Changes in cell surface proteins during normal and vitamin A-inhibited chondrogenesis *in vitro*. *Ann. NY Acad. Sci.*, **312**, 406

19. Lewis, C.A., Pratt, R.M., Pennypacker, J.P. and Hassell, J.R. (1978). Inhibition of limb chondrogenesis *in vitro* by vitamin A:alterations in cell surface characteristics. *Dev. Biol.*, **64**, 31

20. Patt, L.M., Itaya, K. and Hakomori, S.I. (1978). Retinol induces density dependent growth inhibition and changes in glycolipids and LETS. *Nature* (London), **273**, 379

21. New, D.A.T. (1963). Effects of excess vitamin A on cultures of skin and buccal epithelium of the embryonic rat and mouse. *Br. J. Dermatol.*, **75**, 320

22. Hardy, M.H. (1974). Epithelial-mesenchymal interactions *in vitro* altered by vitamin A and some implications. *In Vitro*, **10**, 358

23. Peck, G.L., Elias, P.M. and Wetzler, B. (1977). Effects of retinoic acid on embryonic chick skin. *J. Invest. Dermatol.*, **69**, 463

24. Hardy, M.H., Sweeny, P.R. and Bellows, C.G. (1978). The effects of vitamin A on the epidermis of the fetal mouse in organ culture – an ultrastructural study. *J. Ultrastr. Res.*, **64**, 246

25. Hardy, M.H. Sonstegard, K.S. and Sweeny, P.R. (1973). Light and electron microscopic studies of the reprogramming of epidermis and vibrissa follicles by excess vitamin A in organ culture. *In Vitro*, **8**, 405

26. Banerjee, S.D., Cohen, R.H. and Bernfield, M.R. (1977). Basal lamina of embryonic salivary epithelia. Production by the epithelium and role in maintaining lobular morphology. *J. Cell. Biol.*, **73**, 445

27. Prutkin, L. (1975). Mucous metaplasia and gap junctions in the vitamin A acid-treated tumor, keratoacanthoma. *Cancer Res.*, **35**, 364

28. Elias, P.M., Grayson, S., Caldwell, T.M. and McNutt, N.S. (1980). Gap junction proliferation in retinoic acid-treated human basal cell carcinoma. *Lab. Invest.*, **42**, 469

29. Caputo, R., Gasparini, G., Contini, D. and Berti, E. (1981). Freeze fracture study of psoriatic lesions after oral administration of retinoid. In Orfanos, C.E., Braun-Falco, O., Farber, E.M., Grupper, Ch., Polano, M.K. and Schuppli, R. (eds.). *Retinoids: Advances in Basic Research and Therapy.* pp. 325–329. (Berlin, Heidelberg, New York: Springer-Verlag)

30. McNutt, N.S. (1977). Freeze-fracture techniques and application to the structural analysis of the mammalian plasma membrane. In Poste, G. and Nicolson, G.L. (eds.). *Cell Surface Reviews.* pp. 75–126. (Amsterdam: North Holland Publishing Co.)

14
Further Observations on the Pharmacology of Retinoids

A. VAHLQUIST and O. ROLLMAN

Introduction

Although retinoids are structurally related, their biological activity and pharmacokinetics may differ. Vitamin A, the natural retinoid, is essential not only for the proper functioning of vision and reproduction, but also for the maintenance of epithelia. Its metabolism is strictly controlled and involves a transport protein, retinol binding protein (RBP), and at least two types of intra-cellular receptor proteins.[1] Etretinate, an aromatic analogue of vitamin A acid, exerts vitamin A-like activity in epithelial tissues and its main metabolite binds to one of the intra-cellular receptor proteins.[2] However, it is not transported by serum RBP[3] and it is not stored in the liver of experimental animals, at least not to the same extent as vitamin A.[4]

Clinical trials have revealed, that etretinate accumulates somewhere in a deep compartment resulting in a dramatically increased apparent $T_{1/2}$ of the drug after prolonged therapy.[3,5] We recently reported high concentrations of etretinate in subcutaneous fat and proposed that the drug is stored in the fat tissue.[6] Other synthetic retinoids, such as isotretinoin, do not seem to suffer from this drawback[7] but are, on the other hand, less efficient remedies for various diseases.[8] For the continued clinical use of etretinate, it appeared essential, therefore,to elucidate further the tissue storage of the drug. Another aim of our study was to investigate the possible interference of etretinate therapy with endogenous vitamin A levels of the skin.

Material and Methods

Patients

Altogether 36 patients were studied, 27 of whom have been earlier reported.[6] The remaining nine patients are described in Tables 1 and 2 and Figures 1–3. All patients received or had received etretinate (Tigason) 0.5–1mg/kg/day for various periods of time. Superficial skin samples from the back were obtained by shave biopsy[9] and are referred to as epidermis. Specimens of subcutaneous fat were obtained from the buttock as described elsewhere.[6] Needle biopsy of the liver (kindly performed by Dr L. Lööf) provided samples for retinoid analysis and routine histology. Autopsy material (kindly supplied by Drs A. Eriksson and S. Jagell) was sent from the University Hospital, Umeå, in boxes packed with dry ice.

Analysis

Tissue specimens (2–20mg) or serum (150μl) were hydrolysed in KOH ethanol at 80°C and the retinoids extracted stepwise as described earlier.[6,10] By this procedure, etretinate is quantitively converted to Ro 10-1670 (the free carboxylic acid of the drug) and retinyl esters to retinol. The extracts were analysed by high-performance liquid chromatography (HPLC) and the retinoids quantitated with the aid of internal standards. In a few experiments, an alternative approach was used whereby, in order to distinguish Ro 10-9359 and Ro 10-1670, the hydrolysis was omitted.[6] This approach yielded semi-quantitative data.

Results and Discussion

Table 1 shows the etretinate concentrations in epidermis and subcutis of patients receiving Tigason for various periods of time. Therapeutic concentrations are attained in epidermis within 1 week of treatment and

Table 1. Concentrations of etretinate (including its main metabolite) in epidermis and subcutis of Tigason-treated patients (mean ± SD).

Duration	Number*	Epidermis (ng/g)	Number	Subcutis (ng/g)
1 week	6	192 ± 108	5	670 ± 425
1 month	7	231 ± 62	7	3657 ± 3542
2–4 months	6	185 ± 142	1	4594
5–13 months	6	282 ± 155	3	4530 ± 5074
14–35 months	6	251 ± 157	6	9207 ± 4600

*Number of samples from 22 different patients; dosage: 0.5–1.0mg/kg/day.

there is no sign of further cumulation. The drug does, however, accumulate in the subcutis and, after 1 month the concentrations are almost 20 times higher than those in epidermis. Thereafter, the etretinate values in subcutis level off, although in patients treated continuously for 1–3 years higher values are occasionally found (max 16,000ng/g). The accumulation of etretinate in fat tissue indicates storage and the clearance of the drug from this tissue is exceedingly slow. Figure 1 shows the results of a cross-sectional study of subcutis from patients who had previously received etretinate therapy. The $T_{1/2}$ of the adjusted exponential is approximately 100 days.

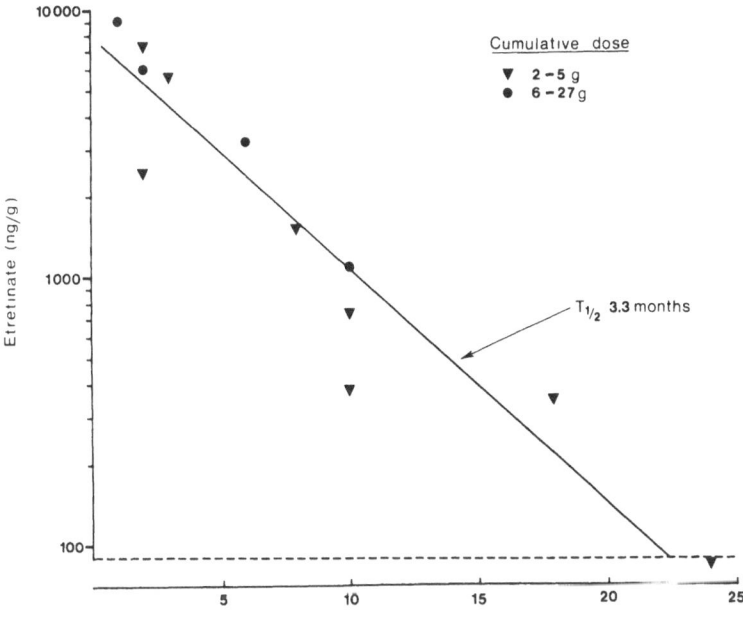

Figure 1. Disappearance of etretinate from subcutaneous fat after withdrawal of treatment. Cross-sectional study of 11 patients. Indicated in the Figure are the cumulative doses received before stopping treatment. The interrupted line indicates the sensitivity limits of the assay. The full-drawn exponential approximately fits the data (adapted from *Br. J. Dermatol.*[6] by permission of the editor).

Assuming a uniform distribution of etretinate in fat tissues, the amount of drug stored by a patient of normal weight during a course of treatment would be about 100mg. This is the amount usually administered over 1–3 days. The transfer of etretinate from fat tissue to plasma is presumably more efficient than the uptake of an orally administered dose. It may be calculated that immediately after stopping treatment, the input of etretinate from body fat to plasma would be approximately 500μg daily. After 6 months, the daily input would be about 100μg. The plasma concentration of the drug is usually 10–40ng/ml at this time corresponding to a total amount in plasma of about 50μg. Since the plasma $T_{1/2}$ of etretinate is 5–10 h after a single dose, a daily net input of 100μg from the fat may theoretically account for the observed plasma concentration of the drug. However, these calculations do not take into account other plausible storage compartments for etretinate.

The liver, which is the principle storage organ for vitamin A, has also been implicated in the storage of etretinate.[5] Liver biopsy provides a means for studying this possibility. Three of our patients underwent a thorough examination because of elevated serum transaminases. These patients had been off etretinate treatment for 1–210 days. The results of the liver biopsies are given in Table 2 together with values of etretinate in serum and subcutis. It can be seen that the etretinate concentration in subcutis always exceeds those in liver and serum. The difference is smallest in patient GP who had been without treatment for only 1 day. The liver vitamin A concentrations, which fall within the normal range, are 200–5,000 times higher than those of etretinate. Incidentally, the liver histology did not reveal any signs of hepatotoxicity attributable to etretinate therapy.

In an autopsy case treated with Tigason for nearly 3 years, samples were available from several organs. Figure 2 confirms that the etretinate level is highest in body fat followed by the liver. The data also show that the tissue distributions of etretinate and vitamin A are different. Whereas the liver

Table 2. Biopsy data from three patients at different intervals after interrupting Tigason treatment. The etretinate concentrations refer to the sum of the parent drug and its main metabolite.

	GP	AL	GB
Diagnosis	Mb Darier	Psoriasis vulgaris	Psoriasis vulgaris
Age/sex	47/♂	36/♂	60/♀
Duration of treatment (weeks)	150	2	8
Time off treatment (weeks)	0.2	3	30
Etretinate concentration in serum (ng/ml)	299	27	26
Etretinate concentration in subcutis (ng/g)	11,800*	1,744	2,991
Etretinate concentration in liver (ng/g)	2,428	64	102
Vitamin A concentration in liver (μg/g)†	520	350	328

*A previous biopsy 1 year earlier showed a value of 5832ng/g.
†Normal range 50–600μg/g. (Vahlquist, unpublished).

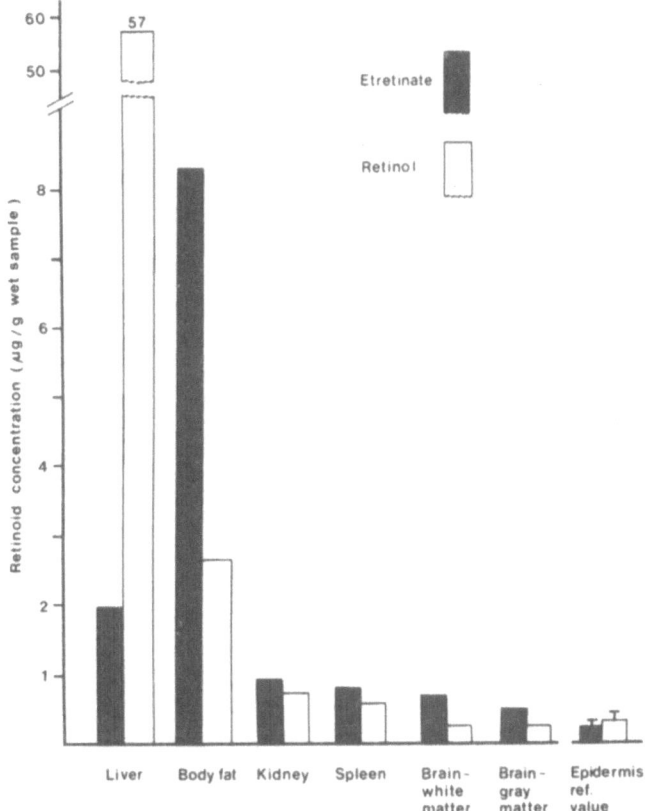

Figure 2. Autopsy data on tissue concentrations of etretinate and vitamin A in a patient treated for 3 years. The patient, who suffered from the Sjögren–Larsson syndrome, was cachectic and died from pneumonia at the age of 27. Etretinate treatment (0.5mg/kg/day) was continued until the day of death. Fat tissue was obtained from the retro-ocular space. Skin samples were not available. The normal epidermal concentrations observed during etretinate treatment are indicated for reference. Values for etretinate and retinol were obtained by the hydrolytic procedure (see under Methods).

contains 30 times more vitamin A than etretinate, the subcutis contains three times more etretinate. In other organs, the distributions of the two retinoids are more consistent and the concentrations are similar to those found previously for epidermis (shown separately in Figure 2).

The autopsy material was also used to analyse the distribution of the parent compound (Ro 10-9359) and the main metabolite (Ro 10-1670). For this purpose, the hydrolysis was omitted from the analytical procedure. Figure 3 shows the chromatograms obtained with extracts of homogenized kidney, spleen, brain, liver and body fat. The HPLC profiles indicate that in body fat virtually all of the drug is in its parent form (Ro 10-9359) thus corroborating previous findings.[6] In liver and brain Ro 10-1670 predominates over Ro 10-9359. Intermediate distributions are seen in the

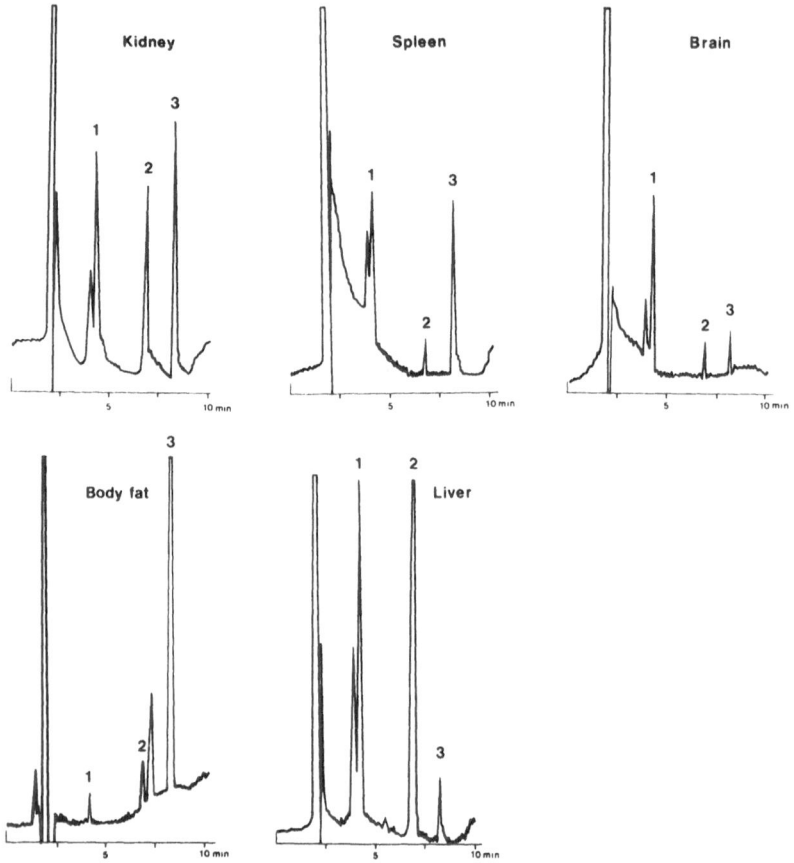

Figure 3. HPLC separation of (1) Ro 10-1670, (2) retinol, and (3) Ro 10-9359 in extracts of five different tissues. The material was the same as in Figure 2 except that hydrolysis was omitted from the analysis. Column: 200 × 4.6mm i.d., ODS-Nucleosil (5μ). Mobile phase: 90:10:0.5 acetonitrile–water–acetic acid at 1.2ml/min. Detection 340nm. No internal standards added. Retinyl fatty-acyl-esters were retained by the column.

spleen and kidney. Previous analyses have shown similar amounts of Ro 10-9359 and Ro 10-1670 also in serum and epidermis.[6]

It is plausible that Ro 10-9359 and Ro 10-1670 bind to different components in the tissues since in serum the former binds primarily to lipoproteins and the latter to albumin[3]. The more lipophilic nature of the ester Ro 10-9359 would accommodate its accumulation in fat tissues and would suggest that this compound is primarily involved in the storage of the drug. The unesterified Ro 10-1670 is less lipophilic and plays an essential role in the biological action, metabolism and excretion of the drug. The accumulation of Ro 10-1670 in the liver suggests that this material is intended for conjugation and biliary excretion. The different distributions of Ro 10-9359 and Ro 10-1670 in the tissues would serve to explain why the drug disappears rather rapidly from the liver while persisting in the fat tissue when the treatment is discontinued. Preliminary results from our laboratory indicate that the distribution of isotretinoin, which is also an unesterified carboxylic acid, is similar to that of Ro 10-1670 and is therefore not stored in the body fat.

The structural relationship and the similar concentrations of etretinate and vitamin A in several peripheral tissues (see Figure 2) suggest that the two compounds may interact metabolically. In fact, indirect evidence has been adduced showing that the vitamin A composition of uninvolved psoriatic skin is affected by etretinate treatment[6] while the serum transport of the two compounds is apparently independent.[3]

Abnormalities in the vitamin A composition of lesional epidermis have been reported in several skin disorders known to respond to etretinate therapy.[11-13] If these abnormalities were corrected by the therapy, then further studies of the pharmacodynamics of the drug would be desirable. For this purpose repeated skin biopsies were obtained from five patients. Figure 4 shows the relative proportions of two epidermal retinoids (retinol

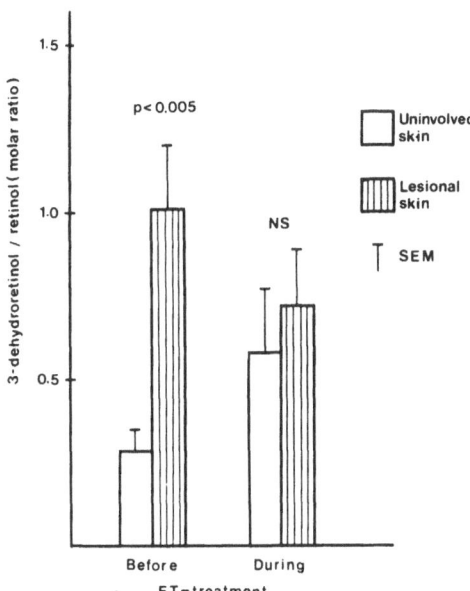

Figure 4. Relative proportions (ratio) of 3-dehydroretinol and retinol in extract of uninvolved and involved epidermis before and during etretinate treatment. Five patients participated (Psoriasis vulgaris 2, Mb Darier 2, Discoid lupus erythematosus 1). Repeated samples were obtained at intervals of 2–4 weeks.

and 3-dehydroretinol) in univolved and lesional skin, respectively. Before etretinate therapy, the retinoid ratios are significantly different ($p < 0.005$). During therapy, the ratio increases in uninvolved skin and decreases in lesional skin, resulting, after a few weeks of therapy, in almost equal ratios. Although the results may seem contradictory, they are consistent with observations made on the proliferative response to etretinate therapy.[14] Etretinate stimulates the epidermal proliferation rate in normal appearing skin while impeding the rate in hyperproliferative skin lesions. We cannot attribute the different responses in normal and diseased skin to differences in the tissue concentrations of the drug since these are virtually identical (mean 220 and 240ng/g in uninvolved and lesional skin, respectively).

Whether the etretinate-induced change in the epidermal vitamin A composition is due to direct metabolic interference or is a result of changes in keratinocyte proliferation and differentiation cannot, at present, be resolved. Ongoing *in vitro* studies will hopefully clarify the underlying mechanism and may thus contribute to the understanding of the biological action of etretinate.

Acknowledgement

This study was supported by grants from the Swedish Medical Research Council (03X-05174), the Welander Foundation and the Swedish Psoriasis Association.

The skilful technical assistance by Mrs S. Gebre-Medhin and I. Pihl-Lundin is gratefully acknowledged.

References

1.   Goodman, D.S. (1980). Vitamin A metabolism. *Fed. Proc.*, **39**, 2716
2.   Sani, B.P., Titus, B.C. and Banerjee, C.K. (1978). Determination of binding affinities of retinoids to retinoic acid-binding protein and serum albumin. *Biochem. J.*, **171**, 711
3.   Vahlquist, A., Michaëlsson, G., Kober, A., Sjöholm, I., Palmskog, G. and Pettersson, U. (1981). Retinoid-binding proteins and the plasma transport of etretinate (Ro 10-9359) in man. In Orfanos, C.E. *et al.* (eds.). *Retinoids: Advances in Basic Research and Therapy.* p. 109. (Berlin, Heidelberg, New York: Springer-Verlag)
4.   Hänni, R. (1978) Pharmacokinetic and metabolic pathways of systemically applied retinoids. *Dermatologica*, **157**, (suppl. 1), 5
5.   Paravicini, U. (1981). Pharmacokinetics and metabolism of oral aromatic retinoids. In Orfanos, C.E. *et al.* (eds.). *Retinoids: Advances in Basic Research and Therapy* p. 13. (Berlin, Heidelberg, New York: Springer-Verlag)
6.   Rollman, O. and Vahlquist, A. (1983). Retinoid concentrations in skin, serum and adipose tissue of patients treated with etretinate (Ro 10-9359). *Br. J. Dermatol.* (In press)
7.   Brazzel, R.K. and Colburn, W.A. (1982). Pharmacokinetics of the retinoids isotretinoin and etretinate. *J. Am. Acad. Dermatol.*, **6**, 643
8.   Peck, G.L. (1980). Retinoids in dermatology. *Arch. Dermatol.*, **116**, 283
9.   Vahlquist, A., Lee, J.B., Michaëlsson, G. and Rollman, O. (1982). Vitamin A in

human skin. II. Concentrations of carotene, retinol and dehydroretinol in various components of normal skin. *J. Invest. Dermatol.*, **79**, 94

10.   Vahlquist, A. (1982). Vitamin A in human skin. I. Detection and identification of retinoids in normal epidermis. *J. Invest. Dermatol.*, **79**, 89

11.   Vahlquist, A. (1980). The identification of dehydroretinol (vitamin A_2) in human skin. *Experientia,* **36**, 317

12.   Rollman, O. and Vahlquist, A. (1981). Cutaneous vitamin A levels in seborrhoic keratosis, actinic keratosis and basal cell carcinoma. *Arch. Dermatol. Res.*, **270**, 193

13.   Vahlquist, A., Lee, J.B. and Michaëlsson, G. (1982). Darier's disease and vitamin A. Concentrations of retinoids in serum and epidermis of untreated patients. *Arch. Dermatol.*, **118**, 389

14.   Fritsch, P.O., Pohlin, G., Längle, U. and Elias, P. (1981). Response of epidermal cell proliferation to orally administered aromatic retinoid. *J. Invest. Dermatol.*, **77**, 287

15
The Effects of Etretinate on Angiogenic Capability and Cytoxic Activity of Peripheral Blood Lymphocytes in Psoriasis

M.J. KAMIŃSKI, A. SZMURLO, S. MAJEWSKI, S. JABLOŃSKA and M. PAWIŃSKA

Introduction

The efficacy of Ro 10-9359 (etretinate) in the therapy of extensive psoriasis, especially of the pustular and erythrodermic forms has been clearly documented.[1,2] The mechanism of etretinate action on the clearing of the psoriatic lesion is, however, not understood. Different targets for the action of this drug may be considered, as keratinocytes, vascular endothelial cells (VEC) and immunocompetent and inflammatory cells.[3]

In non-treated psoriasis, blood vessel alterations were observed[4] and immunoregulatory imbalances, especially involving the T-cell system have been found by some investigators but denied by others (cf. ref. 5). There is a close relationship between the immune response and the vascular system.[6] Lymphoid cells have been shown to produce factors that stimulate the proliferation and migration of vascular endothelial cells.[7,8] In 1975 Sidky and Auerbach introduced a so called 'lymphocyte-induced angiogenesis' (LIA) assay, in which both the cell-mediated immunity (CMI) and vascular changes are measured *in vivo*.[9] In this assay an intra-dermal injection of incompatible lymphocytes into mouse skin results in new blood vessel formation at the injection site. The number of newly formed blood vessels corresponds to the number and immunocompetence of the injected cells. The interaction of lymphocytes and VEC is, however a more complex phenomenon, since besides the stimulatory effects, the lymphoid cells may exert a cytotoxic activity against endothelium.

The present study was aimed at assessing the immunocompetence of psoriatic peripheral blood lymphocytes as measured by their capability to induce new blood vessel formation in the *in vivo* LIA assay. We have studied the effect of etretinate therapy on angiogenic capabilities of lymphocytes from patients with different forms of psoriasis. *In vitro* studies involved the effect of etretinate on cytotoxic activity of psoriatic lymphocytes against human vascular endothelium.

Material and Methods

Patients

Twenty patients with psoriasis (13 with psoriasis vulgaris, three with generalized pustular psoriasis of von Zumbusch type and four with pustular psoriasis palmo-plantaris) were included in the study. Eight patients were studied before and after treatment with etretinte (1mg/kg body-weight to a total daily doses of 50–75mg). All patients were followed by a standard clinical and laboratory protocol.[13] The control group consisted of 20 healthy individuals, matched according to age and sex (all were blood donors to the Blood Transfusion Centre).

Preparation of Mononuclear Cell Suspension

Samples of 10–15ml of heparinized blood were diluted 1:1 with PBS and layered onto Ficoll–Uropoline mixture.[10] Isolated cells consisted of 92–97 per cent lymphocytes and 3–8 per cent monocytes as identified by myeloperoxidase staining.

Lymphocyte-Induced Angiogenesis Assay

Balb/c inbred female mice, 4–5 months old, were used as recipients of lymphocytes. In order to prevent the rejection of human cells, the mice were immunosuppressed by a total-body X-ray irradiation (600 R exposure, Müller RT 1100 apparatus, 100 R per min in air, filter Al 1.25mm, irradiation at 10mA, 70kV). 2 hours after irradiation the mice were anaesthetized with chloral hydrate (3.6mg/10mg body-weight) and both their flanks were shaved. The tested lymphocytes in a dose of 10^6 viable cells in 0.1ml of 199 TC medium were then injected intradermally. Each recipient was injected with at least two different inocula. Each kind of inoculum was injected in different flank locations on different recipients. After 3 days the mice were killed by cervical dislocation, their skin was dissected from the underlying muscles and its inner surface was inspected at 32 × magnification, using the green filter. All blood vessels directed towards the injection site were counted according to morphological criteria.[9] These vessels differed from the background vasculature due to their tortuosity and divarications. All counting was blind and performed by the same person.

Isolation and Culture of Human Endothelial Cells

Endothelium was isolated from umbilical veins by digestion with 0.075 per cent collagenase (Type 1 Sigma with slight modifications of original method described by Jaffe.[11]) Isolated cells were cultured in 199 TC medium with 20 per cent fetal calf serum, supplemented with 20mmol/l Hepes, 1.6mmol/l glutamine and $100\mu g/ml$ of gentamicin. The endothelial nature of cultured cells was checked by the immunofluorescence test using specific anti-factor VIII antigen antibodies.

Cytotoxicity Assay

Lymphocytes employed in the cytotoxicity assay originated from patients with active psoriasis vulgaris. Four of eight patients were treated with etretinate for 2–4 weeks. Control lymphocytes were isolated from healthy individuals (blood donors), and additionally in two experiments also from patients with active SLE (a negative control), since natural cytotoxicity in SLE has been reported to be low.[12]

Target cells in the assay were human vascular endothelial cells of 1–2 passage. Cells were cultured in Linbro multi-well trays covered with gelatin, and grown until confluence. Then they were labelled with ^{51}Cr for 1 h, rinsed three times with the culture medium and finally the lymphocytes were added in ratio 30:1. After 4 h incubation, the radioactivity of supernatants was counted in gamma-counter. Cytotoxicity indices were calculated according to the formula:

$$\frac{\text{exp. release} - \text{spontaneous release}}{\text{max. release} - \text{spontaneous release}} \times 100.$$

In additional experiments K562 erythroleukaemic cells were used as targets. The effect of etretinate on *in vitro* cytotoxicity of psoriatic and control lymphocytes against K562 was studied. Etretinate was dissolved in DMSO and further in culture medium to obtain concentrations 1, 10 and $100\mu g/ml$. A cytotoxicity test was performed for 18 h at 30:1 effector: target ratio. The solvent alone did not evoke ^{51}Cr release as compared to spontaneous isotope release using the culture medium alone.

Results

The results are shown in Figures 1–3 and Table 1.

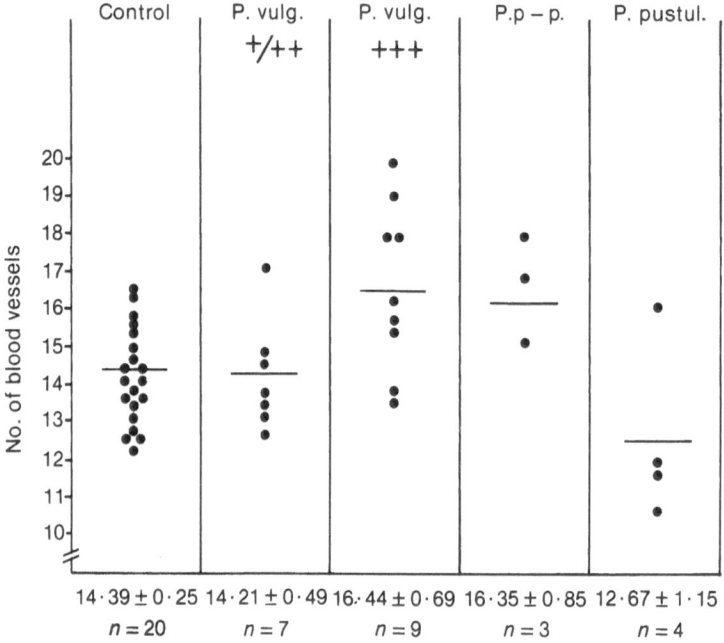

Figure 1. Angiogenic capability of lymphocytes.

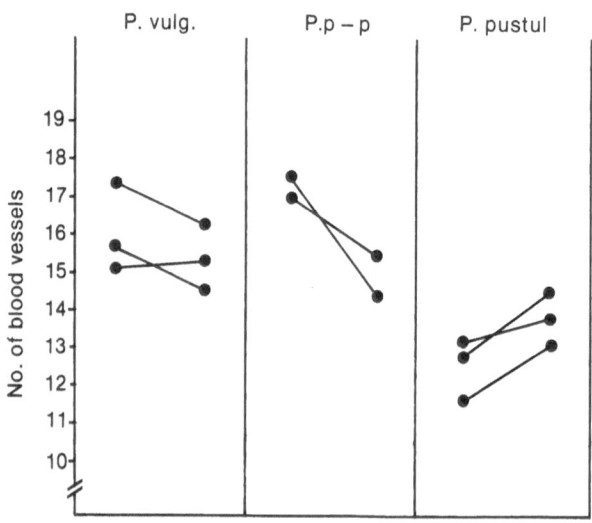

Figure 2. Modulation of lymphocyte angiogenic capability by Ro 10-9359.

148

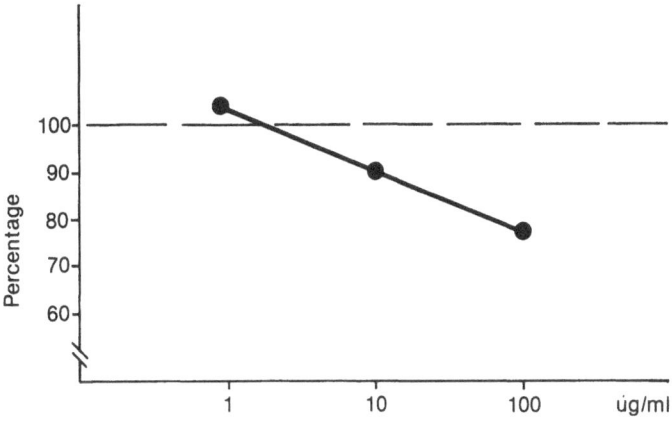

Figure 3. Effect of Ro 10-9359 on natural killer cell activity in vitro.

Table 1. Decrease natural killer cell activity against VEC in psoriasis vulgaris. Ratios of cytoxicity index in p. vulgaris and controls.

1.	0.62
2.	0.44
3.	0.32
4.	0.87
5.	0.50
6.	0.28
7.	0.65
8.	0.81

Discussion

The results showed that angiogenic capability of lymphocytes differs in different forms of psoriasis. If psoriasis vulgaris patients are considered as a whole single group, no significant differences in angiogenic capabilities of their lymphocytes are found as compared to controls. However, if psoriasis is divided into active (eruptive with pin-point lesions) and stationary, the angiogenic capability of lymphocytes in the former but not in the latter is significantly higher than that in control group. In stationary psoriasis no differences from control were found irrespective of the extent of the skin involvement. In pustular psoriasis (von Zumbusch type) the lymphocyte angiogenic capability is decreased, whereas in pustular psoriasis palmoplantaris it seems to be increased. Since angiogenic reaction is dose-

149

dependent, one can calculate that the number of cells required to evoke the same number of blood vessels is about ten times higher in pustular psoriasis (von Zumbusch) than in active common psoriasis. The etretinate treatment affected the angiogenic capability of peripheral blood lymphocytes. This effect was observed 2–4 weeks after starting the treatment. The angiogenic capability of lymphocytes in etretinate-treated patients showed a tendency to return to the baseline; it decreased in active common psoriasis and increased in generalized pustular psoriasis (slowly however in the former).

The increased angiogenic capability in active psoriasis vulgaris and pustular psoriasis palmo-plantaris might by caused by either the decrease of suppressor cell activity (resulting in excessive production of angiogenic lymphokines by T-cell subsets) or by direct stimulation of cells being the effectors in the induction of angiogenesis. The most potent cells in evoking angiogenesis are T cells with high and with moderate affinity receptors for sheep red blood cells.[10] These two subsets are active when tested separately but exert inhibitory effects on each other when mixed.

The observed inhibition of angiogenic capabilities might be caused by the increase of suppressor cell activity or by the decreased activity of effector cells. In humans, T cells with Fcγ receptors may exert suppressive and/or cytotoxic functions. The decrease of FcγR-cell activity might be responsible for the increased angiogenic capability of lymphocytes in active psoriasis vulgaris and might be also responsible for a decrease in cytotoxicity against various targets. Etretinate affected only angiogenic capabilities and not cytotoxic activities and therefore the mechanisms of its action would be rather related to the cells directly involved in induction of angiogenesis.

Conclusions

The angiogenic capability of peripheral blood lymphocytes from psoriatic patients differs from that of healthy controls. This capability is increased in active but not in stationary psoriasis vulgaris, decreased in pustular psoriasis (von Zumbusch type) and seems to be increased in pustular psoriasis palmo-plantaris.

After etretinate treatment for 2–4 weeks (depending on the psoriasis form), the angiogenic capability of lymphocytes shows a tendency to return to the baseline. Lymphocytes from psoriasis vulgaris (active form) exert lower cytotoxicity against human endothelial cells or K562 erthroleukaemic cells as compared to controls. Etretinate treatment has no effect on this cytotoxic activity.

When etretinate is added *in vitro* during 18h cytotoxicity assay with the use of psoriatic or control lymphocytes, the cytotoxicity is decreased only at higher ($100\mu g/ml$) drug concentration.

References

1. Peck, G.L. (1981). Retinoids in clinical dermatology. In Fleischmajer, R. (ed.). *Progress in Disease of the Skin.* Vol 1, p. 227. (New York: Grune and Stratton)
2. Farber, E.M. and Nall, L. (1981). The use of oral retinoids aromatic in psoriasis therapy: an overview of past, present and future developments. In Orfanos, C.E. *et al.* (eds.). *Retinoids: Advances in Basic Research and Therapy.* Vol. 1, p.515. (Berlin, Heidelberg, New York: Springer-Verlag)
3. Tsambaos, D. and Orfanos, C.E. (1981). Effects of oral retinoids on dermal components in human and animal skin. In Orfanos, C.E. *et al.* (eds.). *Retinoids: Advances in Basic Research and Therapy.* p.99. (Berlin, Heidelberg, New York: Springer-Verlag)
4. Braverman, I.M. (1977). Microcirculation in psoriasis. In Cox, A.J. and Farber, E.M. (eds.). *Psoriasis: Proc. 2nd Int. Symp.* p.28. (New York: Yorke Medical)
5. Clot, J. and Guilhou, J.J. (1982). Studies on cellular aspects of the immune response in psoriasis. In Beutner, E.H. (ed.). *Autoimmunity in Psoriasis.* p.241 (Boca Raton, Florida: CRC Press)
6. Burrger, D.R. and Vetto, R.M. (1982). Vascular endothelium as a major participant in T-lymphocyte immunity. *Cell. Immunol.*, **70**, 357
7. Zetter, B.R. (1980). Migration of capillary endothelial cells is stimulated by tumor-derived factors. *Nature (London)*, **285**, 41
8. Auerbach, R. (1981). Angiogenesis-inducing factors: a review. *Lymphokines*, **4**, 69
9. Sidky, Y.A. and Auerbach, R. (1975). Lymphocyte-induced angiogenesis: a qualtative and sensitive assay of graft-vs-host reaction. *J. Exp. Med.*, **141**, 1084
10. Kamiński, M.J., Nowacyk, M., Skopińska-Rózewska, E., Kamińska, G. and Bem, W. (1981). Human peripheral blood lymphocyte subpopulations isolated on the basis of their affinity for SRBC differ in angiogenesis-inducing capability. *Clin. Exp. Immunol.*, **46**, 327
11. Jaffe, E.A. (1980). Culture of human endothelial cells. *Transpl. Proc.*, **12** suppl. 1, 49
12. Tsokos, G.C., Rook, A.H., Djeu, J.R. and Balow, J.E. (1982). Natural killer cells and interferon responses in patients with SLE. *Clin. Exp. Immunol.*, **50**, 239
13. Wolska, *et al.* (1983). *J. Am. Acad. Dermatol.* (In press)

16
The Effect of Etretinate on Chemotactic Activity of Polymorphonuclear Leukocytes in Various Forms of Psoriasis

A. LANGNER, M. FRACZYKOWSKA, S. JABLOŃSKA, J. SZYMAŃCZYK and T. CHORZELSKI

Introduction

There are many data supporting the view that polymorphonuclears (PMNs) may play a major role in the pathogenesis of psoriasis. PMNs are a constant finding in the stratum corneum (Munro microabscesses) in fully developed lesions, and appear also in the corium of earliest psoriatic papules.[1,2] Increased activity of PMNs in psoriasis, as measured by chemotaxis assay,[3,4] enzyme level,[5] superoxide anion production,[6,7] and enhanced adherence favour their direct involvement in the formation of skin lesions.

It is generally recognized that etretinate is effective in the treatment of certain forms of psoriasis, particularly in pustular and erythrodermic psoriasis. The mechanism of the action remains, however, unknown.

One of the earliest histopathological events during the treatment with etretinate is the disappearance of PMNs infiltrate[2,8] and the reduction of their migration from the vessels into the dermis,[9] observed also by Dubertret et al.[10] using the skin chamber technique.

In our preliminary studies,[11] we have shown a striking inhibition of PMNs chemotactic activity in psoriatic patients treated with etretinate as well as in vitro conditions. Similar results have been obtained in independent study by Pigatto.[12] The aim of the present work was to evaluate the influence of etretinate on the chemotactic activity of PMNs in various forms of psoriasis in relation to the clinical response.

Material

Following cases were included in the study: six generalized erythrodermic and/or very widespread psoriasis, three generalized pustular psoriasis and eight pustular palmo-plantar psoriasis, treated with etretinate, as well as four erythrodermic and/or very widespread cases treated with etretinate and PUVA (Re-PUVA). The drug was given in a daily dosage of 0.8–1.0mg/kg body-weight until complete clearing of cutaneous lesions (6–9 weeks).

The chemotaxis assay was performed regularly every 3 weeks, until 9 weeks.

Patients treated with Re-PUVA received at the beginning only etretinate, in a dosage as in the former groups for 1 week and, after introduction of PUVA, in a reduced dose 0.5mg/kg body-weight. The irradiations were carried out three times weekly in a single dosage of UVA 1.7J/cm^2, jointly 17-20, 4J/cm^2.

Biochemical examinations, specifically of triglycerides, alkaline phosphatase, transaminases, etc. were carried out before, during and after completion of the treatment.

Methods

Chemotactic activity was determined by the modified Boyden chamber assay.[13] Neutrophils were isolated from peripheral blood following the technique of Henson[14] and Diaz-Perez.[15]

In brief, freshly drawn blood was mixed with 0.085mol/l trisodium citrate, 0.065mol/l citric acid and 2 per cent dextran in distilled water. After centrifugation (550 × g, 20 min at room temperature), the plasma as well as the buffer coat were removed. The remaining erythrocytes and PMNs were resuspended in 2.5 per cent gelatin in saline. Erythrocytes were allowed to sediment and the supernatant was removed, centrifuged (40 × g 10 min at room temperature). The remaining erythrocytes were lysed in 0.83 per cent NH$_4$Cl and the PMNs were washed in medium TC-199, twice. The concentration of cells was adjusted to 2 × 10^6 cell/ml. Giemsa staining revealed 99–95 per cent PMNs in each experiment. The cell viability was consistently between 93 and 98 per cent, as measured by trypan blue exclusion.

For chemotaxis assay, standardized chambers were used. One filter (Sartorius Membranfilter Pore size 50.0 μm) separated two compartments. The upper compartment was filled with 2 × 10^6 PMNs in 0.5ml TC-199 and the lower compartment with chemoattractant. Casein in concentration 5mg/ml and autologous serum diluted 1:1 with TC-199 served as chemoattractants. Chambers were incubated in 37°C for 3 hrs. The filters were fixed with methanol, stained with haematoxylin and cleared with xylene. All tests were performed in duplicate. The number of cells which had migrated through the filters was determined in 20 high power fields per filter.

Results

The results are presented in Tables 1-4. In the erythrodermic and wide-

Table 1. Erythrodermic and widespread psoriasis, including arthropathic variety.

| Number of cases | Before treatment | After treatment | | |
		3 weeks	6 weeks	9 weeks
Casein $n = 6$	80.38 ± 17.98 N 19.5 ± 6.6	41.83 ± 25.32	28.63 ± 23.71	21.88 ± 17.6
Serum $n = 6$	37.54 ± 14.73 N 55.7 ± 33.0	22.59 ± 15.49	8.05 ± 7.52	9.13 ± 8.13

spread psoriasis (Table 1) response to the casein as a chemoattractant was considerably increased before the treatment (80.38 vs. 19.5 in the control group), and progressively decreased reaching a normal level within 6–9 weeks, parallel to the clinical improvement observed in all cases. Response to the autologous serum was slightly diminished before the treatment (37.54 vs. 55.7 in the control group), decreased markedly during the first 3 weeks, and dramatically (8.05–9.13) after 6 weeks of the therapy.

Table 2. Generalized pustular psoriasis.

| Number of cases | Before treatment | After treatment | | |
		3 weeks	6 weeks	9 weeks
Casein $n = 3$	84.2 ± 6.63 N 19.5 ± 6.6	54.6 ± 20.75	35.36 ± 12.92	32.5 ± 12.55
Serum $n = 3$	37.83 ± 12.0 N 55.7 ± 33.0	21.33 ± 18.1	19.11 ± 16.49	9.87 ± 6.18

In generalized pustular psoriasis (Table 2), the initial values of chemotaxis to both chemoattractants were analogous to those in the erythrodermic form. The decrease of chemotactic response to the casein was progressive, but did not reach values in the control group after 9 weeks in spite of great improvement or clearing of the lesions.

The decrease of the response to the autologous serum was the same as in the former group.

Table 3. Pustular palmo-plantar psoriasis.

Number of cases	Before treatment	After treatment		
		3 weeks	6 weeks	9 weeks
Good response				
Casein	108.8 ± 27.79	95.1 ± 31.8	41.25 ± 11.58	27.1 ± 20.3
n = 6	N 19.5			
Serum	35.84 ± 20.6	31.75 ± 15.99	17.6 ± 5.88	13.58 ± 7.39
n = 6	N 55.7			
Poor response				
Casein	36.37 ± 9.58	46.07 ± 19.69	32 ± 8.48	37.25 ± 3.88
n = 2	N 19.5			
Serum	15.85 ± 5.16	8.57 ± 5.5	17.3 ± 0.98	20.25 ± 3.18
n = 2	N 55.7			

In the group of palmo-plantar pustular psoriasis (Table 3), the response to the therapy was good in six cases and poor in two. Chemotactic activity towards casein, initially very markedly increased in six cases, progressively normalized. The activity towards autologous serum, initially somewhat below the normal values, considerably decreased, parallel to the regression of pustular lesions.

In two cases, in whom the response to the therapy was not satisfactory, chemotactic activity towards casein and autologous serum did not change within 9 weeks.

Table 4. Chemotaxis in patients treated by Re-PUVA.

Number of cases	Before treatment	After treatment	
		3 weeks	6 weeks
Casein	81.87 ± 23.18	44.92 ± 23.74	28.7 ± 29.8
n = 4	N 19.5		
	± 6.6		
Serum	34.62 ± 16.92	19.88 ± 11.34	9.0 ± 9.1
n = 4	N 55.7		
	± 33		

Re-PUVA applied to generalized or widespread psoriasis (Table 4) produced excellent clinical effects in all four cases within 6 weeks. The initial chemotactic activity towards casein and autologous serum was analogous to that in the first group (Table 1), so was also the activity after 3 and 6 weeks of therapy.

Discussion

In this series were included cases of widespread generalized and/or pustular psoriasis, all with increased chemotactic activity towards casein. In all cases, except two with pustular palmo-plantar psoriasis, clinical results were very satisfactory, i.e. great improvement or complete clearing of skin lesions were noted within 6–9 weeks of the therapy. The degree of chemotactic activity towards casein was progressive and paralleled clinical improvement. In two cases of pustular palmo-plantar psoriasis, which did not respond to the treatment, chemotactic activity against casein remained unchanged. This is in agreement with our previous findings in patients treated with anthralin[16] and PUVA[16,17] and those of others.[18–20]

A most striking finding in the present study is a dramatic decrease of chemoattractive activity of autologous serum after 6 weeks of the treatment with etretinate. This phenomenon was repeatedly observed in all groups, especially after 6–9 weeks of the therapy. It was less pronounced in palmo-plantar pustular psoriasis not responsive to the treatment.

In our own unpublished investigations, we did not observe any effect of etretinate on chemotaxis, when given in a single dose. Camisa et al.[8] did not notice any effect of retinoids on PMNs chemotaxis but it is not clear how long their patients were treated at the time the chemotaxis was studied. Conceivably, the effect is time dependent. The mechanism of this phenomenon is unclear, and is currently under investigation. It seems probable that a favourable response to etretinate is related to a dramatic decrease of chemoattractive activity of autologous serum in patients with severe psoriasis treated for 6–9 weeks.

Summary

Studies on chemotactic activity on PMNs were performed in 21 patients with various forms of psoriasis (erythrodermic and/or widespread, generalized pustular, and palmo-plantar pustular psoriasis), treated with etretinate. In all, except two cases of pustular palmo-plantar psoriasis, the results were very good, i.e. within 9 weeks there was a complete clearing of cutaneous lesions and/or great improvement. The chemotactic activity of PMNs towards casein, initially markedly increased, progressively decreased and became normal. However, PMNs chemotaxis towards autologous serum, initially slightly diminished, decreased dramatically in all groups during the treatment and was extremely low after completion of the therapy. The significance of this phenomenon for the mechanism of clearing of psoriatic lesions under etretinate treatment is still unclear.

References

1. Chowaniec, O. and Jablonska, S. (1979). Pre-pin-point papules changes preceding pin-point lesions of psoriasis. *Acta Dermatovenero*, **59**, 39
2. Jablonska, S., Wolska, H., Dabrowski, J., Haftek, M., Groniowska, M. and Jarzabek-Chorzelska, M. (1981). Aromatic retinoids in psoriasis: clinical, histological, histochemical, electron microscopical and immunological investigations. In Orfanos, C.E. et al. (eds.). *Retinoids: Advances in Basic Research and Therapy*. p. 165. (Berlin, Heidelberg, New York: Springer-Verlag)

3. Wahba, A., Cohen, H.A., Bar-Eli, M. and Callity, R. (1978). Enhanced chemotactic and phagocytic activities of leukocytes in psoriasis. *J. Invest. Dermatol.*, **71**, 186

4. Kawohl, G., Szperalski, B., Schröder, J.M. and Christophers, E. (1980). Polymorphonuclear leukocyte chemotaxis in psoriasis: enhancement by self activated serum. *Br. J. Dermatol.*, **103**, 527

5. Gliński, W., Jablonska, S., Zarembska, Z., Beutner, E.H. and Jarzabek-Chorzelska, M. (1981). Role of blood-bone factors in psoriasis. In Marks, R. and Christophers, E. (eds.). *The Epidermis in Disease.* (Lancaster: MTP Press)

6. Sedgwick, J.B., Bergstresser, P.R. and Hurd, E.R. (1980). Increased granulocyte adherence in psoriasis and psoriatic arthritis. *J. Invest. Dermatol.*, **75**, 187

7. Sedgwick J.B., Bergstresser, P.R. and Hurd, E.R. (1981). Increased superoxide generation by normal granulocytes incubated in sera from patients with psoriasis. *J. Invest. Dermatol.*, **76**, 158

8. Camisa, Ch., Eisenstat, B., Ragaz, A. and Weissmann, G. (1982). The effects of retinoids on netrophil function in vitro. *J. Am. Acad. Dermatol.*, **6**, 620

9. Tsambaos, D. and Orfanos, C.E. (1981). Effects of oral retinoid on dermal components in human and animal skin. In Orfanos, C.E. *et al.* (eds.). *Retinoids: Advances in Basic Research and Therapy.* p. 99. (Berlin, Heidelberg, New York: Springer-Verlag)

10. Piegetto, P. (1983). Effect of etretinate on the neutrophil chemataxis in pustular and in vulgar psoriasis. *Proceedings of the XVI International Dermatology Congress, Tokyo 24-28 May, 1982.* (In Press)

11. Langner, A., Chorzelski, T.P., Fraczykowska, M., Jablonska, S. and Szymańczyk, J. (1983). Is chemotactic activity of polymorphonuclear leukocytes increased in psoriasis? *Arch. Dermatol. Res.* (In press)

12. Dubertret, L., Lebreton, B.A. and Touraine, R. (1982). Neutrophil studies in psoriasis: in vivo migration, phagocytosis and bacterial killing. *J. Invest. Dermatol.*, **79**, 74

13. Langer, A. and Christophers, E. (1977). Leukocyte chemotaxis after *in vitro* treatment with 8-methoxypsoralen and UV-A. *Arch. Dermatol. Res.* **260**, 51

14. Henson, P.M. (1971). The immunologic release of constituets from neutrophil leukocytes. The role of antibody and complement on nonphagocytosable surfaces or phagocytosable particles. *J. Immunol.*, **107**, 1535

15. Diaz-Perez, J.L., Goldyne, M.E. and Winkelmann, R.K. (1976). Prostaglandins and chemotaxis: enhancement of polymorphonuclear leukocyte chemotaxis by prostaglandin F_2. *J. Invest. Dermatol.*, **66**, 149

16. Langner, A., Chorzelski, T.P., Frączkowska, M., Beutner, E.H. and Jablonska, S. (1981). Effect of anthnalin on stratum corneum antigenicity and polymorphonuclear leucocyte chemotaxis. *Br. J. Dermatol.*, **105** Suppl. 20, 62

17. Langner, A. and Christophers, E. (1981). Chemotactic activity of polymorphonuclear leukocytes in psoriasis. In Marks, R. and Christophers, E. (eds.) *The Epidermis in Disease.* (Lancaster: MTP Press)

18. Michaëlson, G. (1980). Increased chemotactic activity of neutrophil leukocytes in psoriasis. *Br. J. Dermatol.*, **103**, 351

19. Wahba, A., Cohen, H.A., Bar-Eli, M. and Gallily, R. (1979). Neutrophil chemotaxis in psoriasis. *Acta Dermatovener.*, **59**, 411

20. Jablonska, S., Chowaniec, O. and Maciejewska, E. (1982). Histology of psoriasis. The role of polymorphonuclear neutrophils. In Beutner, E. H. (ed.). *Autoimmunity in Psoriasis.* (Boca Raton, Florida: CRC Press)

Section 3

Special Examinations with the Retinoids

17
Spermatological Examinations in Males Treated with Etretinate

L. TÖRÖK

Introduction

Both the various vitamin A derivatives and the aromatic retinoids have opened up new possibilities in dermato-therapy. In recent years the new derivatives have been applied in numerous indications and on an ever increasing number of patients.[1] Meanwhile, clinical and laboratory side-effects of the aromatic retinoids have become known. To date, relatively little attention have been paid to the effects of the new products on the gonads. This may be of particular importance, since these morbostatic preparations are generally administered over long periods.[2]

The present publication gives an account of our spermatological examinations on males treated with aromatic retinoid.

Patients and Method

Eleven male patients aged 22–59 years (average 31 years) took part in the examinations. Seven of them suffered from plaque-type psoriasis, three from M. Darier, and one from keratoderma of both palms and soles. Examinations of ejaculate were carried out under standard conditions immediately before and after retinoid treatment. The following spermatological parameters were assessed: sperm concentration (million/ml), total sperm count (million/ejaculate), absolute and progressive motility (per cent) and sperm morphology (per cent). For treatment of their basic disease, during the first 4 weeks the patients received 25mg aromatic retinoid Ro 10-9359 (Tigason) daily, for the next 8 weeks 50mg of the same preparation daily.

The statistical examinations were made with the paired Student t-test.

Results

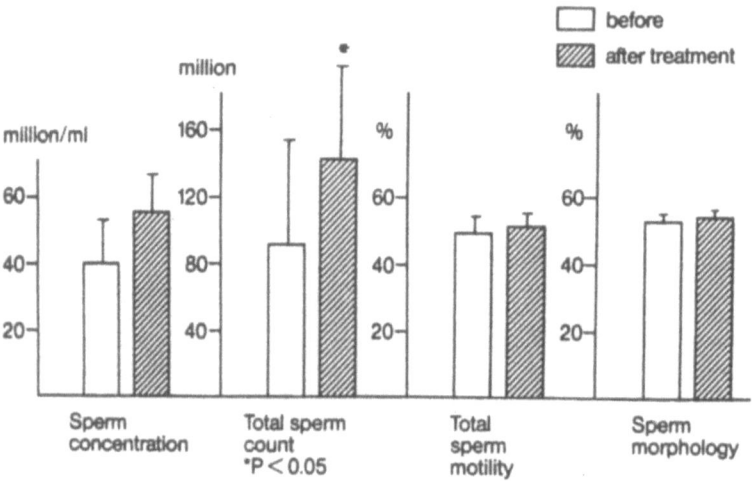

Figure 1. Spermatological parameters of 11 patients before and after Tigason treatment. Values are expressed as mean ± SE.

The variations in the ejaculation parameters examined during treatment are shown in Figure 1. The total sperm count disclosed a significant increase after treatment. The sperm concentration was likewise increased; although this was not mathematically significant, the result was very close to the comparative value (2.219 as against 2.228; number of increases = 8). No essential change was observed either in the sperm morphology, or in the absolute and progressive motility. During the Tigason treatment the wife of one patient conceived and gave birth to a healthy baby.

Discussion

The effects of the aromatic retinoids on spermatogenesis are hardly known at present. Retinoid (Tigason) administration in a high dose to guinea pigs was observed by Tsambaos et al.[3] to lead to a reversible decrease in the diameter of the tubule, to desquamation and disorganization of the germinal epithelium, and to a deficiency of mature spermatoza. Schütte et al.[4] have found a reversible decrease in spermatogenesis in a few cases while administering toxic doses of etretinate to rats. This shows that the reaction to retinoid also depends on the species. With regard to humans, the first spermatological examinations were reported by Plewig *et al.*[5] in connection with a systematic treatment with vitamin A acid (tretinoin). With the exception of a significant increase in the volume of the ejaculate, no changes were found in the other spermatological parameters during the treatment of 12 patients suffering from acne vulgaris. Similarly, no changes were detected in the acrosin activity of the seminal plasma and the spermatoza. Schill *et al.*[2] carried out spermatological examinations on 12 patients treated with aromatic retinoid (Tigason). After treatment for 3 months, no impairment was observed in the spermatological parameters; indeed, the sperm count was significantly elevated, in parallel with a rise in the total sperm count, though this did not prove mathematically significant.

Our own investigations support the observations of Schill *et al.*,[2] in that we did not detect any deterioration in the sperm concentration, the total sperm count, the motility or morphology. In contrast with the findings of Tsambaos *et al.*,[3] we did not observe an unfavourable effect of Tigason on spermatogenesis when administered at a therapeutic dose to humans. On the contrary, and in agreement with Schill *et al.*[2] we experienced a beneficial effect, namely an increase in the total sperm count.

The investigations to date indicate that the oral retinoid Tigason, in the customary therapeutic dose, does not cause chromosomal instability and does not lead to sister chromatid exchange.[6] No mutagenic effect was detected, and the known teratogenic effect appears to be independent of this.[7] We would consider that it could be of value if other authors confirm the favourable effect on spermatogenesis, for it might be possible to develop a drug which had a beneficial influence on the proliferative and differentiating processes of the germinal epithelium. It is conceivable that this effect may turn out to be even more marked with new derivatives; this should stimulate the preparation of further, more selective derivatives, acting only on the germinal epithelium.

Acknowledgement

The author wishes to express his thanks to F. Hoffmann-La Roche and Co. Ltd, Basle, Switzerland, for making available the aromatic retinoid.

References

1. Orfanos, C.E. (ed.) (1981). *Retinoids: Advances in Basic Research and Therapy.* (Berlin, Heidelberg, New York: Springer-Verlag)

2. Schill, W.-B., Wagner, A., Nikolowski, J. and Plewig, G. (1981). Aromatic retinoid and 13-*cis*-retinoic acid: spermatological investigations. In Orfanos, C.E. *et al.* (eds.) *Retinoids: Advances in Basic Research and Therapy.* pp. 389–395. (Berlin, Heidelberg, New York: Springer-Verlag)

3. Tsambaos, D., Hundeiker, M., Mahrle, G. and Orfanos, C.E. (1980). Reversible Spermatogenesestörung durch aromatisches Retinoid bei Meerschweinchen. *Arch. Dermatol. Res.*, **267**, 153–9

4. Schütte, B. and Kuhlwein, A. (1983). Experimentelle Untersuchungen Zum Einfluss des aromatischen Retinoids auf die Spermatogenese bei Ratten. *Z. Hautkr Res.*, **58**, 439

5. Plewig, G., Schill, W.-B. and Hofmann, C. (1979). *Orale* Behandlung mit Tretinoin. *Arch. Dermatol. Res.*, **265**, 37–47

6. Happle, R. and Niedworok, A. (1981). Cytogenetic studies in patients treated with oral retinoid Ro 10-9359. In Orfanos, C.E. *et al.* (eds.) *Retinoids: Advances in Basic Research and Therapy.* pp 61–5. (Berlin, Heidelberg, New York: Springer-Verlag)

7. Obe, G. and Tsambaos, D. (1981). Chromosomal analysis in patients treated with the aromatic retinoid Ro 10-9359. In Orfanos, C.E. *et al.* (eds.) *Retinoids: Advances in Basic Research and Therapy.* pp. 67–70. (Berlin, Heidelberg, New York: Springer-Verlag)

18
Effects of Oral Retinoids on Enzyme Activities of Rat Intestinal and Kidney Tubular Epithelium

S. GUTSCHMIDT and D. TSAMBAOS

Introduction

The profound influence of retinoids on the differentiation and proliferation of epidermis is well established.[1,2] Large numbers of clinical trials have demonstrated the dramatic efficacy of retinoids in the management of keratinizing disorders.[3] Retinoids, as most fat-soluble compounds, are probably absorbed at the proximal small intestine, whereas their metabolites are excreted via bile and urine.[4,5] However, surprisingly little is known about the effects of retinoids on the intestine and the kidneys. In this paper we present a review of our recent work on the alterations in the enzymatic and morphological features of both the rat intestinal and the kidney tubular epithelium under oral treatment with etretinate and the arotinoid Ro 13-6298. Additionally, we report the results of further histological investigations on the liver of the treated animals in order to detect any possible, gross morphological changes in this organ, which reveals the highest uptake of systemically applied retinoids.[6]

Materials and Methods

Experimental Animals and Treatment Schedule

Four different experiments were performed, which are listed in Table 1. In each case daily doses of either etretinate (Ro 10-9359) or arotinoid (Ro 13-6298) dissolved in arachis oil were administered to adult female Wistar

Table 1. Treatment schedule.

Retinoid	Daily dose per kg	Treatment (days)	Number of rats
Experiment 1			
Ro 10-9359	3mg	10	5
–	arachis oil	10	5
Experiment 2			
Ro 10-9359	10mg	10	5
Ro 10-9359	20mg	10	5
–	arachis oil	10	5
Experiment 3			
Ro 10-9359	1mg	10	5
Ro 13-6298	0.002mg	10	5
Ro 13-6298	0.04mg	10	5
–	arachis oil	10	5
Experiment 4			
Ro 10-9359	20mg	17	2 (3)*
Ro 13-6298	0.002mg	17	4 (1)*
Ro 10-9359	1mg	30	5
–	arachis oil	30	5

(n)* = Numbers of animals which died before the end of the treatment period.

rats, whereas litter mates receiving corresponding quantities of arachis oil served as controls. The body-weight of all rats was registered at the beginning and the end of the treatment period. Samples obtained from the jejunum (about 5cm distal to the lig. of Treitz), ileum (about 10cm proximal to Bauhin's valve), ascending and descending colon, from the kidneys and from the liver were processed for morphological and/or enzymatic investigation.

Morphological Investigations

Unfixed cyostat specimens from the different intestinal segments and from the kidneys were used for either routine histological investigation (HE, PAS and Gallocyanin chromealum[7]) or quantitative enzyme measurements *in situ*. Ethanol/acetic acid-fixed intestinal samples were prepared for microdissection[8] and morphometry. In the case of the jejunum and ileum, the villus height, the breadth at the base and apex and the width were measured by means of a graduated eyepiece (see Figure 1b, evaluation of at least ten villus/crypt units per sample). From these data the mean villus surface[9] and the entire mucosal (villus) surface area per unit serosal area were calculated taking into account the number of villi per unit serosal area, which had been counted on photographs according to a standardized method. A similar procedure was applied to the colonic

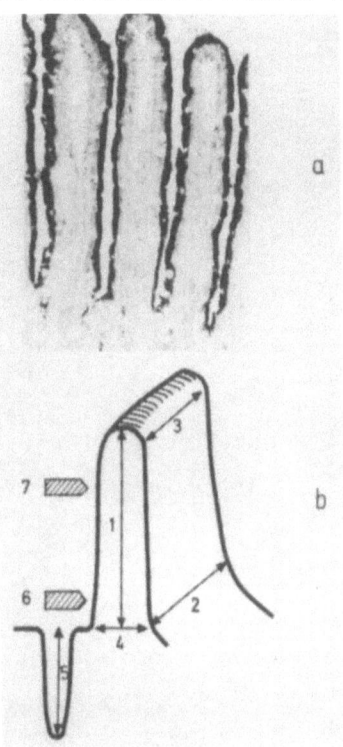

Figure 1. Quantitative assay of brush border enzymes *in situ* and three-dimensional analysis of intestinal villi. (a) Azo-dye in the brush border region (alkaline phosphatase × 24). (b) Schematic presentation of the morphometric parameters registered; 1:villus height; 2,3:villus breadth (base, apex); 4:villus width; 5:crypt length; 6,7; basal, apical measuring position for the kinetic enzyme analysis *in situ*.

mucosa, where numbers of crypts per unit area (Figure 2a) and the corresponding parameters of the microdissected (Figure 2b) crypts were determined.[10] In homogenates of scraped intestinal mucosa and of the kidneys the protein,[11] DNA and RNA[12] content were measured.

Paraffin-embedded liver specimens were stained with haematoxylin–eosin (HE), periodic acid schiff (PAS) and trichrom–masson–goldner and examined by Prof Dr G. Klöppel (Pathol. Institut der Universität Hamburg).

Enzymatic Techniques

The specific activities (mU/mg protein) of neutral α-glucosidase[13] (with sucrose and/or 2-naphthyl-α-D-glucoside), lactase-β-glucosidase,[14] un-

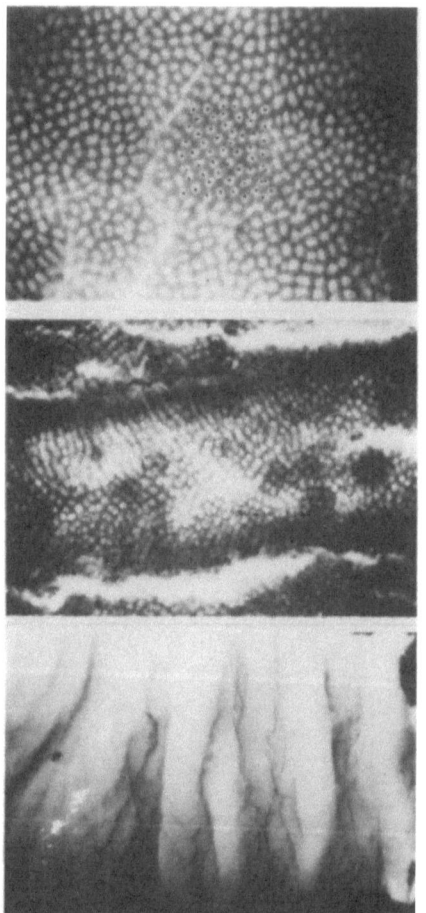

Fig 2. (a)

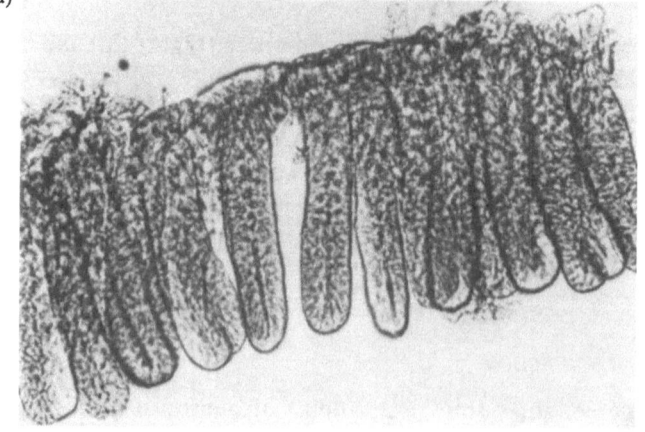

Fig 2. (b)

specific alkaline phosphatase[15] and acid β-galactosidase[16] were determined on the intestinal mucosa and kidneys.

In tissue sections the corresponding *in situ* activities of these enzymes were determined either at the two 'respresentative' villus sites (normally revealing minimal and maximal app. V_{max}[18]) in the brush border region (disaccharidase, alkaline phosphatase), or in the apical cytoplasm of the crypt epithelium[16] (acid β-galactosidase), or in the epithelium at the convoluted part of the proximal kidney tubulus (Figure 3a). In the latter case alkaline phosphatase (Figure 3b) and an additional membrane protease, the dipeptidylpeptidase IV[18], were measured in the brush border region, whereas the neutral α-glucosidase (using a membrane technique) was determined in the apical and the acid β-galactosidase in the basal part of the cytoplasm. In this region also the succinate-dehydrogenase[19] was measured under 'non-kinetic' conditions (Figure 3b).

Statistical Evaluation

Analysis of variance (followed by t tests) and the Kruskal–Wallis test (followed by Wilcoxon $W_{(n)}$ tests) were used in the statistical analysis of the means of each parameter per animal.

Results

Rats treated with the highest dosages of both retinoids developed conjunctivitis, hair loss, desquamation of the skin, erythema and swelling of the snout region. Three animals under Ro 10-9357, 20mg/kg/day, and one animal under Ro 13-6298, 0.002mg/kg/day, which died before the 17th day (see Table 1) were not included in the study. After a 10-day-treatment a significant ($p < 5$ per cent) decrease in body-weight as compared to controls could be found only in the animals treated with 0.04mg/kg/day Ro 13-6298. After 17 days there was a trend for body-weight to decrease after both Ro 10-9357 (20mg/kg/day) and Ro 13-6298 (0.002mg/kg/day). A 30-day-treatment with Ro 10-9357 1mg/kg/day did not significantly influence this parameter.

Intestine

In the first experiment[20] (R 10 3mg/kg/day over a 10-day period, Table 1) a significant increase in the basal and apical villus breadth was found in the ileum, leading to an overall increase in the mucosal surface per unit

Figure 2. Morphometric analysis of colonic mucosa. (a) Submucosal folds (bottom) with the orifices of the crypts (middle), which were counted per unit area (top, dots in the orifices, $\times$ 6.3). (b) Group of crypts after microdissection.

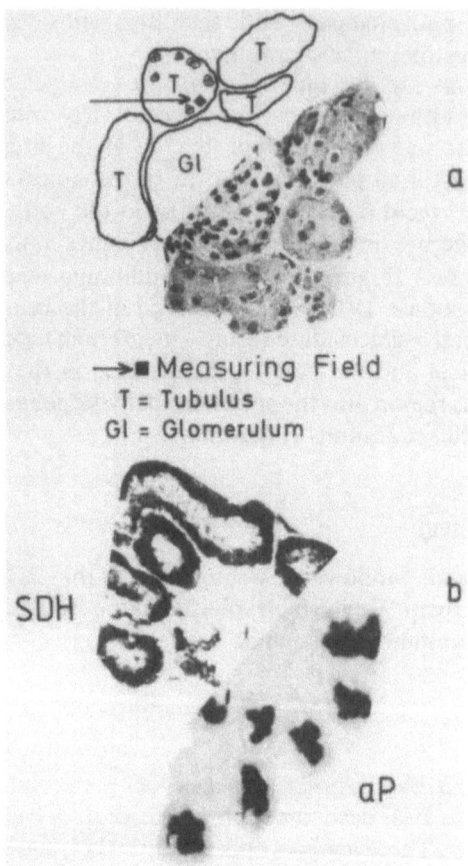

Measuring Field
T = Tubulus
GI = Glomerulum

SDH

Figure 3. *In situ* enzymatic measurements at the proximal kidney tubulus. (a) Semi-schematic presentation of a glomerulum and the adjacent convoluted part of the proximal tubulus. (b) Enzyme reactions at the basal (SDH = succinate dehydrogenase) and apical (aP = alkaline phosphatase) cytoplasm of the tubular epithelium ($\times$ 24).

serosal area (Figure 4a). This increase was accompanied by a significant increase in the specific sucrase activity (Figure 4b), paralleled by a trend of the basal and apical *in situ* V_{max} values of this enzyme to increase.

The results of experiments 2, 3 and 4 clearly show[21], that significant morphological changes occurred in the small intestine, but not in the colon. As Figure 5 shows, therapeutic doses of Ro 13-6298 (0.0002mg/kg/daily) induced an increase in jejunal mucosal surface after 17 days, whereas toxic doses of Ro 10-9359 (10mg/kg/daily) led to a decrease of this parameter in that segment after 10 days. Since in these experiments the other doses did not exert comparable effects and since 3mg (experiment 1) affected only the ileum, no clear dose- or time-dependent of the morphological changes in the

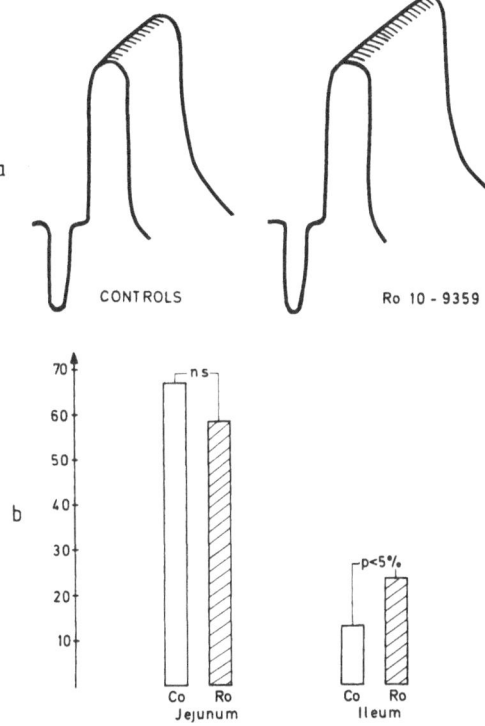

Figure 4. Morphometric and enzymatic changes at the intestinal mucosa after 3mg/kg/day etretinate (Ro 10-9359) over 10 days (experiment 1). (a) Significant increase in ileal villus breadth (base and apex, compare Figure 1) resulting in an overall significant increase in the mucosal surface per serosal area (mm^2/mm^2) in the *ileum*. (b) Significant increase in specific sucrase activity (mU/mg protein, abscissa) in the *ileum*.

small intestinal mucosa in response to oral retinoids could be detected. This is also the case when referring to the specific enzyme activities (Figure 6). The brush border enzymes, however, revealed under both retinoids, regardless of the administered dose, a marked increase in their specific activities in the ileum (hatched bars), but a decrease in the jejunum (filled bars). No significant changes could be detected in the nucleic acid and protein content of the homogenates (per mg wet weight) during this series of experiments.

Kidney

The histological features of the tubular epithelium, the nucleic acid and protein content (per mg wet weight) of the kidneys of animals treated with both retinoids remained unaltered, in experiments 2 and 3.

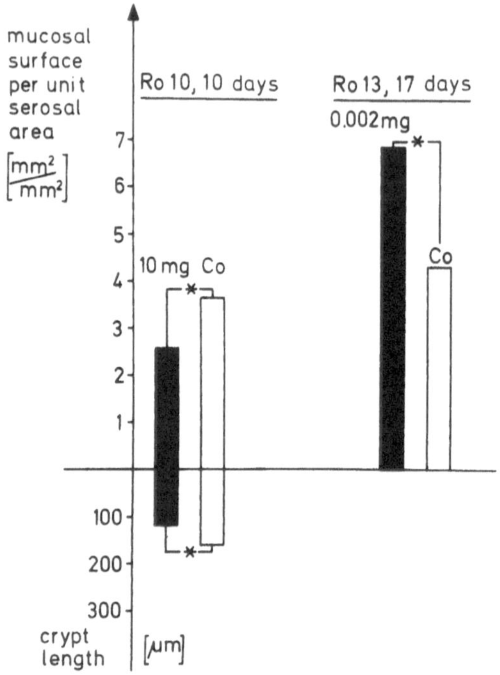

Figure 5. Significant changes in intestinal mucosal architecture. Results of the experiments 2,3 and 4.

During experiment 2 (see Table 1) only the specific neutral α-glucosidase activity (homogenate) and *in situ* acid β-glucosidase activity (tissue section) were significantly increased.[22] Discrete and partially opposite alterations in specific enzyme activities were obtained in experiment 3 (Figure 7). Alkaline phosphatase was decreased after therapeutic doses of etretinate (1mg/kg/day) and after therapeutic and toxic doses, as well, of arotinoid (0.002 and 0.04mg/kg/day), whereas under toxic doses of Ro 13-6298 acid β- galactosidase was decreased and neutral α-glucosidase activity was increased. In the tissue section, however, high doses of arotinoid affected only the *in situ* V_{max} of alkaline phosphatase leading to a decrease after 10 days (Figure 8). Interestingly, the *in situ* activity of a brush border membrane protease, the dipeptidylpeptidase IV, but also the other lysosomal (acid β-galactosidase) and mitochondrial (succinate-dehydrogenase) marker enzymes of the tubular epithelium remained unaltered.

Liver

No histological changes were found in the liver of the treated animals.

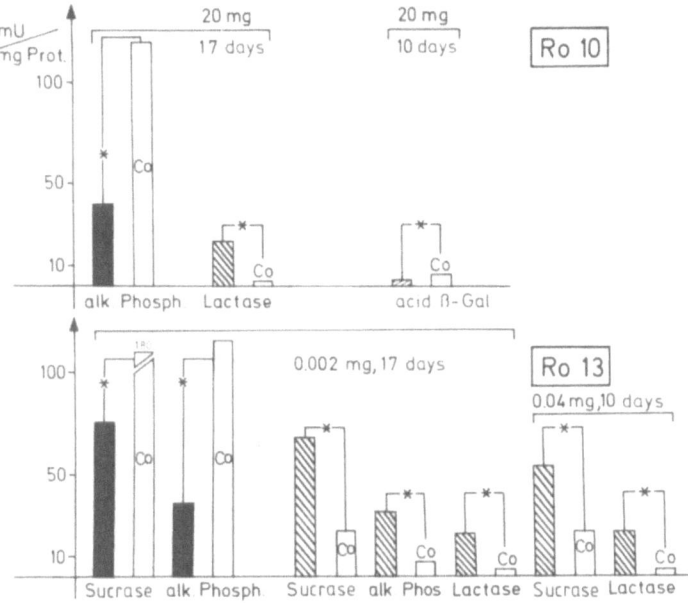

Figure 6. Significant changes in enzyme activities (mU/mg protein in mucosal homo-genates). Results of experiments 2,3 and 4. Etretinate (Ro 10-9359), arotinoid (Ro 13-6298).

Discussion

As shown in this paper, the retinoid-induced changes in the three-dimensional mucosal architecture are not combined with alterations in the histological features of the epithelium, e.g. height of the columnar cells, basophilia. Although the increase and the decrease of mucosal surface are not always accompanied by corresponding changes in crypt length, it seems most likely that hyperproliferation and hypoproliferation of the crypt cell compartment are the underlying phenomena respectively. Since the morphological changes (i.e. mucosal surface) are not paralleled by corresponding enzymatic (specific activity) alterations, it seems likely that the brush-border membrane is the target of the pharmacological action of retinoids. The question as to whether these changes represent direct or indirect retinoid effects on the intestinal mucosa remains to be elucidated. One could assume, for example, that the uniform increase in ileal enzyme activity is an adaptive response to the retinoid-induced decrease of enzyme activity in the jejunum, which probably represents the main absorptive site for the retinoids.

With regard to the kidneys, it should be noted that the physiological importance of the enzyme activities, e.g. the alkaline phosphatase,[23] in the tubular system has not yet been clearly established. Nevertheless, a

173

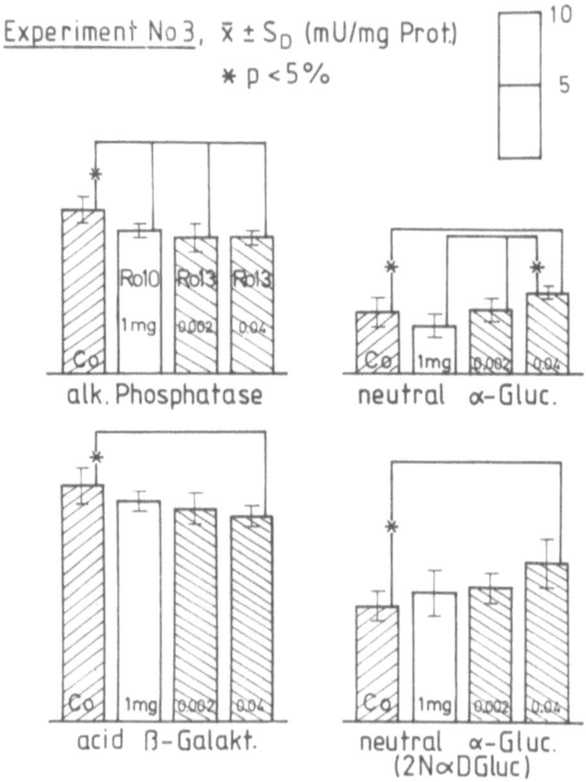

Figure 7. Specific activities (mU/mg protein, homogenate) of kidney tubular enzymes. Results of experiment 3. Etretinate (Ro 10-9359); arotinoid (Ro 13-6298); two different α-glucosidase substrates, saccharose and 2-naphthol-α-glucoside (Sacchar, 2NαDGluc).

decrease of the enzyme activities *in situ*[24,25] or their increase in the urine[26-28] are thought to reflect an impairment of the kidney tubular function. The discrete enzyme alterations observed after treatment with oral retinoids were not uniformly expressed in the epithelium of the proximal tubulus. The brush border alkaline phosphatase was decreased, whereas the *in situ* activity of another brush border enzyme, the membrane protease dipeptidylpeptidase IV, remained unaltered; finally, there was no additional enzymatic or histological evidence for tubular cellular damage.

In conclusion, the results discussed here indicate that etretinate and the arotinoid Ro 13-6298, apart from their influence on the keratinizing epidermis, are capable of exerting distinct effects on the non-keratinizing epithelia of the intestine and of the kidney tubles. Though several effects of vitamin A and retinoids on extracutaneous tissues have been previously

Experiment No 3, $\bar{x} \pm S_D$ (AU), $*$ p < 5 %

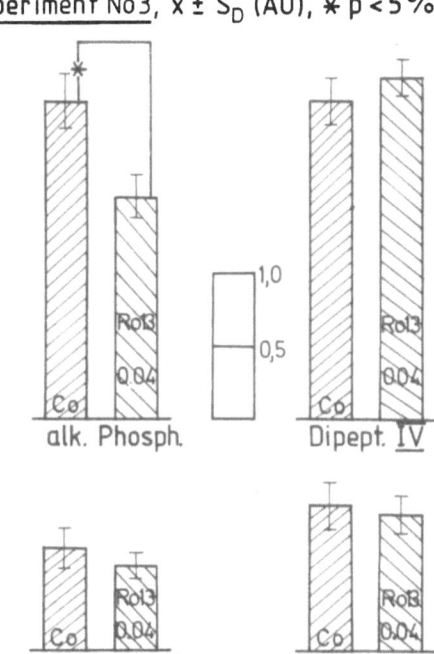

Figure 8. *In situ* activities (AU = absorbance units) of kidney tubular enzymes. Results of experiment 3. Arotinoid (Ro 13); dipeptidylpeptidase IV (Dipept IV); succinate dehydrogenase (Suc. Dehyd.).

reported,[29,30] it is the first time that retinoid-induced alterations of enzyme activities in the intestine and the kidneys have been described. The possible significance of these alterations for the functional integrity of the intestinal and kidney tubular epithelium remains to be elucidated. However, though it is not known whether these retinoid effects can be extrapolated to humans, it seems essential at this time to closely monitor the functional parameters of these organ systems under retinoid therapy, particularly in patients with pre-existing intestinal and kidney disorders.

Acknowledgements

We are indebted to Prof Dr G. Klöppel for the histological examination of the liver sections, to Mrs Ch. Brunn, Mrs U. Feldmann, Mrs M.L. Hanski and Mrs S. Stein for skilful technical assistance, to Mr F. Sandforth for assistance in the statistical evaluation and to Mrs Ch. Brunn for secretarial aid. This study was supported by the Deutsche Forschungsgemeinschaft,

Grants Gu 184/1 and 184/2–2. Part of the results has been presented at the 33rd meeting of the German Dermatological Society, September 30th to October 3rd, Vienna, 1982 and at the second meeting of the North-West German Dermatologists, March 19th, Göttingen, 1983.

References

1. Sporn, M.B., Dunlop, W.M., Newton, D.L. and Smith, J.M. (1976). Prevention of chemical carcinogenesis by vitamin A and its synthetic analogs (retinoids). *Fed. Proc.*, **35**, 1332

2. Elias, P.M. and Williams, M.L. (1981). Retinoids, cancer and the skin. *Arch. Dermatol.*, **117**, 160

3. Orfanos, C.E., Braun-Falco, O., Farber, E.M., Grupper, Ch., Polano, M.K. and Schuppli, R. (1981). *Retinoids: Advances in Basic Research and Therapy.* (Berlin, Heidelberg, New York: Springer-Verlag)

4. Mayer, H., Bollag, W., Hänni, R. and Rüegg, R. (1978). Retinoids, a new class of compounds with prophylactic and therapeutic activities in oncology and dermatology. *Experientia*, **34**, 1105

5. Paravicini, U. (1981). Pharamcokinetics and metabolism of oral aromatic retinoids. In Orfanos, C.E. *et al.* (eds.). *Retinoids: Advances in Basic Research and Therapy.* pp. 13–20. (Berlin, Heidelberg, New York: Springer-Verlag)

6. Hänni, R. (1978). Pharmacokinetic and metabolic pathways of systemically applied retinoids. *Dermatologica*, **157** (Suppl. 1), 5

7. Einarson, L. (1951). On the theory of gallocyanin chromalum staining and its application for quantitative estimation of basophilia. A selective staining of exquisite progressivity. *Acta Pathol. Microbiol. Scand.*, **28**, 82

8. Clarke, R.M. (1970). Mucosal architecture and epithelial cell production rate in the small intestine of the albino rat. *J. Anat.*, **107**, 519

9. Lorenz-Meyer, H., Köhn, R. and Riecken, E.O. (1976). Vergleich verschiedener morphometrischer Methoden zur Erfassung der Schleimhautoberfläche des Rattendünndarmes und deren Beziehung zur Funktion. *Histochemistry*, **49**, 123

10. Gutschmidt, S., Sandforth, R. and Riecken, E.O. (1983). Segmental variation in surface parameters of the normal rat colonic mucosa. *Virchows Arch. B.* In press

11. Lowry, O.H., Rosebrough, N.J., Farr, A.L. and Randall, R.J. (1951). Protein measurements with the folin phenol reagent. *J. Biol. Chem.*, **193** 265

12. Munro, H.N. and Fleck, A. (1966). Recent developments in the measurement of nucleic acids in biological materials. *Analyst*, **91**, 78

13. Gutschmidt, S., Kaul, W. and Riecken, E.O. (1979). A quantitative histochemical technique for the characterization of α-glucosidase in the brush border membrane of rat jejunum. *Histochemistry*, **63**, 81

14. Gutschmidt, S. (1981). *In situ* determinations of apparent K_m and V_{max} of brush border disaccharidases along the villi of normal human jejunal biopsy specimens. *Histochemistry*, **71**, 451

15. Gutschmidt, S., Lange, U. and Riecken, E.O. (1980). Kinetic characterization of unspecific alkaline phosphatase at different villus sites of rat jejunum. A quantitative histochemical study. *Histochemistry*, **69**, 189

16. Gutschmidt, S. (1983). *Die in situ Charakterisierung von Enzymen des intestinalen Resorptionsepithels. Methodik und Befunde in Korrelation zu morphometrischen Parametern der Mucosaarchitektur.* Habilitationschrift, Fachbereich Medizin, Klinikum Steglitz der FU Berlin

17. Gutschmidt, S., Emde, C. and Riecken, E.O. (1980). Quantification of α-glucosidases along the villus of the small intestine in man. Introduction of a computerized histochemical method. *Histochemistry*, **67**, 85

18. Gutschmidt, S. and Gossrau, R. (1981). A quantitative histochemical study of dipeptidylpeptidase IV (DPPIV). *Histochemistry*, **73**, 285

19. Lojda, Z., Gossrau, R. and Schiebler, T.H. (1979). *Enzyme Histochemistry. A Laboratory Manual.* (Berlin, Heidelberg, New York: Springer-Verlag)
20. Gutschmidt, S. and Tsambaos, D. (1982). Effects of aromatic retinoid on non-keratinizing (intestinal) epithelium: biochemical and morphological studies. *Arch. Dermatol. Res.*, **273**, 85
21. Gutschmidt, S. and Tsambaos, D. (1983). Einfluss oraler aromatischer Retinoide auf das Darmepithel im Tierexperiment. *Hautarzt* In Press
22. Gutschmidt, S. and Tsambaos, D. (1982). Effects of large doses of etretinate (Tigason) on enzymes of the rat kidney. *Br. J. Dermatol.*, **107**, 251
23. Tenenhouse, H.S., Scriver, C.R. and Vizel, E.J. (1980). Alkaline phosphatase activity does not mediate phosphate transport in the renal-cortical brush-border membrane. *Biochem. J.*, **190**, 473
24. Wachsmuth, E.D. (1981). Quantification of nephrotoxicity in rabbits by automated morphometry of alkaline phosphatase stained kidney sections. *Histochemistry*, **71**, 235
25. Wellwood, J.M., Lovell, D., Thompson, A.E. and Tighe, J.R. (1976). Renal damage caused by gentamycin: a study of the effects on renal morphology and urinary enzyme excretion. *J. Pathol.*, **118**, 171
26. Dubach, U.C. and Schmidt, U. (1979). *Diagnostic Significance of Enzymes and Proteins in Urine.* (Bern, Stuttgart, Wien: Hans Huber Publishers)
27. Adelman, R.D., Counzelman, G., Spangler, W. and Ishizaki, G. (1976). Enzymuria: an early sign of gentamycin (GN) nephrotoxicity. *Kidney Int.*, **10**, 493
28. Price, R.G., Dance, N. and Robinson, D. (1971). A comparison of the β-glucosidase excretion during kidney damage induced by 4-nitrophenylarsenic acid and by rabbit anti-rat kidney antibodies. *Eur. J. Clin. Invest.*, **2**, 47
29. Tsambaos, D. and Orfanos, C.E. (1981). Chemotherapy of psoriasis and other skin disorders with oral retinoids. *Pharmac. Ther.*, **14**, 355
30. Lotan, R. (1980). Effects of vitamin A and its analogs (retinoids) on normal and neoplastic cells. *Biochim. Biophys. Acta*, **605**, 33

177

Section 4

Retinoids and Neoplasia

19
Detection of Precancerous Bronchial Metaplasia in Heavy Smokers and its Regression after Treatment with a Retinoid

G. MATHÉ, G. SANTELLI, J. GOUVEIA, G. LEMAIGRE, J.L. MISSET, F. GROS, J.P. HOMASSON, B. KIM and M.C. SUDRE. STATISTICAL ANALYSIS: H. GAGET

Introduction

Tobacco is by far the most common bronchial carcinogen.[1] The malignant bronchial tumours are often preceded by squamous metaplasia which can be followed by dysplasia.

It is well known that vitamin A deficiency can induce metaplasia of the bronchial mucosa.[2] Retinoids, natural and synthetic derivatives of vitamin A, have been shown to be able to prevent or to cure precancerous lesions and chemically-induced cancer in *in vitro* and *in vivo* experiments.[3-5]

Etretinate, a vitamin A derivative, has proved *in vivo* to be able to prevent chemically-induced papillomas and carcinomas in mice,[6] and to amplify some immune reactions (T lymphocytes, macrophage activity, antibody-dependent cytotoxicity[7]). It was able to restore the *in vitro* tracheo-epithelial metaplasia caused by vitamin A deficiency or induced by chemical carcinogens.[8]

We looked for HLA phenotypes loci A and B in most of our patients.

This study is an evaluation of bronchial metaplasia in heavy smokers and its favourable evolution under ctrctinate treatment.

Patients and Methods

We attempted to detect and quantify bronchial squamous metaplasia in heavy smokers by endoscopic examinations. Patients were referred by doctors from public, private, university or regional hospitals who collaborated in this study. All patients included in this study were heavy smokers with a rate of intoxication of at least 15 packet-year (product of the number of cigarette packs smoked daily by the number of years of intoxication duration). Patients with the following characteristics were excluded from the study:

(1) severe organic disease that was not controlled by treatment,
(2) pregnancy,
(3) women who were not practising birth control.

132 smokers underwent a first bronchoscopy, with careful and complete macroscopic exploration of all the bronchial tree, and biopsies were taken from each of the ten following sites: carina, right upper lobe bifurcation, middle lobe bifurcation, bifurcation of superior (apical) segment bronchus of right lower lobe, trifurcation of right basal bronchi, bifurcation of left upper lobe, bifurcation of lingula, bifurcation of superior (apical) segment bronchus of left lower lobe, and bronchi at the level of left basal segment (two samples). Specimens were also taken from all doubtful lesions. Each biopsy specimen was placed in a labelled bottle containing Bouin fixative and it was cut into 10 serial sections 4μm thick. All specimens were stained with haematoxylin and eosin for histopathological examination.

An index of metaplasia (MI), expressed as a percentage, was calculated as follows:

$$MI = \frac{\text{number of sections with metaplasia}}{\text{number of sections examined}} \times 100.$$

At this stage of the study, 61 patients (48 males and 13 females) out of the 132 included in this study had an MI less than 15 per cent without any treatment. One patient was excluded from the study for another reason (see below).

Seventy patients whose MI was more than 15 per cent were treated with etretinate (Figure 1) at a daily dose of 25mg per os for 6 months. Each volunteer was followed up by a member of our team (either hospital physicians or private practitioners, all members of the 'Groupe Français de Prévention Pharmacologique des Cancers') who looked carefully for any side-effects.

Follow-up consisted of clinical examination, liver function tests (SGOT, SGPT, alkaline phosphatase), serum creatinine and electrocardiograms before the beginning of treatment and on the 30th, 90th and 180th day of treatment.

After 6 months, the patients were submitted to a second bronchoscopy

CH3O — COOC2H5

ethyl 9-(4-methoxy-2,3,6-trimethylphenyl)-3,7-dimethyl-
2,4,6,8-nonatetraenoate (Ro 10-9359)

Figure 1. Chemical formula of etretinate.

with the same method as the first. Results yielded a second metaplasia index.

HLA phenotypes loci A and B were studied in 74 of our patients at the blood bank of the Hôpital Paul-Brousse. The samples were carried out before the first fibroscopy and before starting treatment.

Results

132 patients underwent 196 fibroscopies without any morbidity. 61 patients were not treated because their MI was less than 15 per cent. One cancer *in situ* was discovered and the patient was excluded from the study and submitted to surgery. 70 patients entered a 6-month treatment period with etretinate; 35 of them were evaluated because they finished the course of treatment and underwent a second fibroscopy. 15 patients were lost during the folow-up period. Two were not evaluated because they failed to follow the protocol of treatment. Four stopped smoking during treatment. Two stopped treatment because of toxicity (see below). 12 are under treatment

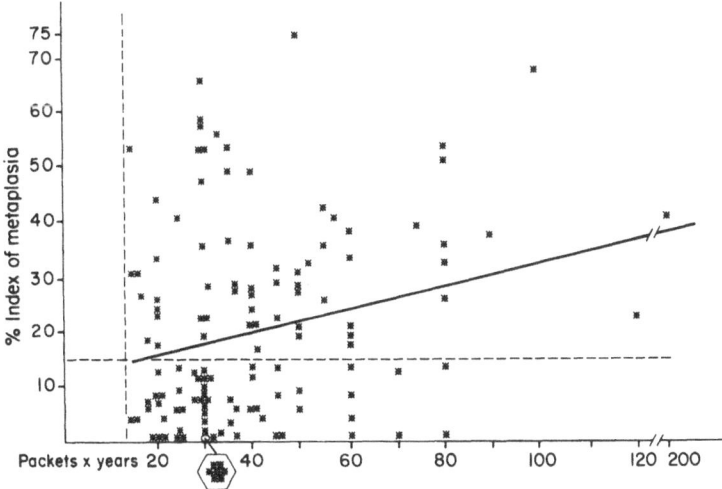

Figure 2. Index of metaplasia (MI in relation to the number of cigarettes smoked expressed in packet-year).

183

and will be evaluable later.

Histological studies of the biopsy fragments of the 131 patients allowed us to establish a positive correlation between MI and tobacco intoxication. This correlation follows a correlation line (Figure 2). High frequency of MI more than 15 per cent is statistically significant ($p < 0.01$).

Bronchial metaplasia is statistically more severe in men than in women although mean values of age and total tobacco consumption are not different.

37 patients were treated. Of them, two stopped treatment because of side-effects (one had cutaneous toxicity after accidental overdose and the other had transient abnormalities of liver functions, but he was an alcholic). One patient whose MI was about 12 per cent before treatment was erroneously included. His MI dropped down to 3 per cent. The MI of other patients treated for 6 months dropped from 34.57 per cent down to 26.96 per cent, corresponding to a mean of 40.6 packet-year. This difference in MI is statistically significant with $p < 0.001$ (Figure 3).

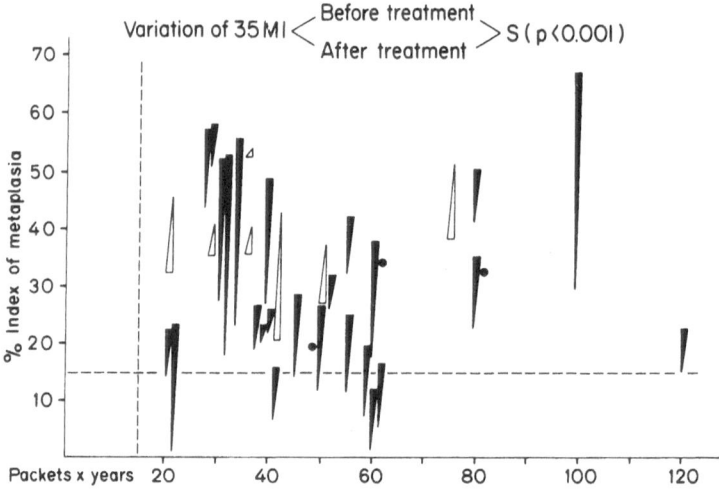

Figure 3. Variation of MI in 35 volunteers after 6-month treatment with a retinoid. Δ : increase of metaplasia; ▼ : decrease of metaplasia.

Moreover, four patients stopped smoking during treatment. They were, of course, excluded from the study on the effect of etretinate but it is worth noting that their MI, which were 19 per cent, 74 per cent, 40 per cent and 40 per cent respectively at initiation of therapy, dropped to 0 per cent in the patients after 6 months, which was far quicker than expected.[9]

A widespread HLA phenotype loci B associated with a small population sample did not permit us to draw further conclusions. The loci A distribution was, in our group of patients, comparable to the distribution of a control group[10] (Table 1).

Table 1. Percentage of genic frequencies.

Groups Loci A	Heavy smokers $MI > 0$ per cent, $n = 74$ (per cent)	Control group[10] $n = 304$ (per cent)	Heavy smokers $MI = 0$ per cent, $n = 10$ (per cent)
A 1	0.11	0.12	0.05
A 2	0.23	0.26	0.25
A 3	0.13	0.13	0.10
A 9	0.11	0.10	0.10
A 10	0.07	0.05	0.05
A 11	0.07	0.06	0.10
A 19.2	0.13	0.07	0.05

The MI of ten of our patients was 0 per cent in spite of their high tobacco intoxication (mean value: 34 packet-year). We could not find any significant difference between the loci A distribution in this subgroup and the control group. The locus A 1 distribution was 0.12 per cent in the control group; it was 0.05 per cent in the heavy smoker group (MI = 0 per cent). The p value (0.46) was not significant.

Discussion

It appears clearly from our trial that it is possible to perform bronchoscopic examination and take several biopsy specimens-from the patients without causing any morbidity. The treatment protocol was easily accepted by the patients.

Our aim was not to detect bronchial cancer, although we discovered one case during this trial.

We can assert a positive correlation between the extent of tobacco intoxication and the degree of bronchial metaplasia.

The degree of MI in our trial seems to be sex-related. 66 per cent of women had a MI less than 15 per cent. When we compared the female group with the male group, which had similar tobacco intoxication (mean values: 41.7 and 32.4 packet-year respectively), we found a statistically significant increase of MI in the male group. This might be related with the lower frequency of women's bronchial cancer. When heavy smokers are informed about their precancerous bronchial lesions, this can incite them to stop cigarette intoxication.

Bronchial MI dropped significantly with a p value less than 0.001 in the 35 patients who completed the whole protocol course.

Our goal is to evaluate the efficacy of a long-term administration of etretinate on bronchial metaplasia and we intend to carry on this trial further. We believe it would be interesting to study a group of patients who have stopped smoking, since they are still at high risk of cancer for up to 13 years after giving up smoking.[11]

References

1. Wynder, E.L., Hoffman, P. and Gori, G.B. (1975). *Proc. 3rd World Conference on Smoking and Health*, DHEW, No 76.1221 (NIH). (Washington: Government Printing Office)
2. Mayer, H. Unpublished results. Cited by Mayer, H., Bollag, W., Hanna, R. and Rüegg, R. (1978). Retinoids, a new class of compounds with prophylactic and therapeutic activities in oncology and dermatology. *Experientia*, **14**, 1105
3. Auerbach, O., Stout, A.P., Hammond, E.C. and Garfinkel, L. (1961). Changes in bronchial epithelium in relation to cigarette smoking and in relation to lung cancer. *N. Engl. J. Med.*, **265**, 253
4. Auerbach, O., Stout, A.P., Hammond, E.C. and Garfinkel, L. (1962). Bronchial epithelium in former smokers. *N. Engl. J. Med.*, **267**, 119
5. Auerbach, O., Stout, A.P., Hammond, E.C. and Garfinkel, L. (1962). Changes in relation to sex, age, residence, smoking and pneumonia. *N. Engl. J. Med.*, **267**, 111
6. Bollag, W. (1974). Therapeutic effect of aromatic retinoid acid analog on chemically induced skin papillomas and carcinomas in mice. *Eur. J. Cancer*, **10**, 731
7. Bruley-Rosset, M., Hercend, T., Martinez, J., Rappaport, H. and Mathé, G. (1981). Prevention of spontaneous tumours of aged mice by immunopharmacological manipulation: study of immune antitumor mechanisms. *J. Natl. Cancer Inst.*, **66**, 1113
8. Clamon, G.H., Sporn, M.B., Smith, J.M. and Saffiotti, U. (1974). α and β retinyl acetate reverse metaplasias of vitamin A deficiency in hamster trachea in organ culture. *Nature (London)*, **250**, 64
9. Bertram, J.F. and Rogers, A.W. (1981). Recovery of bronchial epithelium on stopping smoking. *Br. Med. J.*, **283**, 1567
10. Dausset, J. (1982). *HLA 1982, Complexes Majeur d'Histocompatibilité de l'Homme*. p. 93. (Paris: Flammarion)
11. Mathé, G. and Cattan, A. (1976). *Cancérologie à l'Usage du Praticien et de l'Etudiant*. p. 972. (Paris: Expansion Scientifique Française)

20
Cutaneous Neoplasia and Etretinate

B. BERRETTI and CH. GRUPPER

Development of synthetic vitamin A derivatives (synthetic retinoids) for prophylaxis and treatment of epithelial neoplasia has been underway for the last 10 years;[1-14] since 1971, retinoids have been reported to be effective as both prophylactic and therapeutic agents in experimental skin cancers. Moreover, clinical therapeutic benefits have been observed in man in some non-pigmented cutaneous and mucous premalignant and malignant disorders.[1-14]

Since 1977, we have treated 80 patients suffering various premalignant or malignant skin conditions with etretinate (aromatic retinoid – Ro 10-9359, Tigason). Preliminary results for our first 36 patients have been reported at the International Symposium on Retinoids held in Berlin in 1980.[6]

Patients

Eighty patients have been treated, 53 males and 27 females with a mean age of 62 years (range from 36 to 84 years). Sixty patients were of skin type I, 12 of type II, five of type III, two of type IV and one of type V.

The following table shows a breakdown of the types of cutaneous disorders represented:

26 multiple actinic keratoses: 23 isolated and 3 associated with basal cell carcinoma (BCC).

17 multiple superficial relapsing basal cell carcinomas associated with actinic keratoses.

20 isolated basal cell carcinomas.

5 Bowen's disease.

4 squamous cell carcinomas (SCC).

2 cases of chronic arsenic intoxication with multiple keratoses and cutaneous carcinomas.

6 keratoacanthomas.

Methods

Therapeutic Management

The mean initial dosage of etretinate was 1mg/kg, taken in two or three divided doses after fat-rich meals. The basic dosage was maintained for 3 months, after which time clinical results were evaluated. Lesions which were not completely cleared after this initial etretinate treatment were treated with conventional destructive methods (electrodesiccation, radiotherapy, surgery or topical antimitotics).

Most patients (58) underwent maintenance treatment: the etretinate dosage was progressively reduced, first to 0.75 and subsequently to 0.50mg/kg/day or less. In most cases, etretinate was withdrawn after 4–5 months of continuous treatment.

Each patient was subjected to laboratory tests before and after treatment in order to detect not only any haematological, hepatic or renal toxicity, but also to check lipoprotein status.

Histological samples were performed for most patients before treatment and, when possible, after the clearing of lesions.

Evaluation of Results

Clinical examinations were performed weekly by the same observer in order to determine clinical results and side-effects of initial treatment.

The 58 patients undergoing maintenance treatment continued to be followed up even after cessation of etretinate treatment: the length of remission as well as chronology, incidence and severity of relapses were noted. This follow-up study ranged between 12 and 36 months in duration.

Results

The results of clearing phase therapy are shown in Table 1, with results of the follow-up study in Table 2.

Examples of the effect of therapy are shown in Figures 1–6. Figures 1 and 2 show examples of before and after therapy (upper and lower respectively) of actinic keratosis and basal cell carcinoma.

Figures 3, 4 and 5 show respectively a squamous cell carcinoma superimposed on X-ray dermatitis; a giant phagedenic keratoacanthoma and Bowen's disease of the glans penis. Figures of before therapy are shown on

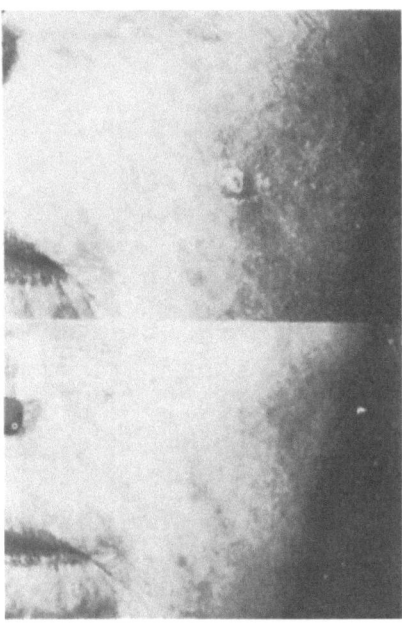

Figure 1. Upper: actinic keratosis on left cheek before therapy; lower: after 2 months therapy.

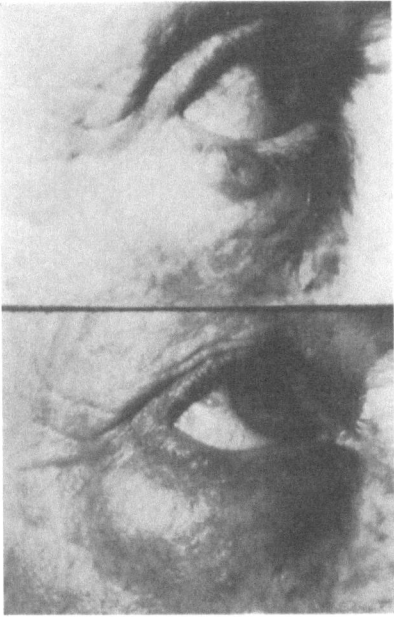

Figure 2. Upper: basal cell carcinoma of lower right eyelid; lower: after 5 weeks therapy showing clinical clearing but histology was still abnormal.

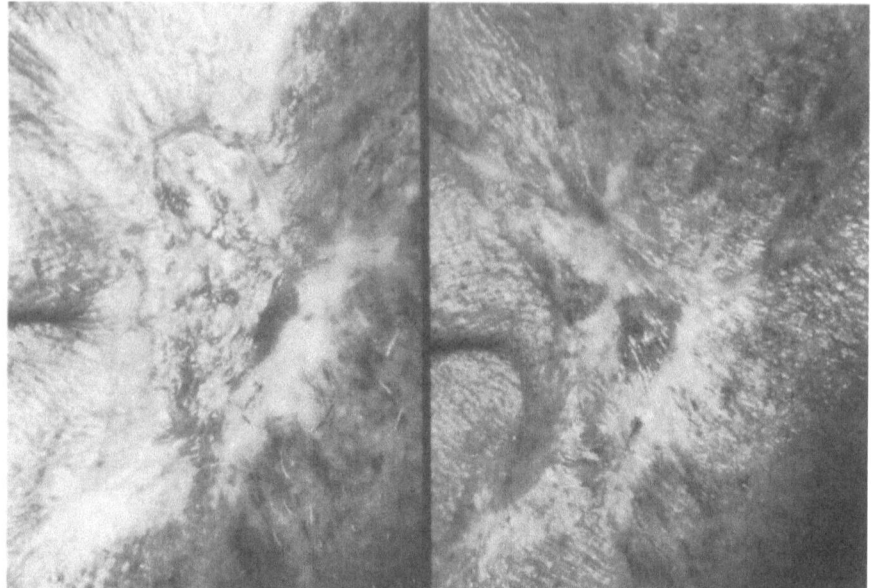

Figure 3. Left: squamous cell carcinoma and surrounding X-ray dermatitis; right: clinical (and histological) clearing after 3 months therapy.

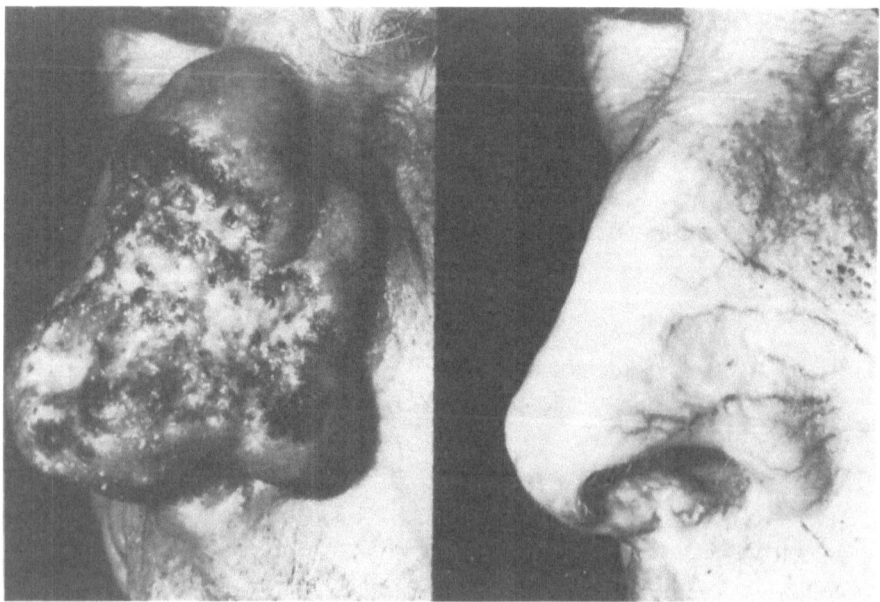

Figure 4. Left: giant phagedenic keratoacanthoma of nose; right: after 3 months therapy.

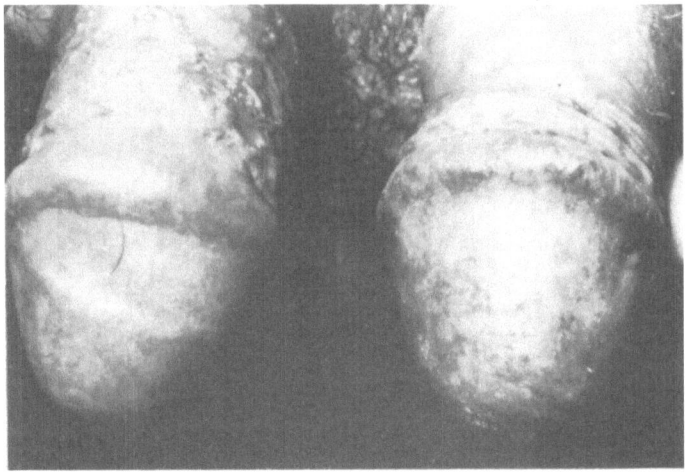

Figure 5. Left: Bowen's disease of glans penis; right: clinical (and histological) clearing after 3 months therapy.

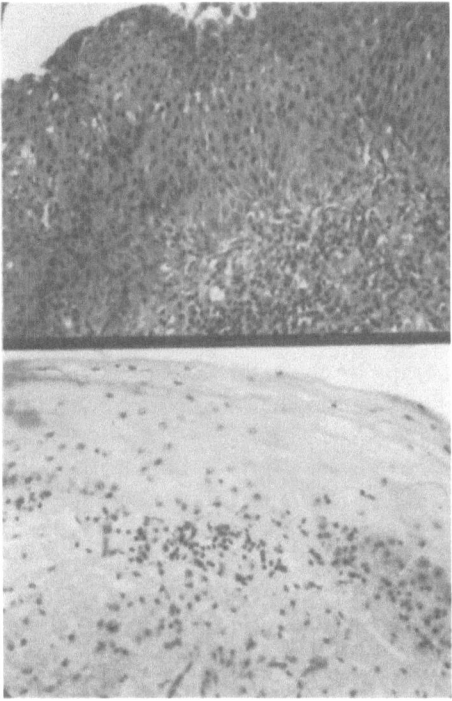

Figure 6. Upper: histology of Figure 5 before therapy; lower: histology after therapy.

Table 1. Results of clearing phase.

Patients	Complete clearing	Good improvement	Limited reduction	No improvement
26 AK	22	3	0	1
20 relapsing multiple AK + BCC				
on AK	13	5	0	2
on BCC	2	7	9	2
20 isolated BCC	1	7	5	7
5 Bowen's disease	1	2	1	1
4 SCC	1	0	1	2
2 cutaneous carcinoma + AS	0	2	0	0
6 keratoacanthoma	6	0	0	0

BCC = basal cell carcinoma, SCC = squamous cell carcinoma, AK = actinic keratoses, AS = arsenical keratoses

Table 2. Follow-up study (12 months after cessation of etretinate).

Patients	Still cleared	Relapsed
20 AK	4	16
14 relaping multiple AK + BCC		
AK	4	10
BCC	2	12
10 isolated BCC	9	1
5 Bowen's disease	5	0
2 SCC	2	0
2 cutaneous carcinoma + AS	0	2
6 keratoacanthoma	5	1

the left and after therapy on the right.

Figure 6 upper shows before therapy and Figure 6 lower after therapy histology.

Like other authors, we observed a number of clinical side-effects attributable to etretinate treatment. Some were frequent, occurring in about 90 per cent of patients: mainly cheilitis with exfoliation, rhagades, stomatitis, glossitis and dryness of the nasal mucosa. Other effects were seen less frequently (transitory alopecia, palmo-plantar lesions with ragged desquamation, thinning of the skin with hyperhidrosis, pruritus and generalized erythema). In a few cases (six patients), side-effects were sufficiently severe to require early cessation of etretinate treatment.

No changes were seen in the laboratory parameters studied.

Discussion

Etretinate proved effective in keratoacanthoma and in actinic keratosis. In the six keratoacanthoma patients, complete clearing was obtained after 1–3 months of treatment; one patient with the severe relapsing phagedenic type situated on the nose, suffered a relapse on the scalp 27 months after withdrawal of etretinate. The other five patients showed no relapses. Of the 46 patients with actinic keratoses (AK), whether or not in association with BCC, complete clearing (clinical and histological) was obtained in 75 per cent, with a good improvement in an additional 20 per cent. These results confirmed both our preliminary report in Berlin[6] and a recently published double-blind study.[9]

Etretinate showed a limited therapeutic effect in cutaneous carcinomas. Of the 42 cases of BCC, either isolated or associated with arsenic intoxication or AK, complete clinical and histological clearing was obtained in only three patients (7 per cent) with a good improvement (obvious reduction in the size and thickness of tumours) in a further 19 (42 per cent). In Bowen's disease and SCC, complete clearing was seen in only two patients, with a good improvement in another two. Of a total of 51 patients initially treated, further treatment with a conventional destructive method was required in 46 (90 per cent).

Our follow-up study shows that relapses occurred at various times after reduction in dosage or cessation of etretinate treatment. This is particularly true for relapsing conditions: multiple actinic keratoses and multiple superficial BCC. BCC recurrences occurred earlier, more frequently, and with greater severity than did recurrences of AK. A maintenance treatment is therefore mandatory, but optimal dosage and duration are still to be determined. Some authors have reported a clear prophylactic effect of etretinate in certain relapsing premalignant or malignant conditions with continuous courses of treatment for 2–4 years.[4,7,8,10] For AK, we adopted an intermittent schedule: a short course of treatment at a daily dosage of 1mg/kg for 2 months annually allowed most patients to remain free of lesions.

Conclusions

Etretinate seems to constitute a novel therapeutic approach to the treatment of cutaneous non-pigmented precancerous and cancerous conditions, partially confirming animal experimental data and other clinical reports.[1-14]

In the treatment of keratoacanthomas and actinic keratoses, etretinate appears to constitute a promising first line of treatment; nevertheless, maintenance dosing is required to avoid relapse; continuous or intermittent dosage schedules may be useful. For cutaneous carcinomas (BCC,

SSC, Bowen's disease), etretinate seems to be of some use, especially as an adjuvant before or after conventional destructive methods, in particular when these methods are only palliative. Additional studies with higher dosages of etretinate should be performed in order to determine the exact susceptibility of cutaneous cancers to a more aggressive dosage schedule.

References

1. Bollag, W. and Hanck, A. (1977). From vitamin A to retinoids : modern trends in the field of oncology and dermatology. *Acta Vitaminol. Enzymol. (Milano)*, **311**, 113
2. Mayer, H., Bollag, W., Hänni, R. and Rüegg, R. (1978). Retinoids, a new class of compounds with prophylactic and therapeutic activities in oncology and dermatology. *Experientia*, **34**, 1105
3. Peck, G.L., Olsen, T.G., Butkus, D. *et al*. (1979). Treatment of basal cell carcinomas with 13-*cis* retinoic acid. *Proc. Am. Assoc. Cancer Res.*, **20**, 56
4. Schnitzler, L., Schubert, B. and Verret, J.L. (1980). Essai de prévention des épithéliomas cutanés par la rétinoïde aromatique. *Ann. Dermatol. Vénéréol.*, **107**, 657
5. Sporn, M.B. and Newton, D.L. (1979). Chemoprevention of cancer with retinoids. *Fed. Proc.*, **38**, 2528
6. Berretti, B., Grupper, C.H., Edelson, Y. and Bermejo, D. (1981). Aromatic retinoid in the treatment of multiple superficial basal cell carcinoma, arsenic keratosis and keratoacanthomes. In Orfanos, C.E. *et al*. (eds.). *Retinoids: Advances in Basic Research and Therapy*. pp. 397–399. (Berlin, Heidelberg, New York: Springer-Verlag)
7. Schnitzler, L. and Verret, J.L. (1981). Retinoid and skin cancer prevention. In Orfanos, C.E. *et al*. (eds.). *Retinoids: Advances in Basic Research and Therapy*. pp. 385–388. (Berlin, Heidelberg, New York: Springer-Verlag)
8. Peck, G.L. (1981). Retinoids in clinical dermatology. In Fleischmajer, R. (ed.). *Progress in Diseases of Skin*. Vol. 1, pp. 227-263. (New York: Grune and Stratton)
9. Moriaty, M., Dunn, J., Darragh, A., Lambe, R. and Brick, I. (1982). Etretinate in the treatment of actinic keratosis. *Lancet*, **1**, 364
10. Peck, G.L., Gross, E.A., Baktus, D. and Di Giovanna, J.L. (1982). Chemoprevention of basal cell carcinoma with isotretinoin. II. Oral retinoids a workshop. *J. Am. Acad. Derm.*, **6**, 815
11. Moon, C.R. and McCormick, D.L. (1982). Inhibition of chemical carcinogenesis by retinoids. II. Oral retinoids a workshop. *J. Am. Acad. Derm.*, **6**, 809
12. Meyskens, F.L. Jr. (1982). Studies of retinoids in the prevention and treatment of cancer. II. Oral retinoids a workshop. *J. Am. Acad. Derm.*, **6**, 824
13. Ehrl, P.A. (1980). Klinische Untersuchungen eines aromatischen Retinoids (Ro 109359) zur Behandlung oraler Hyperkeratosen. *Dtsch Zahnärtzl. Z.* **35**, 554
14. Elias, P.M. and Williams, M.L. (1981). Retinoids, cancer and the skin. *Arch. Dermatol.*, **117**, 160

21
Cutaneous Neoplasia and the Retinoids

T. KINGSTON and R. MARKS

Introduction

There is much evidence from epidemiological studies,[1] *in vitro* studies,[2] and animal experiments[3] that vitamin A and the retinoids reduce the probabability of cutaneous neoplasia. Furthermore, there are also reports suggesting that these drugs have an anti-neoplastic action as well. Basal cell carcinomata have been treated with moderate success with isotretinoin[4] and etretinate.[5] Multiple keratoacanthomata have been suppressed by isotretinoin,[6] and encouraging results in the treatment of multiple solar keratoses have been reported.[7]

We have studies the efficacy of the potent arotinoid ethyl ester Ro 13-6298 and aromatic retinoid etretinate in the treatment of patients with multiple solar keratoses and squamous cell epitheliomata as well as their effects on uninvolved skin.

Methods

16 patients of mean age 67 years were studied. All had multiple solar keratoses (range of duration 2–32 years). Five patients additionally had squamous cell carcinomata and three patients had basal cell carcinomata. The number and area of lesions were recorded in each patient, photographs and biopsies of representative lesions were also taken. To assess the effect of arotinoid on normal skin a further biopsy was taken from a constant reference site on the inner forearm of each subject. After incubation of the skin in tritiated thymidine and subsequent auto-radiography the number of labelled basal and suprabasal cells was

expressed as a proportion of the number of basal cells (labelling index) in each specimen. The mean epidermal thickness (MET) was measured using the Quantimet 720 image analysis system. The densitometer module of the Quantimet was employed to measure the optical density of the Formazan and indigo reaction products after reacting cryostat sections of skin for glucose-6-phosphate dehydrogenase and non-specific esterase activity.[8,9] Each patient was then given arotinoid orally at a dosage of $1\mu g/kg/day$ for 28 days. The patients were then questioned as to the presence of side-effects, the lesions counted and measured and biopsies again taken from lesions and uninvolved skin for the same investigations as previously.

A similar methodology was carried out in two patients given etretinate, 1mg/kg/day for 2 months and three patients given etretinate, 1.5mg/kg/day for 4 weeks then 1mg/kg/day for a further 8 weeks.

Results

With Arotinoid

Ten patients improved, showing a decrease in the number of and the area of the lesions and a reduction in surface scaliness whilst six were unchanged. Table 1 shows the results for all 16 patients. There was a small but significant reduction in mean number and mean total area of the keratoses. There was no effect on the squamous cell carcinomata and the basal cell carcinomata.

Table 1. Mean numbers and area of solar keratoses, basal cell carcinoma and squamous cell carcinomata before and after treatment with Ro 13-6298, in 16 patients.

	Mean number of lesions $\pm SD$	Mean total area of lesions $(mm^2) \pm SD$
Pretreatment	14 ± 9.6	592 ± 312
Post-treatment	11 ± 8.4	439 ± 388
Significance (paired t-test)	$p < 0.02$	$p < 0.001$

Table 2 refers to the normal forearm skin of the subjects. The mean epidermal thickness (MET) was increased significantly after treatment but there was no change in the labelling indices (LI). There was a general increase in the epidermal activity of glucose-6-phosphate dehydrogenase and non-specific esterase from the basal to the granular layer but these results did not achieve significance.

Table 3 shows the side-effects that occurred: cheilitis, pruritus, peeling of the palms and soles or eczema were experienced in 11 cases. No significant change was noted in the blood count, urea and electrolytes, liver

Table 2. Mean epidermal thickness and labelling indices in normal forearm skin before and after treatment with Ro 13-6298, in 16 patients.

	Mean epidermal thickness (μm) ± SD	Labelling indices (per cent) ± SD
Pretreatment	57.22 ± 13.87	5.55 ± 3.02
Post-treatment	75.69 ± 19.17	7.22 ±4.92
Significance	0.05< p< 0.02	NS

Table 3. Side-effects in 16 patients treated with arotinoid (Ro 13-6298).

	Numbers affected
Cheilitis	6
Pruritus	6
Exfoliation of palms and soles	5
Eczema	4

function tests, fasting cholesterol or triglycerides during the course of treatment.

With Etretinate

No improvement was noted in two patients who received etretinate, 1mg/kg/day for 2 months, but there was a marked improvement in the three patients who received 1.5mg/kg/day. However, at this dose level, side-effects of cheilitis, blepharitis and peeling were prominent.

Discussion

Ro 13-6298 has been used previously to treat patients with psoriasis but its use in cutaneous neoplasia has not been properly documented. Although potent on a weight basis, its anti-neoplastic activity is definite but not dramatic after 4 weeks administration. Our experience with etretinate would suggest that more prolonged treatment with arotinoid at a higher dose would be more beneficial.

The way in which retinoids exert their anti-neoplastic effect is unclear. Fritsch[11] has demonstrated changes in the lectin staining pattern of mouse epidermis after administration of etretinate reflecting selective changes in keratinocyte membrane glycoconjugates, which may affect intercellular adhesion and growth control. The anti-neoplastic effect may be in part via immunomodulation as the retinoids can inhibit mitogen stimulation of T lymphocytes,[12] induce stimulation of peritoneal macrophages to inhibit the growth of a cultured tumour cell line and cause a reduction in the number of spontaneously occurring tumours in old age.[13] Furthermore, they have an adjuvant effect.[14]

The effect of retinoids on epidermal cell proliferation seems complex. The lack of change in the labelling index and the normal pattern of auto-radiographically-labelled cells in solar keratoses after treatment does not indicate any profound change in the proliferative process. The retinoids have been shown[15] to inhibit ornithine decarboxylase activity and are in this way inhibitory to the accumulation of polyamines associated with tumour production. Yet another possibility is that their anti-tumour activity results from a cytolytic action on abnormally differentiated cells. Our ultrastructural observations on biopsies of solar keratoses and uninvolved skin removed before and after treatment are similar to those of others[16,17] in that there is an increase in granular material between epidermal cells after retinoid administration. The granular material some-times contains fragments of organelles (see Chapter 11) and we believe that this intercellular material may represent the remains of lysed cells. We have also seen cells in the process of dissolution after treatment with arotinoid (Figure 1). As mentioned previously there is an increase in non-

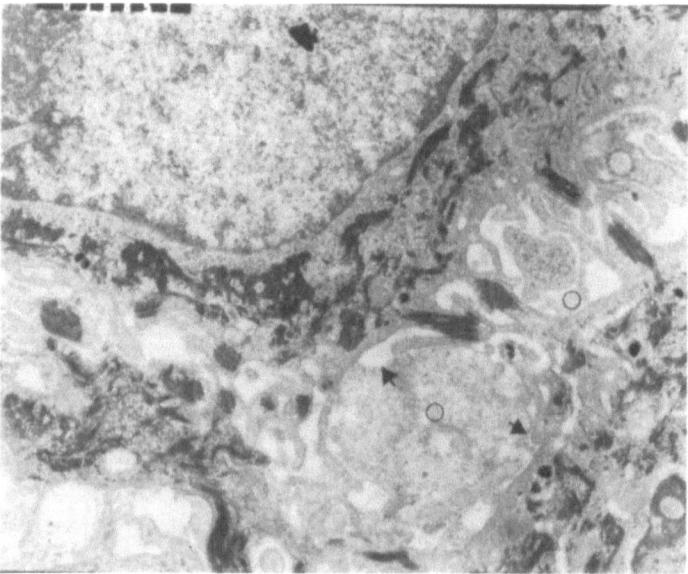

Figure 1. Electron micrograph from the basal region of a solar keratosis lesion after aroten-oid therapy. Fine and coarse granular material is evident between the cells (open circles). This is partially surrounded by plasma membrane in places (arrows). ($\times$ 6200).

specific esterase activity after arotinoid administration. This is an indicator of lysosomal hydrolytic enzyme activity and it must be remembered that labilization of lysosomal membranes is an acknowledged action of vitamin A.

References

1. Kark, J., Smith, A. and Hames, C. (1982). Serum retinol and the inverse relationship between cholesterol and cancer. *Br. Med. J.*, **284**, 152
2. Harisiadis, L., Miller, R., Hall, E. and Borek, C. (1978). A vitamin A analogue inhibits radiation induced autogenic transformation. *Nature*, (*London*), **274**, 487
3. Bollag, W. (1974). Therapeutic effect of an aromatic retinoic acid analog on chemically induced skin papillomas and carcinomas in mice. *Eur. J. Cancer*, **10**, 731
4. Peck, G., Gross, E., Butlaus, M. and Di Giovanna, M. (1982). Chemoprevention of basal cell carcinoma with isotretinoin. *J. Am. Acad. Dermatol.*, **6**, 615
5. Beretti, B., Grupper, Ch., Edelsan, Y. and Bermejo, D. (1981). Aromatic retinoid in the treatment of multiple superficial basal cell carcinoma, arsenical keratoses and keratoacanthoma. In Orfanos, C.E. *et al.* (eds.). *Retinoids: Advances in Basic Research and Therapy*. pp. 397–400. (Berlin, Heidelberg, New York: Springer-Verlag)
6. Hayday, R., Reed, M., Dzubow, and L. Shuprek, J. (1980). Treatment of kerato-acanthomas with oral 13-*cis*-retinoic acid. *N. Engl. J. Med.*, **303**, 560
7. Moriarty, M., Dunn, J., Darragh, A., Lambe, R. and Brick, I. (1982). Etretinate in the treatment of actinic keratoses. *Lancet*, **1**, 364
8. Chayen, J., Bittensky, L., Butcher, R. and Poulter, L. (1972). (eds.). *A Guide to Practical Histochemistry*. pp. 211–214. (Edinburgh: Oliver and Boyd)
9. Holt, S. (1958). Indigogenic staining methods for esterases. In Danielli, J. (ed.). *General Cytochemical Methods*. p.375. (New York: Academic Press)
10. Tsambaos, D. and Orfanos, C. (1981). Chemotherapy of psoriasis and other skin disorders with oral retinoids. *Pharmacol. Ther.*, **14**, 355
11. Fritsch, P., Nemanie, M. and Elias, P. (1982). Perturbations of membrane glycosylation in retinoid treated epidermis. *J. Am. Acad. Dermatol*, **6**, 801
12. Bauer, R. and Orfanos, C.E. (1981). Influence of retinoid on human blood cells *in vitro*. TMMP retinoid inhibits the mutogenic properties of lectins and modulates the lymphocytic response. In Orfanos, C.E. *et al.* (eds.). *Retinoids: Advances in Basic Research and Therapy*. pp. 153–160. (Berlin, Heidelberg, New York: Springer-Verlag)
13. Hercend, Th., Bruley Rosset, M., Florentin, I. and Mathé, G. (1981). *In vivo* immunostimulatory properties of two retinoids: Ro 10-9359 and Ro 13-6298. In Orfanos, C.E. *et al.* (eds.). *Retinoids: Advances in Basic Research and Therapy*. pp. 21–30. (Berlin, Heidelberg, New York: Springer-Verlag)
14. Jurin, M. and Tannock, I. (1972). Influence of vitamin A on immunological response. *Immunology*, **23**, 283
15. Boutwell, R. (1982). Retinoids and inhibition of ornithine decarboxylase activity. *J. Am. Acad. Dermatol.*, **6**, 796
16. Kanerva, L., Niema, K., Lanharanta, J., Juvakoski, T. and Lassus, A. (1981). Electron microscopic characterisation of the mucous-like material before and after retinoid and retinoid-PUVA (RePUVA) treatment of psoriasis. In Orfanos, C.E. *et al.* (eds.). *Retinoids: Advances in Basic Research and Therapy*. pp. 467–472. (Berlin, Heidelberg, New York: Springer-Verlag)
17. Orfanos, C. (1982). Oral retinoid in psoriasis: current clinical experience and possible mechanisms of action. In Farber, E.M. *et al.* (eds.). *Psoriasis*. pp. 197–209. (New York: Grune & Stratton)

Section 5

Isotretinoin – Clinical and Laboratory

22
A Dose Response Study of 13-*cis*-Retinoic Acid Therapy in Cystic Acne

D.H. JONES, W.J. CUNLIFFE, K. KING and A.J. MILLER

Introduction

Peck's[1] original observations in 1979 of the effectiveness of 13-*cis*-retinoic acid in cystic acne have been well supported. In double-blind studies using smaller doses, Farrell,[2] in 15 patients, and Jones,[3] in 76 patients, have confirmed his results. Plewig[4] in an open study on 79 patients has shown similar improvements. Rapini[5] is reporting on a much larger series of 150 patients.

The drug has also been shown to be of use in Gram-negative folliculitis by Plewig[4] and Jones,[6] and in rosacea,[7] but there is debate about its role in hidradenitis suppurativa.[8]

Peck[9] has shown that the drug is not acting as a placebo, and Strauss[10] has confirmed that it is superior to the aromatic retinoid (etretinate).

Methods

Seventy-six patients (Table 1) with severe acne were randomly assigned to three dose groups (1.0, 0.5 and 0.1mg/kg body-weight). Previous acne therapy was discontinued 6 weeks prior to the study. Therapy was prescribed for 16 weeks and follow-up was undertaken for a further 16 weeks. Monthly observations were made of (1) acne grade of the face, back and chest, (2) a count of non-, superficial and deep inflamed lesions on the face, (3) clinical side-effects, (4) haematological and biochemical parameters, (5) sebum excretion rate (SER)[3] by the gravimetric method of

Table 1. Patient demography.

Dose (mg/kg body-weight)	0.1	0.5	1.0
Number of patients	22	30	24
Male	11	18	17
Female	11	12	7
Age (years)	23.7	24.3	24.5
(range)	(17–34)	(16–42)	(14–45)
Weight (kg)	63.3	63.9	64.9
(range)	(50.5–79)	(44–50)	(47–88)
Duration (years)	9.0	10.1	9.4
(range)	(3–21)	(4/12–20)	(18/12–19)
SER ± SE	1.74	1.90	1.95
$\mu g\ cm^{-2}\ min^{-1}$	±0.17	±0.15	±0.20
Acne grade	4.60	4.87	7.35
± SE	±0.77	±0.05	±0.99
Acne lesions	54	54	79
± SE	±10	±10	±10

Strauss and Pochi,[11] and (6) facial skin microflora (Williamson and Kligman scrub technique).[12]

A further visit was made at 44 weeks (28 weeks off therapy) when these observations were repeated.

Statistics

The parametric data were analysed by Student's *t*-test for changes within the groups, and by one-way analysis of variance for comparison between the groups. Wilcoxon's rank-sum test was used for analysis of the non-parametric data.

Results

There was a good attendance during the treatment period (Table 2). The numbers declined during the follow-up period as patients were withdrawn and placed on further therapy for a number of reasons – (1) failure to respond, (2) good response but residual lesions, and (3) relapse of their acne. These individual results will be discussed in a later paper.

Four patients who have not been included in this study's results were withdrawn during therapy. One patient had a marked exacerbation and needed to be treated with a combination of 13-*cis*-retinoic acid and erythromycin. Three patients (one from each dose group) had severe arthralgias, and needed to have their dose reduced. There were only three consistent non-attenders – all between 32 and 44 weeks.

Table 2. Patient numbers.

Weeks	0	4	8	12	16	20	24	28	32	44	
1.0mg/kg body-weight											
Attended	24	24	24	24	24	23	19	18	20	13	
Withdrawn	0	0	0	0	0	1	2	3	3	9	−9
Failed to attend	0	0	0	0	0	0	3	3	1	2	
0.5mg/kg body-weight											
Attended	30	30	29	28	28	26	25	21	23	17	
Withdrawn	0	0	0	0	0	0	1	3	3	7	−12
Failed to attend	0	0	1	2	2	4	4	6	4	6	
0.1mg/kg body-weight											
Attended	22	22	22	20	21	18	12	17	14	9	
Withdrawn	0	0	0	0	0	2	4	5	7	11	−14
Failed to attend	0	0	0	2	1	2	6	0	1	2	

Acne Grade

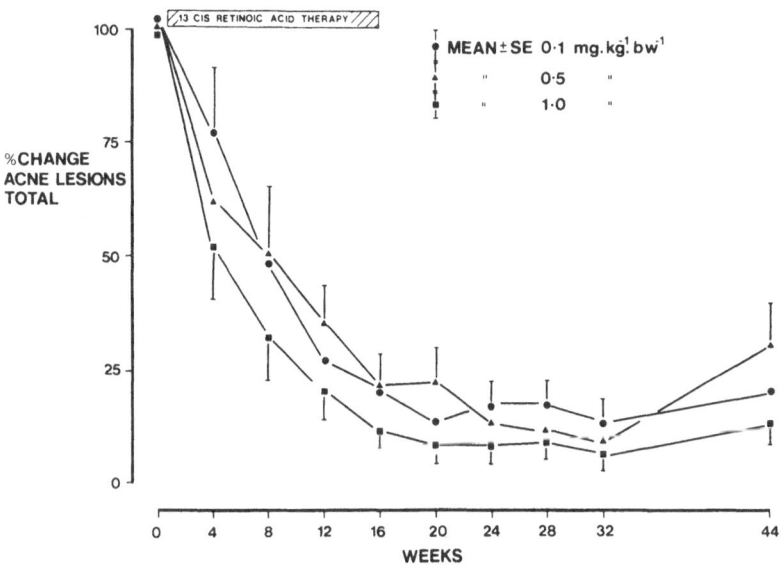

Figure 1. Response of total acne grade vs. time.

There was a steady and significant improvement of 70 per cent in acne grade over the 16 week treatment period ($p < 0.01$) reaching a maximum at 20–24 weeks (Figure 1). There was no significant difference between the dose groups. This improvement is maintained to 28 weeks post-therapy in over half the patients in the 1.0mg/kg body-weight (15 out of 24 patients), and 0.5mg/kg body-weight (18 out of 30 patients) groups, but in only one third of the 0.1mg/kg body-weight (7 out of 22 patients). This difference is significant ($p < 0.01$ chi-squared test).

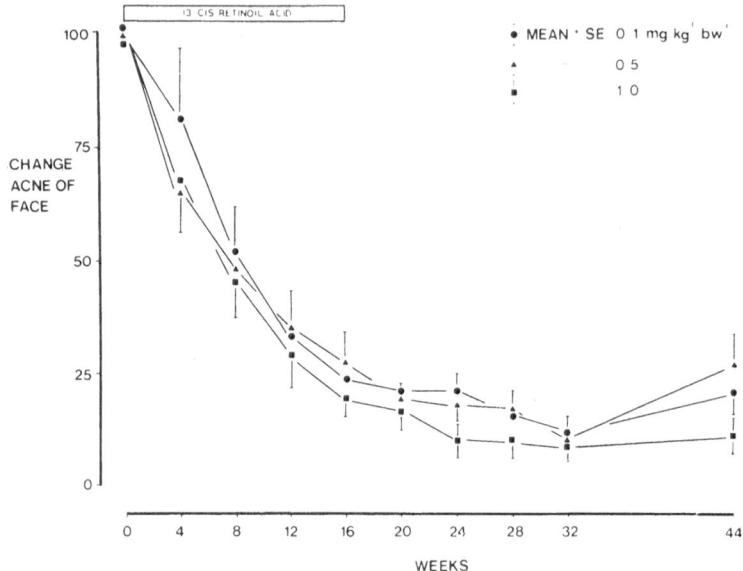

Figure 2. Response of facial acne grade vs. time.

The fluctuation in results from 16–44 weeks is due to patients relapsing and then being withdrawn from the trial for further therapy.

Facial acne (Figure 2) does better than that of the back (Figure 3) or chest (Figure 4). This is probably more characteristic of the site of acne

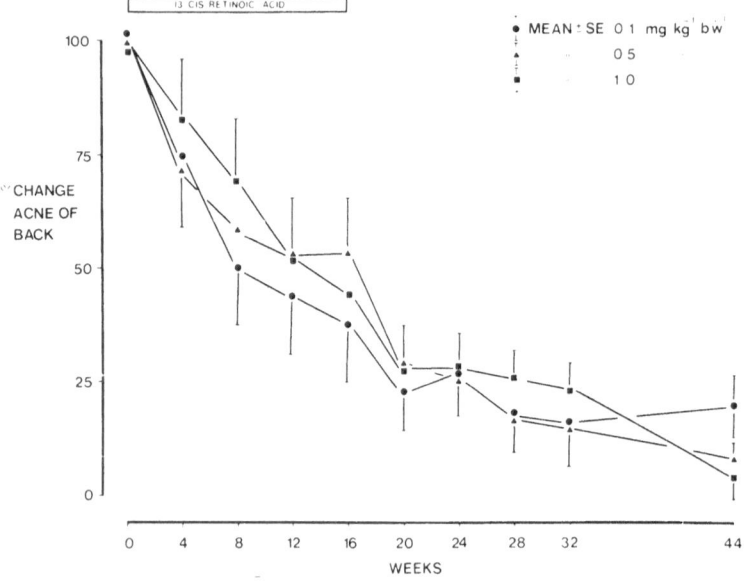

Figure 3. Response of back acne grade vs. time.

DOSE RESPONSE STUDY OF 13-*CIS*-RETINOIC ACID

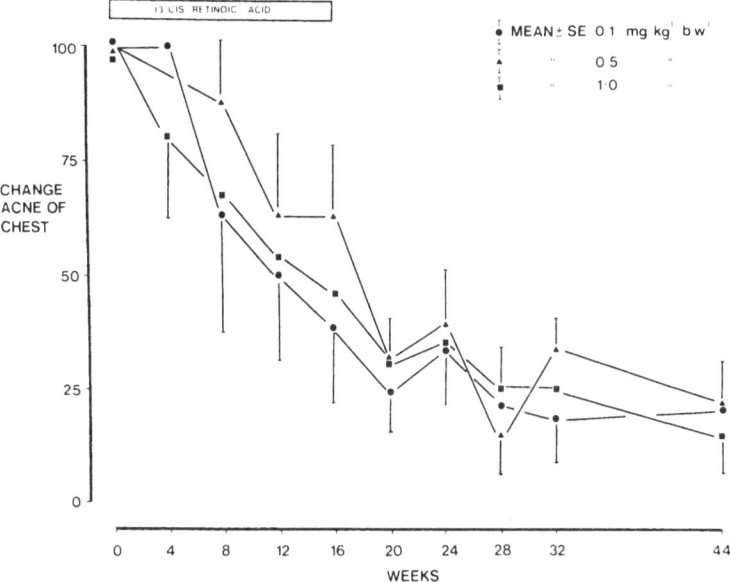

Figure 4. Response of chest acne grade vs. time.

than the drug, as this pattern of response has also been shown to occur with erythromycin by Greenwood *et al.*[13] This pattern is illustrated in the 1.0mg/kg body-weight group (Figure 5) but a similar result is found in other groups.

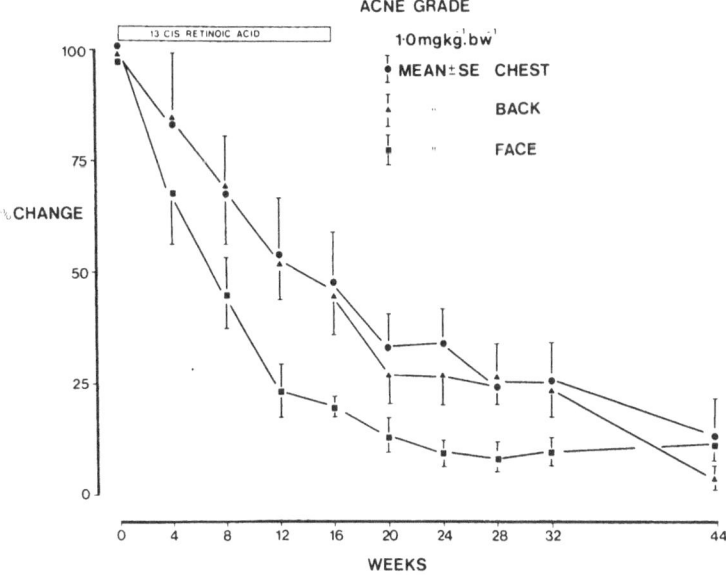

Figure 5. Response of acne grade of three sites vs. time in the 1.0mg/kg body-weight group.

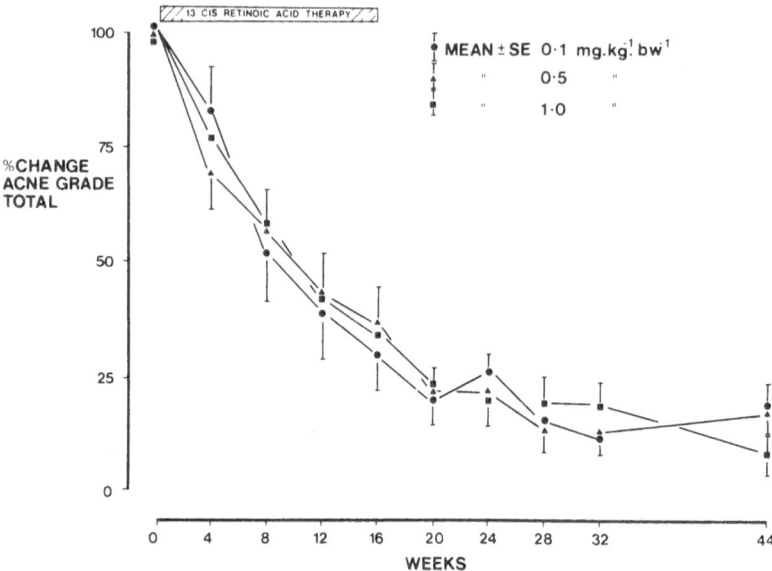

Figure 6. Response of total acne lesions vs. time.

Acne Lesions

The reduction in acne lesions (Figure 6) follows a similar pattern to that of the acne grade. There is a significant response ($p < 0.0005$) of an 80–90

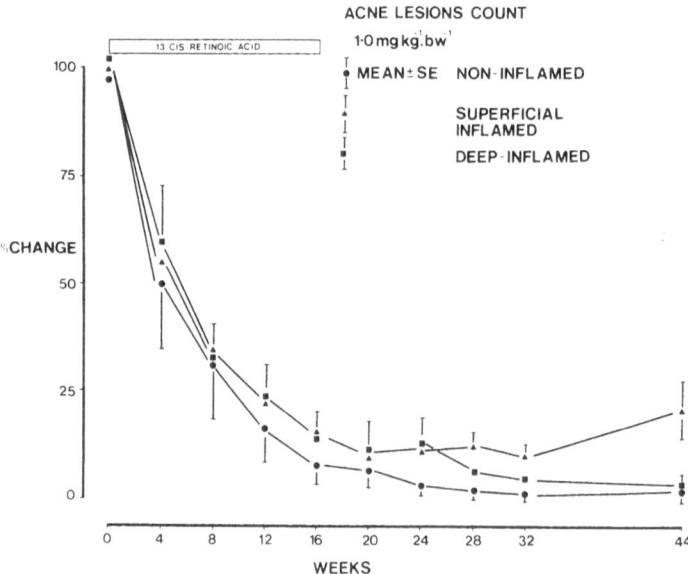

Figure 7. Response of three types of acne lesions vs. time in the 1.0mg/kg body-weight group.

per cent reduction at 16 weeks which is maintained during follow-up.

There is a rise in acne lesion numbers at 44 weeks as four patients in the 0.5m/kg body-weight group and 3 in 0.1mg/kg body-weight group had relapsed.

All types of acne lesions are cleared equally well as illustrated by the pattern of response in the 1.0mg/kg body-weight (Figure 7).

Individual Response

The analysis of the data as mean results of the groups hides individual variations and gives a false impression during the follow-up period. Therefore, the patients were assigned to various categories, with a 50 per-cent improvement being taken as a sign of success. These results have already been touched upon and will be discussed more fully in another paper.

Table 3. Analysis of patients with less than 50 per cent improvement at 16 weeks.

Dose (mg/kg body-weight)	1.0	0.5	0.1
> 50% improvement at 16/52	4	8	4
> 50% improvement at 32/52	1	2	3
Overall result			
Good response	3	5	0
Poor response	1	3	4

However, by these criteria, 16 patients (21 per cent) had failed to respond at 16 weeks (Table 3) but only six of these failed to make this improvement during follow-up, and so the failure rate overall is 12 per cent. These six patients were withdrawn by 32 weeks and received further therapy. One patient received a second course of 13-*cis*-retinoic acid in higher dosage, to which he responded and has had no further problems. Five patients received antibiotics – four have been lost to follow-up and one continues to be troubled by his acne.

The other ten patients had improved to 50 per cent of their pretreatment grade by 24 weeks. Six of these patients were judged a success at 44 weeks and five have maintained their improvement. Three patients were left with residual lesions, and two responded to further therapy. The remaining patient's improvement was brief and she rapidly relapsed and has remained a therapeutic problem.

In summary, there is a definite failure rate with 13-*cis*-retinoic acid therapy, but, of the slow responders, eventually half had a successful outcome.

Table 4. Percentage incidence of clinical side-effects.

Dose (mg/kg body-weight)	0.1	0.5	1.0
Cheilitis	90	97	92
Facial Dermatitis	48	62	76
Epistaxis	29	31	44
Desquamation	29	28	40
Arthralgia	20	17	28
Conjunctivitis	0	14	20
Malaise	5	7	16

Side-Effects

Clinical

The proportion of patients who experienced a particular side-effect at any time during therapy is indicated in Table 4. Though the table suggests a dose response, there is only a statistical difference in the facial dermatitis and conjunctivitis between the 0.1 and 1.0mg/kg body-weight groups ($p <$ 0.05 chi-squared test). The severity also seemed to vary between doses.

Cheilitis and facial dermatitis settled during therapy as the patients treated themselves with lip salves and oily creams. Arthralgias and epistaxes were consistent problems. Conjunctivitis was a late complication. We have not been able to demonstrate that the conjunctivitis is due to a decrease in meibomian secretion.[14]

Biochemical

The only biochemical abnormalities detected were rises in the serum-glutamyl-O-transferase and fasting plasma lipids. A number of patients had a trace of proteinuria on odd occasions (Table 5).

There was a significant rise in the SGOT in the 1.0mg/kg body-weight but not in the other groups ($p <$ 0.0005). These rises tended to occur in the first 4 weeks (Figure 8) and settled during therapy to return to normal post-treatment.

Table 5. The incidence of biochemical side-effects.

Dose (mg/kg body-weight)	1.0	0.5	0.1
Numbers	24	30	22
↑ SGOT	19	13	4
↑ Triglyceride	3	1	1
↑ Cholesterol	1	1	2
Proteinuria	4	6	3

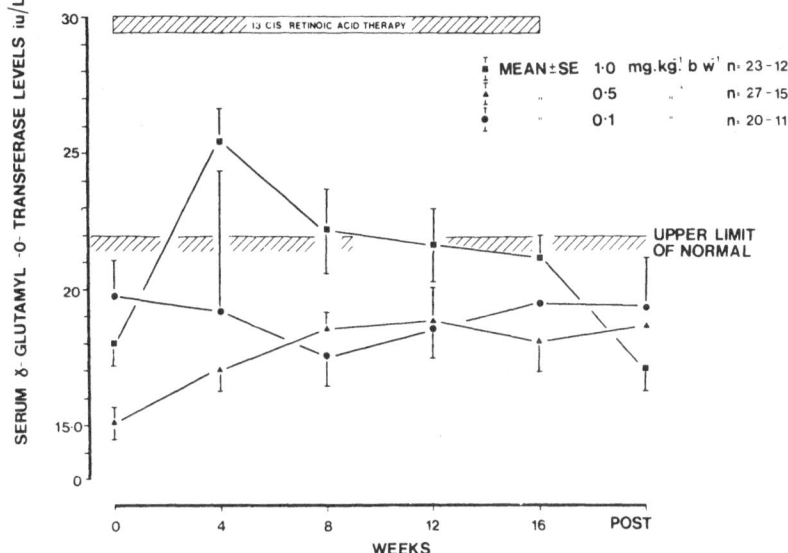

Figure 8. Serum γ-glutamyl-*O*-transferase values in the three dose groups vs. time.

Only a few individuals had abnormal fasting lipids (Table 5). In the groups as a whole, there were significant rises (*p* < 0.005) in the mean level gradually during therapy though this rapidly settled to pretreatment values off therapy. This occurred at all doses (Figure 9).

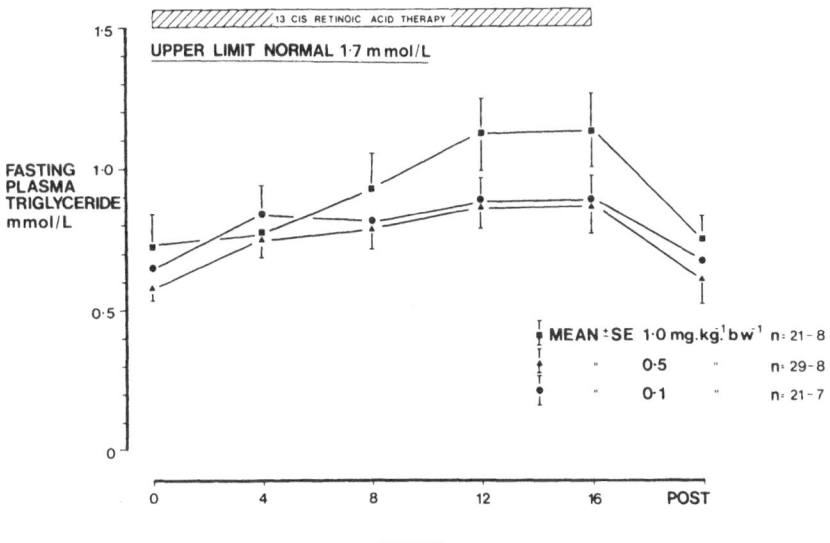

Figure 9. Fasting plasma triglyceride in the three dose groups vs. time.

Discussion

These results confirm those of other workers already cited and an unpublished report from van der Meeren.[15] This drug is certainly effective at all three doses. The clinical side-effects are tolerable in the majority of patients. The lower overall success rate of the 0.1mg/kg body-weight dose at the end of the follow-up suggests it is probably not suitable as a single agent for an initial short course of therapy. The high incidence of biochemical side-effects in the 1.0mg/kg body-weight dose group leads us to recommend the 0.5mg/kg body-weight dose.

It is interesting that our results correspond with other workers, even though the treatment periods vary between 12 and 24 weeks.

Most workers have made unpublished observations that a proportion of patients experience an exacerbation of their acne during the first 2 weeks. Gross[16] has, therefore, treated patients with a loading dose of 2mg/kg body-weight for 2 weeks followed by 0.5mg/kg body-weight for 14 weeks. His study showed that exacerbations do not occur, and that his results at 16 weeks were better than using 0.5mg/kg body-weight throughout.

Firm decisions on the optimal therapeutic regime for this drug cannot therefore be made at this time.

Acknowledgements

We wish to thank Mr R.A. Forster for his advice, Miss V.B. Cmiech for her technical help, Mrs P. Hick for secretarial help and Roche Products Ltd. for their support.

References

1. Peck, G.L., Olsen, T.G., Yoder, F.W., Strauss, J.S., Downing, D.T., Pandya, M., Butkus, D. and Arnaud-Battandier, J. (1979). Prolonged remissions of cystic and conglobate acne with 13-cis-retinoic acid. N. Engl. J. Med., **300**, 329
2. Farrell, L.N., Strauss, J.S. and Stranieri, A.M. (1980). The treatment of severe cystic acne with 13-cis-retinoic acid. J. Am. Acad. Dermatol., **3**, 602
3. Jones, D.H., King, K., Miller, A.J. and Cunliffe, W.J. (1983). A dose response study of 13-cis-retinoic acid in acne vulgaris. Br. J. Dermatol., **108**, 333
4. Plewig, G., Nikolowski, J. and Wolf, H.H. (1982). Action of isotretinoin in acne rosacea and gram-negative folliculitis. J. Am. Acad. Dermatol., **6**, 766
5. Rapini, R.R., Konecky, E.A., Schillinger, B., Comite, H., Exner, J.H., Strauss, J.S., Shalita, A.R. and Pochi, P.E. (1983). Effect of varying dosages of isotretinoin on nodulocystic acne. J. Invest. Dermatol., **80**, 357
6. Jones, D.H., King, K. and Cunliffe, W.J. (1982). Treatment of gram-negative folliculitis with 13-cis-retinoic acid. Br. J. Dermatol., **107**, 253
7. Fulton, R., Dick, D.C. and Mackie, R.M. (1983). The treatment of rosacea with 13-cis-retinoic acid. Br. J. Dermatol., **108**, 243
8. Jones, D.J., King, K. and Cunliffe, W.J. (1982). Hidradenitis suppurtiva – lack of

success with 13-*cis*-retinoic acid. *Br. J. Dermatol.*, **107**, 253

9.   Peck, G.L., Olsen, T.G., Butkus, D., Pandya, M., Arnaud-Battandier, J., Gross, E.G., Windhorst, D.B. and Cheripko, J. (1982). Isotretinoin versus placebo in the treatment of cystic acne. *J. Am. Acad. Dermatol.*, **6**, 735

10. Goldstein, J.A., Socha-Szott, A., Thomsen, R.J., Pochi, P.E., Shalita, A.R. and Strauss, J.S. (1982). Comparative effect of isotretinoin and etretinate on acne and sebaceous gland secretion. *J. Am. Acad. Dermatol.*, **6**, 760

11. Strauss, J.S. and Pochi, P.E. (1961). The quantitative gravimetric determination of sebum production. *J. Invest. Dermatol.*, **36**, 293

12. King, K., Jones, D.H., Daltrey, D. and Cunliffe, W.J. (1982). A double-blind study of the effects of 13-*cis*-retinoic acid on acne, sebum excretion rate and microbial population. *Br. J. Dermatol.*, **107**, 583

13. Greenwood, R. and Cunliffe, W.J. (1982). Rates of response of acne related to sebum excretion rate and antibiotic dosage. *Br. J. Dermatol.*, **107**, Suppl. 22, 24

14. Milson, J., Jones, D.H., King, K. and Cunliffe, W.J. (1982). Ophthalmological effects of 13-*cis*-retinoic acid therapy for acne vulgaris. *Br. J. Dermatol.*, **108**, 333

15. van der Meeren, H.L.M, van der Schroeff, J.G., Stijnen, T., van Duren, J.A., van der Dries, H.A.C. and van Voorst Vader, P.C. (1983). Dose response relationship in isotretinoin therapy for conglobate acne. (Personal communication. Retinoids Symposium, Dutch Dermatological Society)

16. Gross, E.G., Peck, G.L., Gault, P.G. and Wesley, M.N. (1983). Long-term inhibition of quantitative sebum production with isotretinoin. *J. Invest. Dermatol.*, **80**, 357

23
Isotretinoin in the Treatment of Acne

A.R. SHALITA

The introduction of isotretinoin for the treatment of severe, recalcitrant nodulocystic acne has dramatically altered the management of this troublesome and disfiguring disease. Not only has one been able to achieve remarkable improvement in patients with severe inflammatory acne, but also prolonged remissions have been observed in patients treated with this drug. In addition, the change in the emotional status of many of the patients successfully treated with isotretinoin has proved to be one of the most gratifying aspects of this new treatment programme.

Acne is a term used to describe a spectrum of diseases that vary from a few comedones scattered about the face, usually in pre-teenage children, to the severe, destructive nodulocystic variety. In between is a spectrum of disease characterized by varying numbers of inflammatory and non-inflammatory lesions. Although recent health surveys in the United States estimate that at least 80 per cent of the population between the ages of 12 and 25 are afflicted with acne in one of its various forms, the incidence of severe, nodulocystic acne is relatively low. Current estimates suggest that there are approximately 350,000 patients with severe nodulocystic acne in the United States. It is this form of acne for which isotretinoin has become the treatment of choice.

Prior to the introduction of isotretinoin, the treatment of nodulocystic acne achieved modest results at best. Through a combination of high doses of systemic, broad-spectrum antibiotics, topical retinoic acid and antibacterial agents, acne surgery, intra-lesional steroid injections and the occasional use of systemic glucocorticosteroids, nodulocystic acne could be reasonably controlled. In woman, the use of oestrogen, in the form of oral contraceptives, was also beneficial. Typically the patient with nodulocystic acne could expect to be maintained on a treatment programme consisting of one or more of these therapeutic agents for a period of several years. Unpleasant side-effects were common as were frequent exacerbations of the disease, despite the most vigorous therapy.

With the observations of Peck *et al.*[1] that isotretinoin (13-*cis*-retinoic acid) produced marked clearing in patients with nodulocystic acne, a new era in acne treatment began. Even more impressive were the observations by the same authors that not only was dramatic improvement obtained in these patients, but also prolonged remission, sometimes lasting for several years, might be expected. These results were subsequently confirmed by ourselves as well as other investigators in a series of controlled, clinical trials which will be summarized elsewhere in this volume. One of these investigations, however, deserves mention here since it demonstrates a significant difference between retinoids in the therapeutic response in acne. In a multicentre, double-blind study conducted in Boston, Iowa City and New York[2] isotretinoin was compared to etretinate in the treatment of severe nodulocystic acne. Patients were randomly assigned to 1mg/kg/day of one of these two drugs for a period of 8 weeks and observed for another 8 weeks post-treatment. Lesion counts and sebum production were measured at intervals during this study. In this group, totalling 56 patients, there was approximately an 80 per cent reduction in nodulocystic lesions in those patients treated with isotretinoin, whereas those patients treated with etretinate showed only a 20 per cent reduction in lesions. Similarly, isotretinoin produced an almost 90 per cent reduction in sebum production while etretinate produced only about a 20 per cent reduction. Side-effects were similar for the two drugs. Thus it would appear that isotretinoin has a very specific effect in nodulocystic acne and it remains to be determined whether this will hold true when the drug is compared with retinoids other than etretinate.

Clinical Management

The current recommendations for treating nodulocystic acne with isotretinoin suggest a dose of 1–2mg/kg/day for a period of 15–20 weeks. With this dosage regime the overwhelming majority of patients should show an eminently satisfactory response and experience a prolonged remission of their disease. Some patients, however, may require a second course of treatment either because of a relatively unsatisfactory response to the initial treatment or because of a flare-up in the post-treatment period. In either case isotretinoin therapy should not be reinstituted in less than 2 months since there are now considerable data to suggest that continued improvement occurs after therapy has been discontinued and that this improvement continues for at least 2 months. There have been some data to suggest that lower doses of isotretinoin may also be effective in treatment of nodulocystic acne.[3] More recent experience, in a larger clinical trial, however, suggests that while comparable clinical response may be achieved with doses of 0.1, 0.5 or 1.0mg/kg/day of isotretinoin,[4] the relapse rate is considerably higher for the patients on the lower dosage. In addition, preliminary evidence suggests that these lower doses do not produce a significant reduction in side-effects with the possible exception of serum triglycerides.

Thus, it would appear that the dosage of 1–2mg/kg/day should be adhered to.

Within this dosage range patients with nodulocystic acne of the back and chest usually require treatment with the higher dose of 2mg/kg/day as compared to those patients with purely facial acne who appear to respond perfectly well to the lower dose of 1mg/kg/day. It has been a fairly uniform observation among investigators in different countries that the back and chest are slower to repond and require a higher dose for satisfactory reponse than facial lesions. From a practical point of view it has been our practice to start patients with significant involvement of the back and chest on to 2mg/kg/day for at least 8 weeks. It at the end of that time there has been significant improvement (50 per cent or more reduction in lesions), we may then decrease the dose to 1mg/kg/day. Patients with facial acne are maintained on the dose of 1mg/kg/day for the full course of treatment. If a reduction of 70 per cent or more in the lesion count has occurred prior to the completion of a full course of therapy, treatment may be discontinued somewhat earlier. It is our practice, however, not to stop treatment any earlier than 12 weeks since, in our experience, treatment for shorter periods of time results in a higher recurrence rate.

Many patients with severe nodulocystic acne will experience flares of their disease if prior therapy is discontinued upon the institution of isotretinoin therapy. It is, therefore, our recommendation that conventional therapy such as systemic antibiotics be continued during the first month or two of treatment with isotretinoin. Recent information, however, suggests that the combination of isotretinoin and a tetracycline may result in an increased incidence of pseudotumour cerebri. I would therefore, recommend that tetracyclines should not be used in conjunction with isotretinoin. For the time being, at least, it would appear that erythromycin or trimethoprim-sulpha are satisfactory antibiotics for use in conjunction with isotretinoin. We have also observed flares of cystic disease occurring somewhere between 6 and 10 weeks of therapy. We have no good explanation for this phenomenon but it can usually be satisfactorily managed by the intra-lesional injection of corticosteriods or the systemic administration of corticosteroids for short periods of time (1–2 weeks).

Side-Effects

Although isotretinoin produces dramatic improvement and prolonged remission of the disease in patients with severe nodulocystic acne, it is not without significant side-effects. All of the side-effects experienced with isotretinoin have previously been observed with chronic administration of retinol. Those associated with isotretinoin, however, are more closely related to those associated with chronic hypervitaminosis A rather than the acute syndrome which usually produces central nervous system toxicity. These side-effects, therefore, are mostly related to mucocutaneous symptoms. The most prominent among these are cheilitis which has become a virtual hallmark of patients treated with isotretinoin. Other common side-effects are dry, scaly skin, erythema, pruritus, dryness of the mucous membranes and epistaxis. Associated with the dry skin there may be peeling of the palms and soles. These side-effects, for the most part, are easily managed by local symptomatic therapy. We recommend the use of petrolatum for the cheilitis. In those patients who do not respond to this simple treatment a satisfactory response may be achieved with 1 per cent hydrocortisone ointment. Similarly, epistaxis may be reduced by the application of a thin coating of petrolatum to the nasal mucous membranes. The patient should be cautioned, however, not to apply excess amounts of petrolatum in the nose since this may result in aspiration. For the other manifestations of dry skin simple emollient lotions are usually satisfactory. Rarely a conjunctivitis sicca may occur and this may be treated with a combination steroid–antibiotic ointment.

In addition to the mucocutaneous side-effects, bone, joint or muscle discomfort are fairly common. These are usually relieved by the administration of aspirin or a non-steroidal anti-inflammatory agent. Nausea, vomiting and other gastro-intestinal discomfort have been described in approximately 15–30 per cent of patients treated with isotretinoin. A lesser number of patients describe central nervous system symptoms such as headache, fatigue, etc. To my knowledge, bone changes (hyperostoses) have not been reported in patients receiving isotretinoin for acne, but further investigation into this phenomenon is currently being conducted.

A variety of laboratory abnormalities have been observed in patients receiving isotretinoin for the treatment of nodulocystic acne. Most prominent among these are elevations of triglycerides. Since triglyceride elevation appears to be dose-related, it is unlikely that large increases in triglycerides will occur with patients receiving isotretinoin for acne. Nevertheless, patients must be monitored at regular intervals for this laboratory value. It is recommended that serum triglycerides be monitored every week or every two weeks until the response has been established and the triglyceride levels have reached a plateau. In our practice we continue to observe the patient and monitor the triglyceride levels closely when increases of the order of 200–400mg/dl occur. At levels between 400 and 600mg/dl we will place the patient on a strict diet and/or reduce the dose of the drug while continuing to closely monitor the laboratory value. In the range of 600–700mg/dl it is probably advisable to discontinue the drug since one is now approaching the range where an increased risk of pancreatitis occurs. There is no evidence, however, that these increased triglyceride levels, for the period of time that patients are receiving isotretinoin for acne, will produce any increased risk of coronary artery disease.

Other laboratory abnormalities which have been observed include elevation in the sedimentation rate, decreased white cell counts, increased platelet counts, white cells in the urine and an increase in the values reported for liver function tests. In our experience, none of these laboratory value changes has been significant enough to cause discontinuation of therapy.

Of somewhat more concern is the well-known fact that retinoids, in general, and isotretinoin specifically are teratogenic. Although the dose at which isotretinoin is teratogenic in animals is considerably higher than those used in the treatment of cystic acne it is, nevertheless, essential that female patients being treated with isotretinoin practise strict birth control. Should a patient become pregnant during treatment with isotretinoin the desirability of continuing this pregnancy should be discussed with the patient. It should be emphasized, however, that isotretinoin is not mutagenic and that no significant abnormalities in sperm counts or sperm morphology have been observed. Therefore, there is no evidence to suggest that isotretinoin would have any effect on either a patient's ability to conceive or on the integrity of the fetus in a patient who conceives after discontinuance of isotretinoin therapy.

Mechanism of Action

Among the most intriguing aspects of the investigations carried out with isotretinoin in acne patients are the preliminary data concerning its mechanism of action. It would appear from these preliminary observations that isotretinoin affects a variety of the pathogenic events believed to be germane to this disease. Among the most prominent of the effects of the drug is a dramatic inhibition of sebum production.[5] A reduction in size of the sebaceous glands and in sebum production has been observed in both humans[6] and in experimental animals.[7] It would appear that isotretinoin has a specific affect on the proliferating sebaceous epithelium and prevents maturation into lipid-forming cells. Furthermore, preliminary experiments suggest that this is a non-endocrine effect.[7] Although the inhibition of sebum production persists for some time after discontinuance of treatment with isotretinoin, sebum production does eventually return to normal or near normal values. Thus, the effect on the sebaceous gland alone cannot account for the dramatic and prolonged clinical response that has been observed.

Another observation is that isotretinoin treatment results in a profound reduction in the density of *P. acnes*.[8-10] This reduction in *P. acnes* also persists for long periods after discontinuance of treatment with iostretinoin,[11] but probably does not persist for as long as the clinical remission. In all likelihood this reduction in *P. acnes* is directly related to the reduction in sebaceous secretions since this organism uses sebum as a nutrient source.

Although tretinoin has been shown to have a profound effect on the keratinizing epithelium of the follicle, similar results have not yet been observed with oral isotretinoin. Preliminary studies in our laboratory suggest that no significant changes in the follicle wall occur during treatment with isotretinoin. Nevertheless, a reduction in comedones is a frequent clinical observation[12] and a direct effect on the follicular epithelium cannot be excluded.

Of particular interest to our group has been the anti-inflammatory effect of isotretinoin. A variety of immunologic and leukocyte function abnormalities have been described in patients with nodulocystic acne. Among these are increased antibody titres to *P. acnes*,[13] increased blast transformation to antigens extracted from *P. acnes*,[14] hyporesponsiveness to common delayed hypersensitivity antigens[15] and abnormalities of leukocyte chemotaxis and phagocyte function. Specifically we have observed that patients with severe nodulocystic acne may be divided into two subgroups based on the chemotactic properties of their neutrophils. When incubated with standard reference attractants, the neutrophils of these patients are either markedly depressed in their mobility or markedly hyperactive. Of particular interest is that only in those patients whose neutrophils are hyperactive to chemo-attractants can one observe abnormalities of phagocyte function. In these patients neutrophils appear to be capable of engulfing common pathogens such as staphylococci, micrococci and pseudomonas, but appear incapable of ingesting the *P. acnes*. Preliminary data from our laboratories suggest that treatment with isotretinoin significantly reverses these abnormalities of chemotaxis and phagocytosis. Whether this is a result of the clinical improvement and marked decrease in inflammation or a direct effect of the drug on these abnormal leukocytes remains to be determined. Finally, it is important to note that isotretinoin has been demonstrated to inhibit a variety of neutrophil enzymes[16] and may also have a direct inhibitory effect upon neutrophil migration. This may also explain the anti-inflammatory effect of the drug.

Any or all of these mechanisms which are effected by isotretinoin could be invoked to explain the significant clinical response observed. None of them, however, appear to explain the prolonged remission observed after discontinuation of isotretinoin therapy. It is obvious, therefore, that considerably more investigation and long-term follow-up will be required before the precise mechanisms involved in invoking these clinical responses can be resolved.

In summary, isotretinoin has introduced a new era in the therapy of severe nodulocystic acne. Doses of 1–2mg/kg/day result in dramatic clearing of the disease as well as prolonged remission. Although the drug is not without significant clinical side-effects, these are generally well-tolerated by the patient and may be managed by relatively simple measures. Mechanistically, the drug appears to affect all of the pathogenic mechanisms currently thought to play a role in the aetiology of acne. Further investigation, however, is required to establish the precise mechanisms by which this drug exerts its profound effect in acne.

References

1. Peck, G.L., Olsen, T.G., Yoder, F.W. *et al.* (1979). Prolonged remissions of cystic acne with 13-*cis*-retinoic acid. *N. Engl. J. Med.*, **300**, 329
2. Goldstein, J.A., Socha-Szott, A., Thomsen, R.J. *et al.* (1982). Comparative effect of isotretinoin on acne and sebaceous gland secretion. *J. Am. Acad. Dermatol.*, **6**, 760
3. Farrell, L.N., Strauss, J.S. and Stranieri, A. (1980). The treatment of severe cystic acne with 13-*cis* retinoic acid. Evaluation of sebum production and the clinical response in a multiple-dose trial. *J. Am. Acad. Dermatol.*, **3**, 602
4. Rapini, R.P., Konecky, E.A., Schillinger, B. *et al.* (1983). Effect of varying dosages of isotretinoin on nodulocystic acne. *J. Invest Dermatol.* (In preparation)
5. Strauss, J.S. (1983). Oral retinoid therapy for nodulocystic acne. In Shalita, A.R. (ed.). *Dermatologic Clinics: Acne.* (Philadelphia: W.B. Saunders Co.) In press
6. Gomez, E.C. (1982). Actions of isotretinoin and etretination on the pilosebaceous unit. *J. Am. Acad. Dermatol.*, **6**, 746
7. Gomez, E.C. and Moskowitz, R.J. (1980). Effect of 13-*cis* retinoic acid on the hamster flank organ. *J. Invest. Dermatol.*, **74**, 392
8. Leyden, J. and McGinley, K.J. (1982). Effect of 13-*cis* retinoic acid on sebum production and *Propionibacterium acnes* in severe nodulocystic acne. *Arch. Dermatol. Res.*, **272**, 331
9. Plewig, G., Nikolowski, J. and Wolff, H.H. (1982). Action of iostretinoin in acne rosacea and gram-negative folliculitis. *J. Am. Acad. Dermatol.*, **6**, 766
10. Weissman, A., Wagner, A. and Plewig, G. (1981). Reduction of bacterial skin flora during treatment with 13-*cis* retinoic acid. *Arch. Dermatol. Res.*, **270**, 179
11. Leyden, J.J., McGinley, K.J. and Webster, G.F. (1982). Prolonged reductions in *Propionibacterium acnes* in acne conglobata patients treated with 13-*cis* retinoic acid. *J. Invest. Dermatol.*, **78**, 350
12. Plewig, G., Gollnick, H., Meizel, W. *et al.* (1981). 13-*cis* Retinsaure zur oralen Behandlung der Acne conglobata. *Hautarzt.*, **32**, 634
13. Puhvel, S.M., Barfatani, M., Warnick, M. and Sternberg, T.H. (1966). Study of antibody levels to *Corynebacterium acnes*. *Arch. Dermatol.*, **93**, 364
14. Puhvel, S.M., Amirian, D., Weintraub, J. and Reisner, R.M. (1977). Lymphocyte transformation in subjects with nodulocystic acne. *Br. J. Dermatol.*, **97**, 205
15. Shalita, A.R. (1983). Inflammatory acne. In Shalita, A.R. (ed.). *Dermatologic Clinics: Acne.* (Philadelphia: W.B. Saunders Co.) In press
16. Lee, W.L., Shalita, A.R., Sunthralingham, K. and Fikrig, S.M. (1982). Neutrophil chemotaxis by *Propionibacterium acnes* lipase and its inhibition. *Infect. Immun.*, **35**, 71

24
The Overall USA Experience of Retinoids in Acne

W.J. CUNNINGHAM

The overall US experience with 13-*cis*-retinoic acid for treatment of severe, recalcitrant cystic acne has been in general extremely favourable. Many would claim, probably without exaggeration, that the drug is the most important addition to the dermatologic armamentarium in their lifetime for treatment of this physically and psychologically debilitating disease. At this point in time as the drug is becoming available for general use in the UK, Switzerland and Canada as Roaccutane a summary of the US experience adds another perspective.

Isotretinoin (13-*cis*-retinoic acid) has been marketed in the US since September 1982 as Accutane but its history of development traces to the mid-point of this century and that period's use of vitamin A in dermatologic therapy. Neither vitamin A nor its all-*trans*-retinoic acid (tretinoin) possessed an optimum therapeutic ratio with oral administration in treatment of cystic acne, although topically applied tretinoin (Retin A) is widely and beneficially used for acne therapy.

Efficacy of 13-*cis*-Retinoic Acid

13-*cis*-retinoic acid possesses striking efficacy in treatment of cystic acne and also has the ability to induce remission in this formerly recalcitrant disease. An open label pilot study was carried out by Dr. Peck[1] which involved 21 patients with cystic or conglobate acne who previously failed to adequately respond to conventional treatment. Dosing varied with a mean daily dose of 13-*cis*-retinoic acid of 1.5mg/kg/day and a mean duration of first course of therapy of 19 weeks. Only 3 of 21 patients (14%) required a second course of therapy. Prolonged remissions of up to 46 months[2] were experienced by 14 patients.

A randomized double-blind placebo controlled (with placebo cross-over) study of 33 patients[3] tested the efficacy of 13-*cis*-retinoic acid. Initial mean doses of 0.5mg/kg/day were varied during treatment with an overall mean dose of 0.9mg/kg/day. Fifty per cent of patients treated required a second course of therapy, the majority being patients with predominantly truncal acne who had responded only partially to a first course. All patients eventually experienced remission of their disease averaging 38 months in duration. A double-blind, dose-ranging study of doses of 0.1, 0.5 and 1.0mg/kg/day demonstrated efficacy in treatment of cystic acne at doses as low as 0.1mg/kg/day.[4] The small number of patients in the study (12) precluded firm statistical conclusions but in general efficacy appeared to be dose related with mean reduction in cyst count at 8 weeks of 88 per cent, 79 per cent and 56 per cent with doses of 1.0, 0.5, and 0.1 mg/kg/day respectively. Inhibition of sebum production was demonstrated with 88 per cent, 82 per cent and 67 per cent inhibition demonstratable at week 12 of 13-*cis*-retinoic acid therapy at respective doses of 1.0, 0.5 and 0.1mg/kg/day. Sebum production returned to normal values by 8 weeks post therapy in patients treated with the lowest (0.1mg/kg/day) dose. Further study of sebum suppression demonstrated however, that 8 of 20 patients had sebum production below baseline values 30 to 80 weeks after discontinuation of 13-*cis*-retinoic acid; four of the eight had received the 0.1mg/kg/day dosage. Two patients in a separate study obtained 99.0 per cent and 89.5 per cent suppression of sebaceous gland secretion but none-theless did not clinically improve.[5] The relationship of sebaceous gland function to clinical efficacy of 13-*cis*-retinoic acid is thus not yet completely elucidated.

A double-blind comparison of 13-*cis*-retinoic acid and etretinate each administered for 8 weeks at 1mg/kg/day was performed in a study of 56 men with cystic acne.[6] A 42.7 per cent vs. a 7.8 per cent decrease in lesion count respectively clearly demonstrated ($p < 0.05$) the superiority of 13-*cis*-retinoic acid in treatment of cystic acne. Sebaceous gland secretion was suppressed by a mean of 60.1 per cent with 13-*cis*-retinoic acid and by 21.3 per cent by etretinate, again a highly significant difference ($p < 0.001$).

In the USA where 13-*cis*-retinoic acid is indicated for treatment of severe, recalcitrant cystic acne current recommendations include doses of 1–2mg/kg/day for a duration of 15–20 weeks. The drug may be discontinued prior to this time if there is greater than 70 per cent improvement. The clinical response, predominant location of lesions, and appearance and severity of side-effects need to be considered in the dosage choice for an individual patient. The degree and duration of sebum suppression produced by 13-*cis*-retinoic acid appear to be dose related and to correlate to some degree with clinical efficacy. In addition, the best prolonged remission data published to date are those of the pilot study of cystic acne where average maximum dosages of 2.0mg/kg/day were used.[2] Future studies of efficacy of 13-*cis*-retinoic acid should address considerations of severity and predominant location of lesions, rate of improvement during therapy, need for a second course of therapy, incidence and duration of remission, as well as incidence and severity of side-effects in attempts to refine dosage recommendations.

Side-Effects

Administration of therapeutically effective doses of 13-*cis*-retinoic acid nearly invariably produces some clinically noticeable side–effects. These are so common that in their absence one must question adequate compliance or absorption. In treatment of patients with cystic acne they are generally tolerable, being infrequently a reason for discontinuance of therapy and to date have been reversible in nature. As might be predicted, the spectrum of side-effects of administration of 13-*cis*-retinoic acid is similar to that of vitamin A.[7] Within the spectrum however there are differences in frequency and severity of these effects, and because of lack of liver storage of 13-*cis*-retinoic acid, in their temporal features. A summary off the incidence of clinical side-effects observed with 13-*cis*-retinoic acid therapy is presented in Table 1.[8] The patient population included 523 patients treated either for cystic acne or a disorder of keratinization. The high incidence of side-effects relative to drying effects on skin and mucosa may be related to the drug's effect on barrier function. Loss of desmosomes, perturbations of membrane glycosylation, and increased number of gap junctions have been reported to occur in

Table 1. Clinical side-effects in 523 patients treated with isotretinoin in order of decreasing frequency of incidence*.

Findings	Per cent Incidence
Cheilitis, dry lips	90
Conjunctivitis, eye irritation	50
Xerosis; desquamation, especially face	30
Dry mouth	30
Pruritus, itching	25
Epistaxis, petechiae	25
Gastrointestinal symptoms	20
Bone, joint, muscle symptoms	15
Headache	10
Lethargy, fatigue	10
Hair thinning	10
Palmo-plantar desquamation	5

*Adapted from Windhorst and Nigra[8]

epidermis of retinoid treated patients.[9-11]

Meticulous application of barrier type emollients to previously hydrated skin, lips, and nasal mucosa is frequently very helpful. The use of artificial tears similarly is useful in reducing ophthalmic symptoms of dryness.

Bone, joint or muscle pain occur during treatment with 13-*cis*-retinoic acid with a frequency of approximately 15 per cent. While generally these symptoms are mild, a number of individuals experience more severe symptomatology which may require discontinuation of therapy. There have been reports of the observance of skeletal hyperostosis in X-rays of patients receiving 13-*cis*-retinoic acid for treatment of disorders of keratinization. This has not been observed in patients treated with the generally lower doses and shorter durations used in treatment of cystic acne.

A study of vitamin A in treatment of acne found an incidence of headache of 68 per cent.[12] With use of 13-*cis*-retinoic acid this symptom is experienced by only 10 per cent of individuals. Other CNS symptoms such as visual disturbances have similarly a low incidence.

Thinning of hair was reported in 10 per cent of individuals in this series. This reversible symptom is most likely a result of telogen effluvium based on experience with the aromatic retinoid etretinate.[13]

Other phenomena which have occurred during 13-*cis*-retinoic acid treatment include a worsening or flare which may occur within the first month of treatment. Systemic or intra-lesional corticosteroids have been apparently advantageously used by some investigators.[14] The exuberant granulation tissue occasionally seen in healing lesions of cystic acne has been similarly treated with some success.

Laboratory Abnormalities

While a number of laboratory parameters have been observed to be outside normal ranges during treatment with 13-*cis*-retinoic acid the most predictable effect appears to be drug-induced elevation of serum triglycerides in approximately 25 per cent of individuals. Dietary restriction of calories, animal fat and alcohol combined with increased exercise may have triglyceride lowering effects.[15] Most elevations are mild to moderate; rarely levels of over 800mg/dl are reported. The risk of acute pancreatitis is increased at these levels and the drug should be discontinued.

Mild to moderate elevations of SGOT, SGPT, and serum alkaline phosphatase are observed in 10–20 per cent of patients receiving 13-*cis*-retinoic acid. The exact aetiology of these elevations has not been determined but elevations sometimes resolve during continued therapy.[16]

The retinoids in general (including vitamin A) demonstrate teratogenic potential but their relative liabilities vary considerably. The rabbit is the laboratory animal most sensitive to the teratogenic effects of retinoids and in this species 13-*cis*-retinoic acid produces teratogenic effects at a dose of 10mg/kg/day.[17] Vitamin A palmitate, for comparison, produces terato-genic effects at 5mg/kg/day and etretinate at 2mg/kg/day. Direct translation of this information to human experience is not possible, but adequate contraceptive methods are required during and for 1 month after discontinuation of 13-*cis*-retinoic acid therapy. In animals, very high doses of 13-*cis*-retinoic acid have produced decreased spermatogenesis but at therapeutic doses in man these effects have not been observed.[8] In the Ames test, 13-*cis*-retinoic acid is not mutagenic.

Mechanism of Action

The exact mechanism of action of 13-*cis*-retinoic acid is not known. Profound and dose dependent suppression of sebum production has been described. Changes in follicular epithelium, decrease in *P. acnes* density, and striking anti-inflammatory effects have been theorized to play a role in the drug's effect on cystic acne.[18] These promising areas of further research may further elucidate the mechanisms by which this drug produces its dramatic results.

References

1. Peck, G.L., Olsen, T.G., Yoder, F.W., Strauss, J.S., Downing, D.T., Pandya, M., Butkus, D. and Arnaud-Battandier, J. (1979). Prolonged remissions of cystic and conglobate acne with 13-*cis*-retinoic acid. *N. Engl. J. Med.*, **300**, 329
2. Peck, G.L. (1981). Retinoids in clinical dermatology. In Fleischmajer, R. (ed.). *Progress in Diseases of the Skin*, pp. 227–269. (New York: Grune & Stratton, Inc.)
3. Peck, G.L., Olsen, T.G., Butkus, D., Pandya, M., Arnaud-Battandier, J., Gross, E.G., Windhorst, D.B. and Cheripko, J. (1982). Isotretinoin versus placebo in the treatment of cystic acne. *J. Am. Acad. Dermatol.*, **6**, 735
4. Farrell, L.N., Strauss, J.S. and Stranieri, A.M. (1980). The treatment of severe cystic acne with 13-*cis*-retinoic acid. *J. Am. Acad. Dermatol.*, **3**, 602
5. Goldstein, J.A., Comite, H., Mescon, H. and Pochi, P.E. (1982). Isotretinoin in the treatment of acne. *Arch. Dermatol.*, **118**, 555
6. Goldstein, J.A., Socha-Szott, A., Thomsen, R.J., Pochi, P.E., Shalita, A.R. and Strauss, J.S. (1982). Comparative effect of isotretinoin and etretinate on acne and sebaceous gland secretion. *J. Am. Acad. Dermatol.*, **6**, 760
7. Korner, W.F. and Vollm, J. (1975). New aspects of the tolerance of retinol in humans. *Int. J. Vitam. Nutr.*, **45**, 363
8. Windhorst, D.B. and Nigra, T. (1982). General clinical toxicology of oral retinoids. *J. Am. Acad. Dermatol.*, **6**, 675
9. Nemaic, M.K., Fritsch, P.O. and Elias, P.M. (1982). Perturbations of membrane glycosylation in retinoid-treated epidermis. *J. Am. Acad. Dermatol.*, **6**, 801
10. Prutkin, L. (1975). Mucous metaplasia and gap junctions in the vitamin A acid-treated skin tumor, keratoacanthoma. *Cancer Res,*, **35**, 364
11. Paravicini, U. (1981). Pharmacokinetics and metabolism of oral aromatic retinoids. In

Orfanos, C.E. *et al.* (eds.). *Retinoids: Advances in Basic Research and Therapy*, pp. 13–20. (Berlin, Heidelberg, New York: Springer Verlag)

12. Kligman, A.M., Leyden, J.J. and Mills, O. (1981). Oral vitamin A (Retinol) in acne vulgaris. In Orfanos, C.E. *et al.* (eds.). *Retinoids: Advances in Basic Research and Therapy*, pp. 245–253. (Berlin, Heidelberg, New York: Springer-Verlag)

13. Orfanos, C.E. (1980). Oral retinoids – present status. *Br. J. Dermatol.*, **103**, 473

14. Cunningham, W.J. and Ehmann, C.W. (1983). Clinical aspects of the retinoids. *Sem. Dermatol.* (In press).

15. Symposium (1982). *Accutane: A new approach to the treatment of severe, recalcitrant cystic acne.* Sponsored by the State University of New York Downstate Medical Center, October 6.

16. Windhorst, D.B. and Peck, G.L. (1983). The retinoids. In Fitzpatrick, T.B. *et al.* (eds.). *Update: Dermatology in General Medicine*, pp. 226–237. (New York: McGraw-Hill, Inc.)

17. Kamm, J.J. (1982). Toxicology, carcinogenicity, and teratogenicity of some orally administered retinoids. *J. Am. Acad. Dermatol.*, **6**, 652

18. Strauss, J.S. (1982). Systemic retinoids in acne. *Sem. Dermatol.*, **1**, 239

Section 6

Isotretinoin – Duration of Remission of Acne

25
Relapse Rate of Acne Conglobata after Stopping Isotretinoin

H. WOKALEK, R. HENNES, H. SCHELL and H.J. VOGT

13-*cis*-retinoic acid has been shown to possess excellent efficacy in acne conglobata, acne,[1-9] in acne fulminans,[10,11] in severe papular pustular rosacea[12,13] as well as in Gram-negative folliculitis[13,14].

German co-operative multicentre retinoid study group drawn from 19 dermatological departments has recently investigated the optimal oral treatment of acne conglobata with isotretinoin[6,9]. In this three different dose schedules were tested (Table 1). All of these schedules showed clinical efficacy and were nearly dose dependent. Subsequent to this 6-month isotretinoin treatment study, a follow-up by 14 trial centres was started, for which the patients were recruited from the patients of the first investigation. The aim of this follow-up study presented here was to obtain information on the remission and relapse rate of acne after discontinuing the isotretinoin treatment.

There was exclusive isotretinoin treatment over a period of 6 months. Altogether 176 patients with acne conglobata received three different dose-schedules. Figure 1 summarizes the complete study and shows the

Table 1. Dose schedules in acne conglobata treatment (mg/kg body-weight/day).

Dose-group	Start	Modification after 3 months of therapy
I	1.0	0.2
II	0.5	0.2
III	0.2	0.2

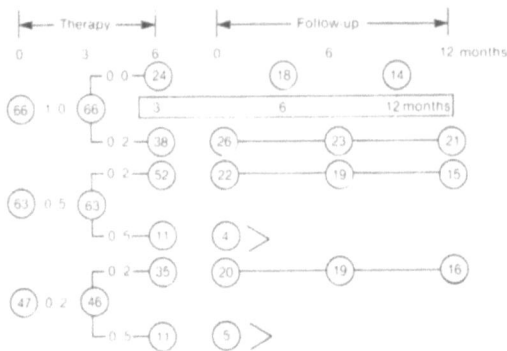

Figure 1. Design of study with number of patients and doses.

therapeutic and follow-up phases. Doses (without circles) and numbers of patients (encircled) are given.

After 3 months of treatment doses were modified according to the clinical success of the treatment. The dose was reduced if clinical improvement (measured by counting the lesions and grading seborrhea) was 66 per cent or more in comparison to the clinical state at the beginning of isotretinoin treatment. No dose reduction was made and a higher dose was not given if the improvement was lower than 66 per cent.

All patients of the dose-group I (1.0mg/kg body-weight) showed over 66 per cent improvement within 3 months. Dose-group I was then divided into two equal subgroups; one group received further treatment with a lower dosage of 0.2mg/kg body-weight/day, the other group received no further treatment at all. This non-treatment group has been followed-up especially to monitor the side-effects of isotretinoin.

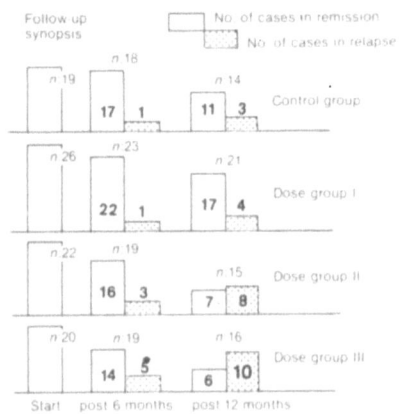

Figure 2. Synopsis of remission and relapse numbers.

Unfortunately not all patients of the treatment period entered the follow-up study, for various reasons.

All patients that could be recruited for the follow-up study showed a 66 per cent improvement within after 3 months. These patients have been followed up over a further period of at least 12 months. No acne treatment at all has been given during this period. Some of the patients terminated the follow-up course early because of relapse and other non-medical reasons.

Parameters

Relapse

A relapse was noted if the physician or the patient asked for acne treatment again.

Lesions

Lesions (open and closed comedones, papules, pustules, and nodes) were counted and registered at every follow-up date.

Seborrhoea

The degree of seborrhoea of skin and hair were registered subjectively by physician and patient and estimated in a score.

Side-Effects

The well known side-effects of isotretinoin treatment (dry lips, dry mucous membranes of the nose, cheilitis, dermatitis facialis and scaling of the skin) were registered by estimating a score for the frequency and intensity per patient.

Results

Figure 2 gives a synopsis of the remission and relapse rate for all dose-groups. The number of remissions and relapses at 6 and 12 months is shown. In the control group and in dose-group I the frequency of remissions and relapses is nearly the same, but in dose-groups II and III a negative dose-dependent augmentation of relapses is evident.

Figure 3 shows, for all three dose-groups, the remissions of every individual patient, including those who have dropped out due to acne relapse. Here, also, a dose-dependent pattern of relapse occurs. In dose-

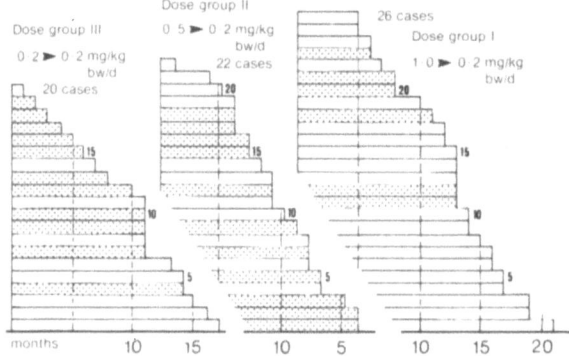

Figure 3. Remissions of individual patients. Shaded patients are those who dropped out owing to acne relapse.

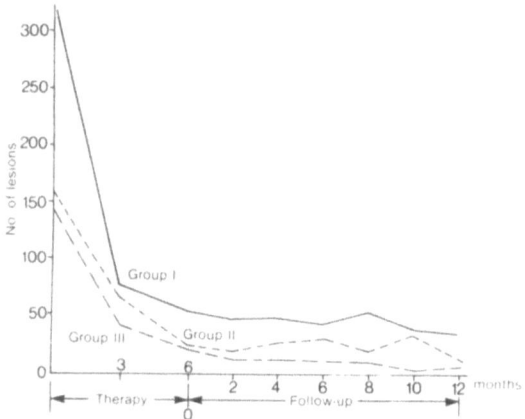

Figure 4. Number of non-inflammatory lesions before, during and after therapy.

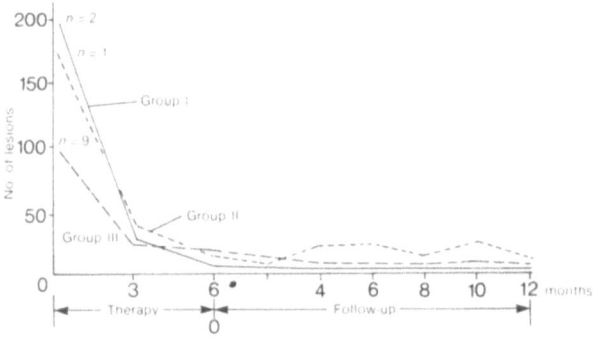

Figure 5. Number of inflammatory lesions before, during and after therapy.

234

group I the earliest relapse occurs after 6 months. In this group, 5 months after the end of therapy all patients are still in remission. In total, six out of 26 patients had to start acne treatment again in this group. In dose-group II the first relapse occurred 5 months after the end of therapy. In dose-group III the first relapse was evident after the second month. On the other hand, some of the patients in this group remained in remission over the total follow-up period of 17 months.

As for the non-inflammatory lesions (open and closed comedones), at the beginning of the follow-up period the trend in each group is nearly parallel with a slightly augmented level in dose-group I patients (Figure 4).

A similar pattern occurs for the inflammatory lesions. In the three dose-groups there is a rather parallel course during the follow-up period (Figure 5).

Because of the similar pattern of all lesions in the different dose-groups we calculated on the one hand the number of non-inflammatory lesions for all patients who remained in remission and on the other hand the number for all patients who relapsed. At the end of the follow-up period the number of lesions in the relapse group corresponds to the number at 3 months. In the remisssion group the therapeutic effect seems to be increasing (Figure 6).

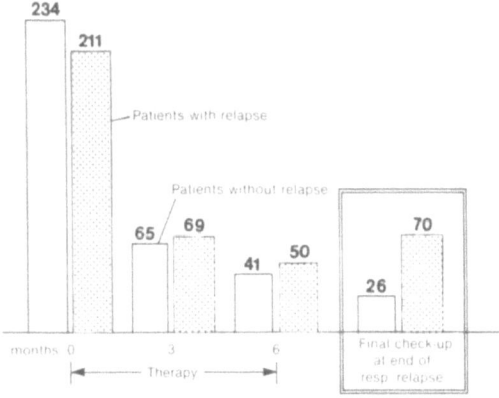

Figure 6. Number of non-inflammatory lesions in patients with and without relapse before and during therapy.

The calculation of the numbers of inflammatory lesions results in a similar pattern. Nevertheless, the number of lesions when relapse occurs exceeds the 3 month value markedly. Here also the therapeutic effect seems to be constant if not increasing in the remission group (Figure 7).

Seborrhoea is an important factor in acne. In Table 2 seborrhoea grading is shown prior to and after therapy as well as at the end of the follow-up

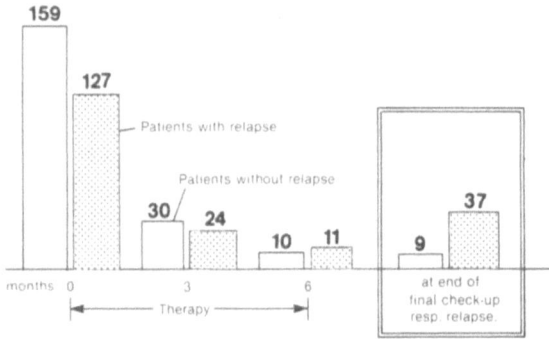

Figure 7. Number of inflammatory lesions in patients with and without relapse before and during therapy.

period. At the end of the therapy period there is no marked difference in the mean score of seborrhoea in all three dose-groups. If we look at the remission and relapse groups we find an augmented score-value for both groups at the end of the follow-up in comparison to the 6 month status. In the relapse group the seborrhoea value is somewhat higher than in the remission group.

Table 2. Degree of seborrhoea before and after therapy.

Dose-group	Number	Therapy Start	End	End of follow-up
I	26	2.3	0.3	
II	22	2.6	0.3	
III	20	2.5	0.2	
Total				
With relapse	29	2.5	0.3	1.7
Without relapse	39	2.4	0.2	1.2

Sixteen patients (dose-group I) were followed up in order to obtain information on side-effects (Figure 8). At the end of the therapy phase all 16 had mucocutaneous side-effects. The mean number of side-effects was five and the mean intensity 1.35 per patient. One month after stopping isotretinoin 12 patients out of 16, 2 months later seven out of 16 and finally 3 months post-therapy three out of 16 patients showed mucocutaneous side-effects. The number of side-effects per patient diminished during the follow-up period and the intensity-score was 'slight'. The most persistent side-effect was dryness of lips and nose as well as dermatitis facialis.

236

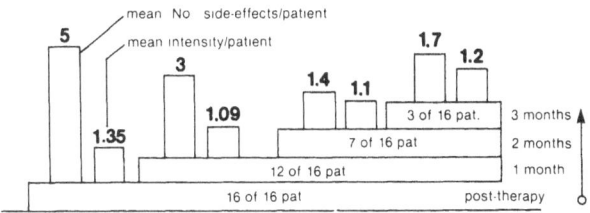

Figure 8. Side-effects in dose-group I patients during and after therapy.

Finally the patterns of triglyceride and cholesterol changes in dose-group I are shown in Figures 9 and 10. We want to focus only on the mean values. At the end of therapy the triglyceride level has risen but is still within the normal range (Figure 9). At the end of the follow-up the mean value reaches the original value. A similar pattern can be shown for cholesterol (Figure 10).

Conclusion

Our follow-up study confirms the results of other groups who have shown that the average number of acne lesions diminishes further after discontinuing isotretinoin for the next 2 month period.[1,2,6-8,15] In dose-

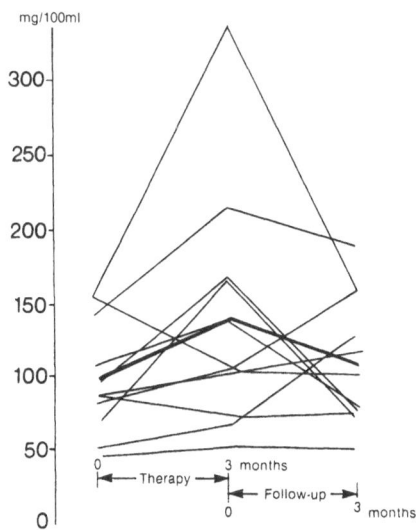

Figure 9. Triglyceride values in serum before, at end of therapy and 3 months after.

237

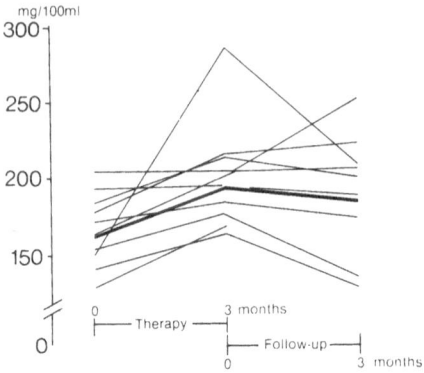

Figure 10. Total cholesterol values in serum before, at end of therapy and 3 months after.

group III relapses appeared relatively early. In dose-group II relapses were distributed over the total relapse period rather equally. In dose-group I relapses appeared markedly less often and if they appeared it occurred later.

It was shown that the number and intensity per patient of side-effects diminished continuously during the follow-up period.

The German multicentre study group recommends an initial therapy of 1.0mg/kg body-weight for the first 3 months of therapy. A dose reduction to 0.5–0.2mg/kg body-weight for a further 3 month period is recommended if the improvement after 3 months is not satisfactory.[6] Our follow-up results obviously support this recommendation.

References

1. Farrell, I.N., Strauss, J.S. and Stranieri, A.M. (1980). The treatment of severe cystic acne with 13-*cis*-retinoic acid. *J. Am. Acad. Dermatol.*, **3**, 602
2. Jones, H., Miller, A.J. and Cunliffe, W.J. (1983). A dose–response study of 13-*cis*-retinoic acid in acne vulgaris. *Br. J. Dermatol.*, **108**, 333
3. Jones, D.H., Cunliffe, W.J. and Cove, J.H. (1981). 13-*cis*-retinoic acid in acne (a double-blind study of dose response). In Orfanos, C.E. *et al.* (eds.). *Retinoids: Advances in Basic Research and Therapy*. pp. 255–258. (Berlin, Heidelberg, New York: Springer-Verlag)
4. Jones, H., Blanc, D. and Cunliffe, W.J. (1980). 13-*cis*-retinoic acid and acne. *Lancet*, **2**, 1048
5. King, K., Jones, D.H., Daltrey, D.C. and Cunliffe, W.J. (1982). A double-blind study of the effects of 13-*cis*-retinoic acid on acne, sebum excretion rate and microbial population. *Br. J. Dermatol.*, **107**, 583
6. Meigel, W., Gollnick, H., Wokalek, H., Plewig, G. *et al.* (1983). Orale Behandlung der Acne conglobata mit 13-*cis*-Retinsäure. Ergebnisse der deutschen multizentrischen Studie nach Therapieschluss. *Hautarzt*, (In press)
7. Peck, G.L., Olsen, T.G., Yoder, F.W., Strauss, J.S., Downing, D.T., Pandya, M., Butkus, D. and Arnaud-Battendier, J. (1979). Prolonged remission of cystic and conglobata acne with 13-*cis*-retinoic acid. *N. Engl. J. Med.*, **300**, 329

8. Plewig, G., Wagner, A. and Braun-Falco, O. (1980). 13-*cis*-Retinsäure. *Münch. Med. Wochenschr.*, **122**, 1287
9. Plewig, G., Gollnick, H., Meigel, W., Wokalek, H. *et al.* (1981). 13–*cis*–Retinsäure zur oralen Behandlung der Acne conglobata. Ergebnisse einer multicentrischen Studie. *Hautarzt*, **32**, 634
10. Plewig, G., Wagner, A. and Braun-Falco, O. (1980). Orale Behandlung schwerster Akneformen mit 13-*cis*-Retinsäure. Klinische Ergebnisse. *Münch. Med. Wochenschr.*, **38**, 1287
11. Wagner, A. and Plewig, G. (1980). 13-*cis*-Retinsäure. *Münch. Med. Wochenschr.*, **122**, 1294
12. Nikolowski, J. and Plewig, G. (1981). Orale Behandlung der Rosacea mit 13-*cis*-Retinsäure. *Hautarzt*, **32**, 575
13. Plewig, G., Nikolowski, J. and Wolff, H.H. (1982). Action of 13-*cis*-retinoic acid (isotretinoin) in acne, rosacea and gramnegative folliculitis. *J. Am. Acad. Dermatol.*, **6**, 766
14. Neubert, U. and Plewig, G. (1980). Gramnegative Follikulitis. Verlaufsbeobachtungen und therapeutische Möglichkeiten. *Zentralbl. Haut. Geschlkr.*, **144**, 38
15. Peck, G.L., Olsen, T.G., Butkus, D., Pandya, M., Arnaud-Battendier, J., Gross, E.G., Windhorst, D.B. and Cheripko, J. (1982). Isotretinoin versus placebo in the treatment of cystic acne. *J. Am. Acad. Dermatol.*, **6**, 735

26
A Follow-up Study of 13-*cis*-Retinoic Acid Therapy in Cystic Acne

D.H. JONES and W.J. CUNLIFFE

Introduction

Strauss,[1] Pochi[2] and Plewig[3] have published data on 13-*cis*-retinoic acid therapy in cystic acne with treatment periods of 12, 16 and 24 weeks, and follow-up periods of 8, 16 and 37 weeks respectively. The response to therapy of the dose-groups as a whole is impressive, as is the continuation of the improvement off therapy. However, analysis of individual results has not been published. The responses of our 76 individual patients have, therefore, been analysed and are now presented.

Methods

The details of the patients' demography, and observations made upon them have been recorded previously.[4]

The patients were divided into three dose-groups – 1.0, 0.5 and 0.1mg/kg body-weight. An arbitary standard of a 50 per cent improvement in acne grade from a pre-treatment baseline has been used to place the patients in various categories at each visit:

(1) Success – greater than 50 per cent improvement,

(2) Partial success – greater than 50 per cent improvement but residual lesions requiring further therapy (usually at 32 weeks),

(3) Failure – less than 50 per cent improvement,

(4) Relapse – (a) Major – greater than 50 per cent improvement but a

return of the acne to 50 per cent or more of the pre-treatment grade,

(b) Minor – greater than 50 per cent improvement but a return of the acne to less than 50 per cent of the pre-treatment grade, and the patients insisted on further therapy.

For the purposes of analysis, patients who failed to attend were assumed to belong to that category in which they had been placed at their last previous visit. Patients withdrawn from the trial remained in the category in which they were placed at the time of withdrawal. Withdrawal occurred because patients were placed on further therapy.

The patients were surveyed by questionnaire 24–30 months post-treatment in order to assess if the improvement had been maintained.

Most of the patients in categories (2)–(4) were placed on second courses of therapy, and their subsequent response to therapy is analysed. Three

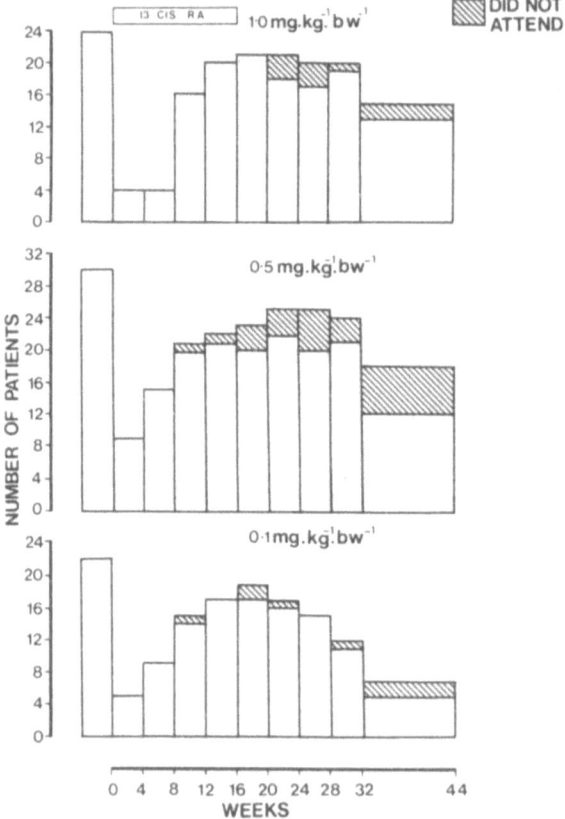

Figure 1. Histogram vs. time of number of successful patients with > 50 per cent improvement which was maintained and no further therapy required.

patients in the 0.1mg/kg body-weight group had a relapse of 50 per cent but wished for no further therapy and had spontaneously improved at the next visit.

Patients in categories (2)–(4) at 44 weeks were classed under the broad heading of 'failures'. The group was widened to include slow responders, i.e. those patients who only achieved a 50 per cent improvement between 16 and 32 weeks. These 'failures' have been compared with the 'successes' with respect to the return of the sebum excretion rate (SER).

Results

The results were analysed statistically by the chi-square test or Fisher's exact probability test if the numbers were too small.

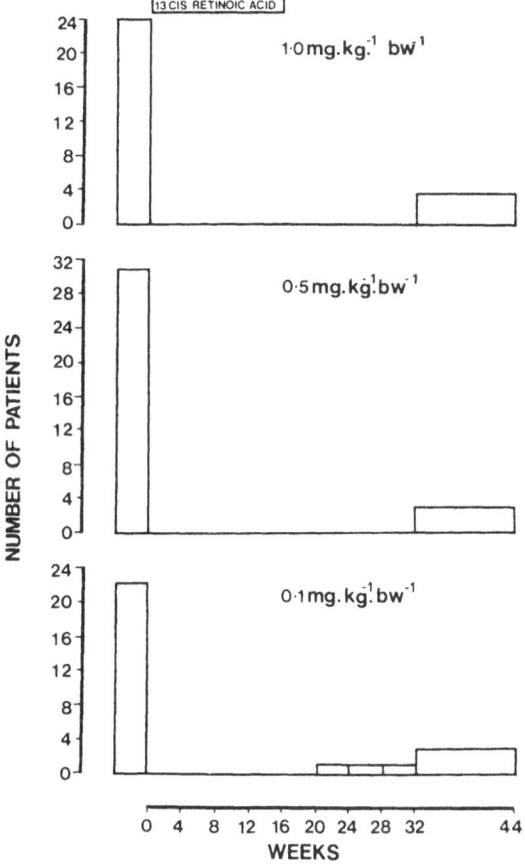

Figure 2. Histogram vs. time of number of partially successful patients with > 50 per cent improvement but failure to clear and therapy given for residual lesions.

Table 1. Patients who replied to the questionnaire and who are now untroubled by their acne.

Dose (mg/kg body-weight)	1.0			0.5			0.1		
Time	44/52	Replied	Now	44/52	Replied	Now	44/52	Replied	Now
Patient categories									
Successes	15	12	11	18	15	12	7	3	1
(After further therapy)									
Residual	4	1	1	3	3	3	3	3	1
Failures	1	1	0	2	2	1	3	1	0
Relapses	4	4	2	7	7	1	9	9	3
Total	24	18	14	30	27	17	22	16	5

Successes (Figure 1)

Twenty-three out of the 24 patients in the 1.0mg/kg body-weight group achieved a 50 per cent improvement, but because of the rapid relapse in two patients, the maximum number seen to improve is 21 patients at 20 and 24 weeks. At 44 weeks, 15 patients had maintained their improvement and required no further therapy. Twelve of these patients replied to the questionnaire and only one patient had relapsed (Table 1).

Twenty-eight out of the 30 patients in the 0.5mg/kg body-weight group achieved a success though the maximum number seen at any one time is 26 patients at 24 weeks. The number at 44 weeks is 18, and 15 of these replied to the questionnaire – 12 were still free of their disease (Table 1).

Nineteen out of 22 patients in the 0.1mg/kg body-weight group achieved a success and this was seen at 20 weeks. However, only seven patients had maintained this at 44 weeks, and of the three who replied, only one patient was untroubled by his acne (Table 1).

There is a significantly smaller success rate at 44 weeks between the 0.1mg/kg body-weight and other two groups ($p < 0.05$).

Partial Successes (Figure 2)

At 32 weeks, four, three and three patients in the 1.0, 0.5 and 0.1mg/kg body-weight groups respectively, had achieved a 50 per cent improvement but felt that they had sufficient residual acne to warrant further therapy. These results are not significantly different. Eight out of the ten patients responded to a second course of therapy (Table 2) – the two non-responders being in the 0.1mg/kg body-weight group. Five out of seven

Table 2. Numbers of patients responding successfully to further therapy after being withdrawn.

Dose (mg/kg body-weight)	1.0		0.5		0.1	
Further therapy	Antib.*	13-Cis†	Antib.*	13-Cis†	Antib.*	13-cis†
Patient category						
Partial success	2	2	3	–	3	–
SUCCESSFUL	2	2	3	–	1	–
Failure	1	–	1	1	3	–
SUCCESSFUL	0	–	0	1	0	–
Relapses						
Major	1	1	1	1	2	1
SUCCESSFUL	0	1	1	1	0	1
Minor	–	2	3	2	5	–
SUCCESSFUL	–	2	2	1	0	–

*Antib. = Antibiotics
†13–Cis = 13-cis-retinoic acid

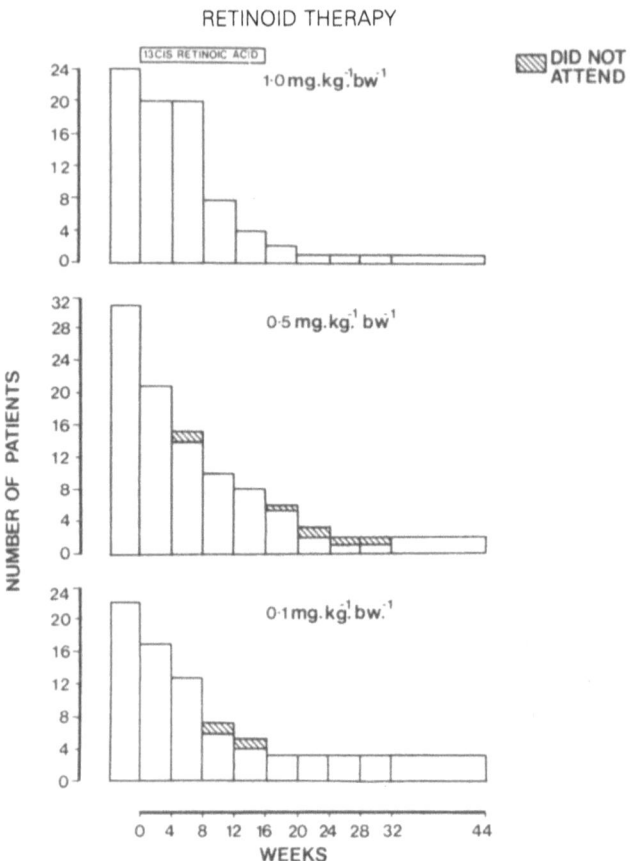

RETINOID THERAPY

Figure 3. Histogram vs. time of number of patients with < 50 per cent improvement.

patients who replied to the questionnaire continue to do well (Table 1). In eight out of the ten patients the residual lesions were on the trunk.

Failures (Figure 3)

This category includes a number of slow responders. Six patients in the 0.5mg/kg body-weight only improved by 50 per cent between 16 and 24 weeks, and there were smaller number in the other two groups. This category of patients has been discussed in an earlier paper. However, at 32 weeks there were only one, two and three patients in the 1.0, 0.5 and 0.1mg/kg body-weight groups respectively, who failed to respond at all. These results are not significantly different.

Only one patient responded to further therapy. The other five patients have continued to be therapeutic problems (Table 2). The failures were not confined to a particular site of the acne.

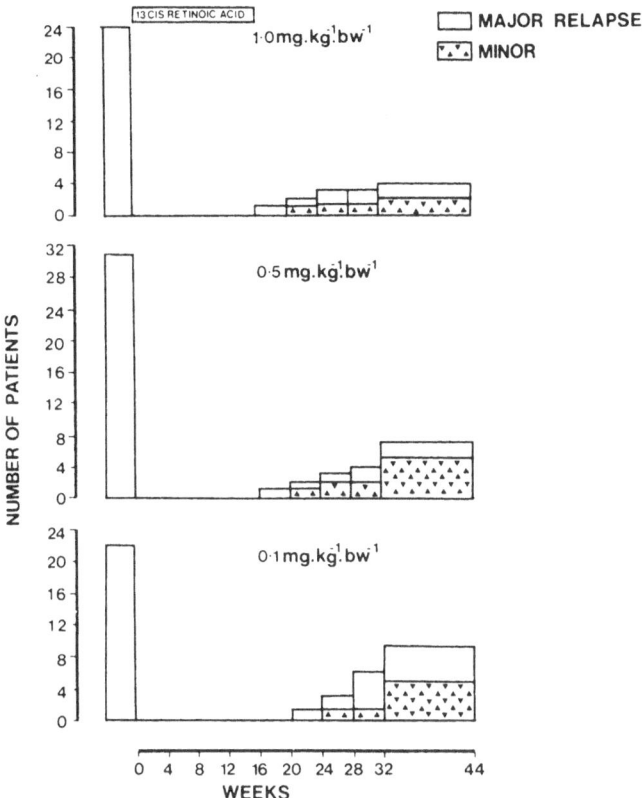

Figure 4. Histogram vs. time of the number of patients in whom the acne relapsed to a major or minor degree.

Relapses (Figure 4)

Twenty-three patients had a relapse of their acne but in three patients this was a single observation at 32 weeks and there had been spontaneous improvement at the next visit. Only eight out of the remaining 20 patients had a relapse of greater than 50 per cent of their pre-treatment grade. Patients relapsed throughout the follow-up period. There was no significant difference between the relapse rate of the 1.0mg/kg body-weight group (four out of 24 patients) and that of the 0.1mg/kg body-weight group (nine out of 22 patients) at 44 weeks.

All of the 20 patients replied to the questionnaire (Table 1), and 14 are continuing to have problems with their acne. 19 out of the 20 patients had been re-treated, and at 44 weeks nine had responded and ten had not (Table 2). There had, therefore, been a further deterioration in four patients after the 28 week follow-up.

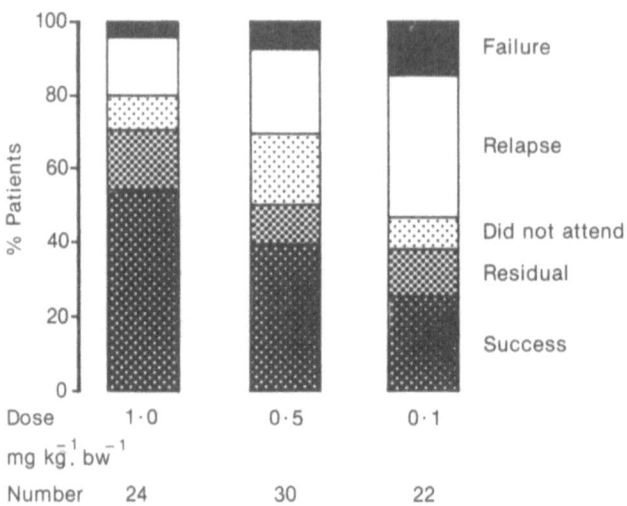

Figure 5. Histogram of percentage of patients in the five categories at 44 weeks.

Summary (Figure 5)

If the proportions of patients in the various categories at 44 weeks are compared, the differences between the doses become more obvious. The patients who did not attend (DNAs) at 44 weeks had all previously been in the successful category. To be fair to 13-*cis*-retinoic acid, these DNAs and those patients with residual lesions could be counted as successes giving minimum and maximum success rates of 55–80 per cent in the 1.0mg/kg body-weight group, 40–70 per cent in the 0.5mg/kg body-weight group and 30–45 per cent in the 0.1mg/kg body-weight group. The long-term results of the 0.1mg/kg body-weight dose are not good with only one patient maintaining his 50 per cent improvement at 24–30 months post-therapy.

In short, a small number of people do not respond to this drug at all. Though a number of people respond only slowly, this does not necessarily imply an unsuccessful outcome. A small proportion will be left with residual lesions on the trunk but will respond to further courses of therapy. The 0.1mg/kg body-weight dose can be discounted in terms of producing a long remission period. There is a relapse rate associated with the two higher doses, but of those patients who achieve and maintain a 50 per cent improvement over a 7 month follow-up period, most will then remain untroubled by their acne.

The results of re-treatment (Table 3) suggest that 13-*cis*-retinoic acid may be used in a second course with good effect.

There was no correlation in the unsuccessful categories between age,

Table 3. Summary of response to further therapy.

Further therapy	Antib.*	13-CIS†	Total
Patients withdrawn	25	10	35
Successful Re-treatments	9	9	18

*Antib. = Antibiotics
†13-CIS = 13-*cis*-retinoic acid

sex, site of the acne or initial SER except eight out of the ten patients with residual lesions had them on the trunk.

Sebum Excretion Rate (Figure 6)

Those patients, who had achieved a 50 per cent improvement within 16 weeks which was maintained and required no further therapy, were compared against all the other patients in each dose-group. It appears that those patients who have done best are those in which the SER returns more slowly towards pre-treatment levels. This does not hold true for the 0.1mg/kg body-weight group, perhaps because there were so few patients in the successful group.

Discussion

The excitement that 13-*cis*-retinoic acid generated was not only due to its efficacy but to the fact that a short course of therapy resulted in prolonged remission. This is certainly true of the high doses used by Peck[5] in his initial trial. Surprisingly, lower doses have been shown to be equally effective.[1-4] Short-term follow-up studies have also suggested significant remission rates with these doses.

In our study if categories (1) and (2) are taken together, the 1.0mg/kg body-weight is associated with a remission of 7 months in 80 per cent patients (19 out of 24), and this is maintained over 24–30 months post-therapy (13 of the 19 replied to the questionnaire and 12 were untroubled).

The 0.5mg/kg body-weight does equally well with a remission in 70 per cent patients (21 out of 30) which is maintained in 15 out of the 18 who replied to the questionnaire.

The 0.1mg/kg body-weight dose fares badly though the response to the questionnaire was poor (six out of ten successful patients from the total 22 replied, and only two patients had no problems from their acne).

Strauss and Plewig have treated their patients for different time periods to ourselves, and so it would be interesting to see whether the length of treatment period is related to the relapse rate. Success does seem to be related to the maintenance of sebum suppression.

One of the therapeutic aims for the use of 13-*cis*-retinoic acid is a short

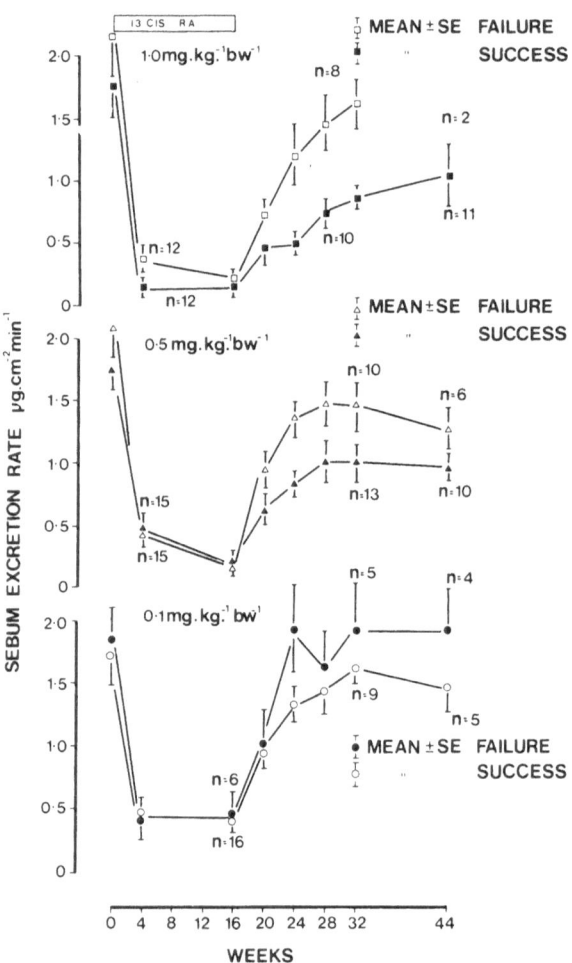

Figure 6. Graph of response of sebum excretion rate in 'Successes' and 'Failures' in the three dose-groups.

course of therapy. The choice, therefore, lies between the 1.0 and 0.5mg/kg body-weight doses. As the 0.1mg/kg body-weight dose did have an 87 per cent success rate at 20 weeks, it might still have a useful role in maintenance therapy.

Acknowledgements

We would like to thank Mr R.A. Forster for his excellent technical advice, Mrs P. Hick for secretarial help and Dr A.J. Miller of Roche Products Limited for his support.

References

1. Farrell, L.N., Strauss, J.S. and Stranieri, A.M. (1980). The treatment of severe cystic acne with 13-*cis*-retinoic acid. *J. Am. Acad. Dermatol.*, **3**, 602
2. Goldstein, J.A., Comite, H., Mescon, M. and Pochi, P.E. (1982). Isotretinoin in the treatment of acne. *Arch. Dermatol.*, **118**, 555
3. Plewig, G., Nikolowski, J. and Wolff, H.H. (1982). Action of isotretinoin in acne rosacea and gram-negative folliculitis. *J. Am. Acad. Dermatol.*, **6**, 766
4. Jones, D.H., King, K., Miller, A.J. and Cunliffe, W.J. (1983). A dose-response study of 13-*cis*-retinoic acid in acne vulgaris. *Br. J. Dermatol.*, **108**, 333
5. Peck, G.L., Olsen, T.G., Yoder, F.W., Strauss, J.S., Downing, D.T., Pandya, M., Butku, D. and Arnaud-Battandier, J. (1979). Prolonged remissions of cystic and conglobate acne with 13-*cis*-retinoic acid. *N. Engl. J. Med.*, **300**, 329

Section 7

Isotretinoin – Mechanism of Action

27
13-*cis*-Retinoic Acid in Acne –
Mechanism of Action

W.J. CUNLIFFE, D.H. JONES, K.T. HOLLAND, S. MILLARD,
and H. AL-BAGHDADI

Introduction

13-*cis*-retinoic acid is of undoubted value in the treatment of patients
with nodular cystic acne and in the treatment of patients with moderately
severe acne, particularly if the patient has failed to respond adequately to
the more conventional treatments.[1-3] The drug has such a dramatic effect
since it influences most of the major factors involved in the aetiology of
acne. Although opinion differs on both sides of the Atlantic as to which is
the prime reason for acne, most Europeans with a few exceptions favour
the view that the main drive to acne is the increased androgen effect on the
sebaceous gland resulting in seborrhoea, a phenomenon which correlates
well with the clinical severity.[4] Kligman and colleagues and others support
the view that hyperkeratinization of the pilosebaceous duct is the main
reason for acne.[5] However it is likely that most opinions favour the view
that bacteria, especially *Propionibacterium acnes (P.acnes)*, are not the
prime role for the development of acne but are important as a secondary
contributing role particularly to the development of inflammation and
possibly with the later development of some of the non-inflamed lesions.[6,7]
The fourth factor in the development of acne is the production of
inflammation. Some data suggest that inflammatory lesions arise
exclusively from non-inflamed lesions[8] but recent histological data in our
own laboratory would support the idea that some inflammatory lesions
may arise from follicles showing no evidence of hyperkeratinization. The
inflammation is undoubtedly due to the diffusion of low molecular weight

biological potent factors which diffuse from the pilosebaceous duct and in turn trigger both complement activation and chemotaxis.[9,10] This chapter will consider the effect of 13-*cis*-retinoic acid on these four factors: sebum production, ductal hyperkeratinization, cutaneous and ductal bacteria and inflammation.

13-*cis*-Retinoic Acid and Sebum Production

Using the established methods of assessing sebum excretion rate[11,12] there is no doubt that this drug has a dramatic effect in reducing sebum excretion rate. All doses so far used (0.05mg–2mg/kg) will reduce sebum production in a dose-dependent way.[1,2,4] Few dermatologists in England, and this includes ourselves, have rarely used doses greater than 1mg. In own laboratories we have investigated the effects of 1.0, 0.5, 0.3, 0.1 and 0.05mg/kg body-weight (Figures 1 and 2). These doses produce a dose-dependent effect which with the 1.0mg and 0.5mg doses has almost reached its maximum reduction of 75–90 per cent by one month. Thereafter there is only a small reduction. There is little difference between the sebum suppressive doses when the patient is given 0.5 and 1.0mg. There is a significant difference between these doses and 0.1mg/kg and 0.05mg (*p* 0.01). In Leeds we have treated patients, usually for 4 months, and have then observed the patients for several months thereafter. The sebum excretion rate slowly rises, reaching its pretreatment level 4 months after

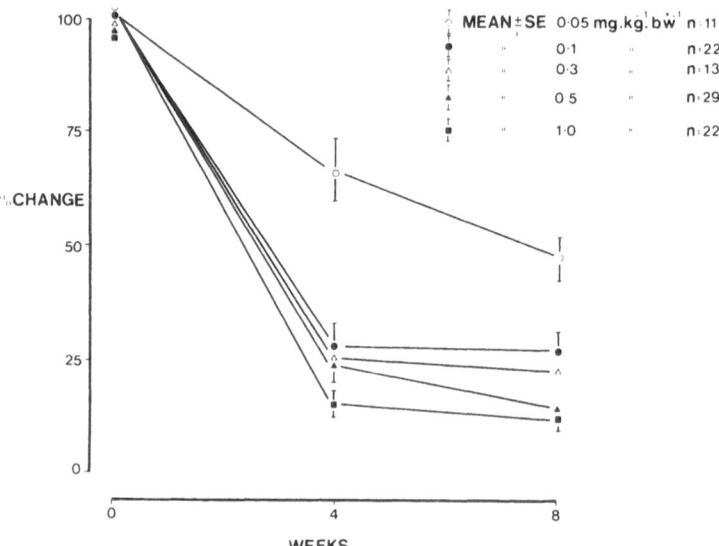

Figure 1. Shows the dose response of sebum excretion during 8-week therapy with various doses of 13-*cis*-retinoic acid treatment.

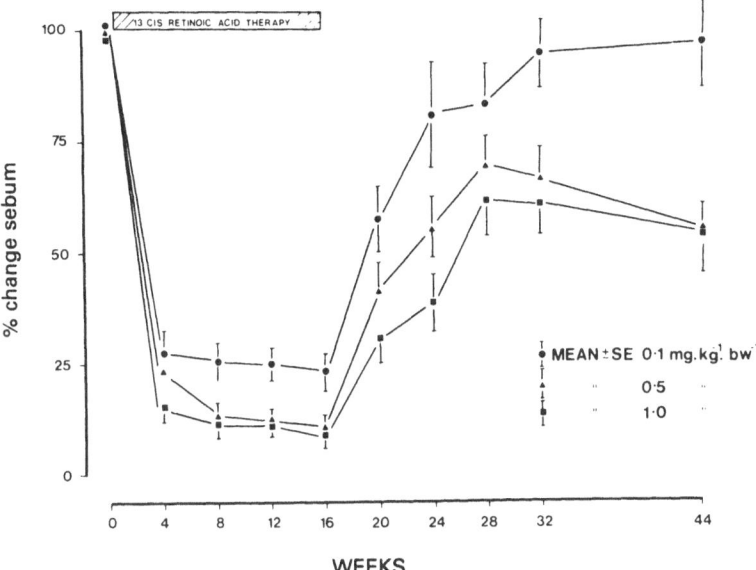

13-*CIS*-RETINOIC ACID IN ACNE – MECHANISM OF ACTION

Figure 2. Shows the sebum excretion rate both during and after discontinuing three doses of 13-*cis*-retinoic acid.

stopping the drug with the 0.1mg dose. (Figure 2). However, in patients treated with 0.5 and 1.0mg doses there is a permanent reduction of the grease levels, the sebum production plateauing out somewhere between 40 and 50 per cent of the pre-treatment level (Figure 2). We have only treated patients with doses of 0.05mg for 8 weeks (Figure 1). In these patients there was a 50 per cent reduction but the sebum excretion had returned to its pre-treatment level within 8 weeks of stopping therapy.

Our results on the effect of the drug on sebum excretion rate are almost identical to those observations made by other clinical research groups.[13,14] Other research groups have experience either with larger doses or with what is called the high dose–low dose studies. In these studies a large dose is given, such as 1–2mg/kg for 2 or 4 weeks, and followed thereafter by a dosage of 0.5mg. We have no such experience, nor have we any experience of using drugs in doses of less than 0.05mg.

Just how the drug produces this dramatic effect is uncertain. Retinoids are known to affect the function of small peptides on endorgans and it is likely that this could be the main action, the drug affecting sebaceous gland differentiation.[15] Support for this observation emanates from the histological appearances of sebaceous glands which undergo dedifferentiation to form an epithelial bud and at times almost completely disappear.[16,17]

The effect of the drug on the sebaceous gland is certainly not hormonally

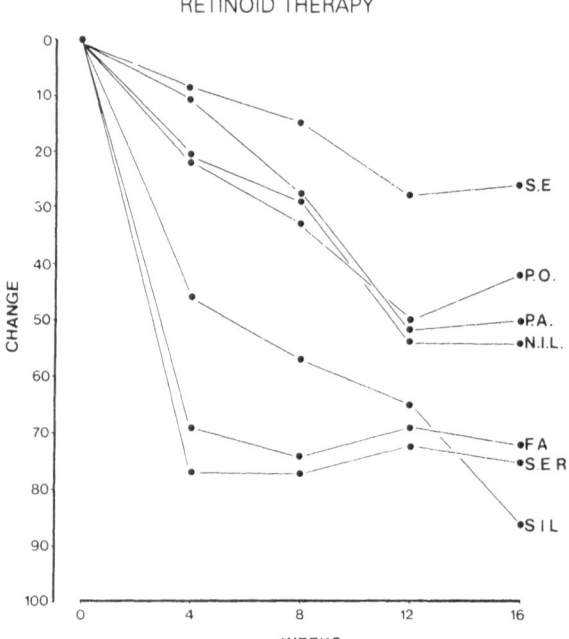

RETINOID THERAPY

Figure 3. Shows the mean reduction in various parameters measured during treatment over a 4-month period with 0.5mg 13-*cis*-retinoic acid. SE = *S. epidermidis*; PO = *P. ovale*; PA = *P. acnes;* NIL = non-inflamed lesions; FA = fatty acids; SER = sebum excretion rate; SIL = small inflamed lesions.

mediated; evidence of this observation comes from studies with the hamster[16] and from several studies in man in which it has been shown that plasma hormones show no change indicating that the drug has no anti-androgenic effect.[18]

13-*cis*-Retinoic Acid and Ductal Hyperkeratinization

Evidence for the effect of the drug on ductal hyperkeratinization comes from two types of observations – clinical and laboratory. Clinically there is a dose-dependent reduction in the number of non-inflamed lesions which parallels the effect on other lesions,[18,19] suggesting that the drug probably acts directly on ductal hyperkeratinization (Figure 3). In contrast to sebum production the reduction is a gradual one paralleling other aspects of clinical improvement, but nevertheless it is one which is also dose-dependent. The reduction in non-inflamed lesions counts at the end of 2 and 4 months on treatment with 0.5mg/kg is 30 and 60 per cent respectively and even 4 months after stopping treatment the reduction in non-inflamed lesions is 30 per cent.

Laboratory evidence of the reduction in ductal hyperkeratinization can

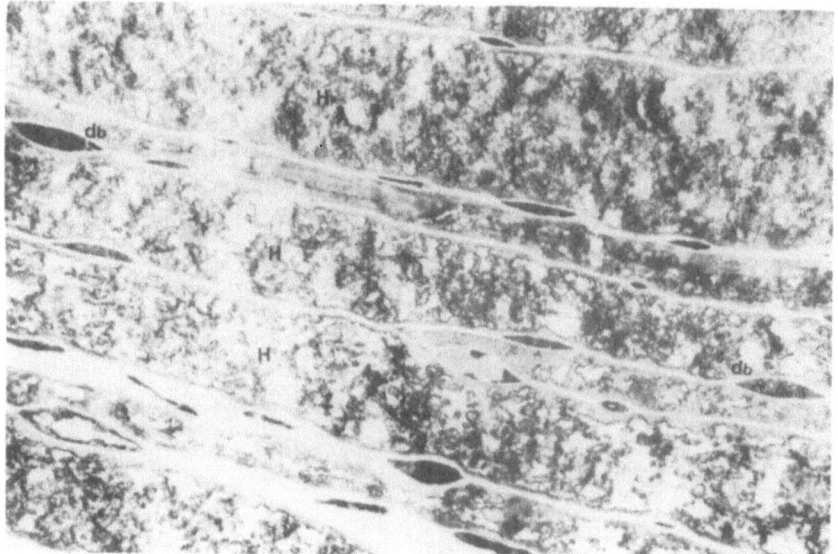

Figure 4. Shows a pre-treatment biopsy of a follicular cast showing the adherent keratinocytes and well formed desmosomal bodies (×22,500).

be demonstrated by using the follicular biopsy technique.[20] In this technique areas of normal looking skin amongst a sea of acne-prone skin are sampled by cyanacrylate gel. This glue is placed on the skin, on top of which is placed a glass slide; after firm pressure for a minute the slide is removed and this takes with it the upper stratum corneum, and the corneocytes material in the upper reaches of the pilosebaceous duct. This latter material can be assessed objectively using a dissecting microscope. As can be seen from Table 1 there is a reduction in ductal hyper-keratinization at 4 months of treatment with 0.5mg/kg.

Electron microscopy of the samples shows several changes. These features are highlighted in Figures 4 and 5. The effect of treatment is to produce some damage to the desmosomes, of which one of the earliest physical signs is vacuolation. Concomitant with this process is the accumulation of an amorphous-like materiai within the intercellular spaces. There are also changes in the character of the corneocytes which become less dense and there is a concomitant associated reduction in the number of bacteria.

13-*cis*-Retinoic Acid and Bacteria

Plewig and his colleague[21] and ourselves[22] have demonstrated that the drug has no effect on the growth of bacteria. More recently we have carried out work in the chemostat, and this again has confirmed no functional effect of the drug on the organism. Nevertheless the drug does produce *in vivo* a reduction in surface *Staphylococcus epidermidis, P. acnes* and *Pityrosporum ovale* bacteria (Figures 6, 7 and 8). The first observation of this effect occurred more or less simultaneously in the German and English literature.[21,22] Subsequently two groups of authors – Leyden and McGinley – have demonstrated a similar reduction in the number of *P.acnes*. There is a hint of some dose relationship although the effect is not as clear cut as

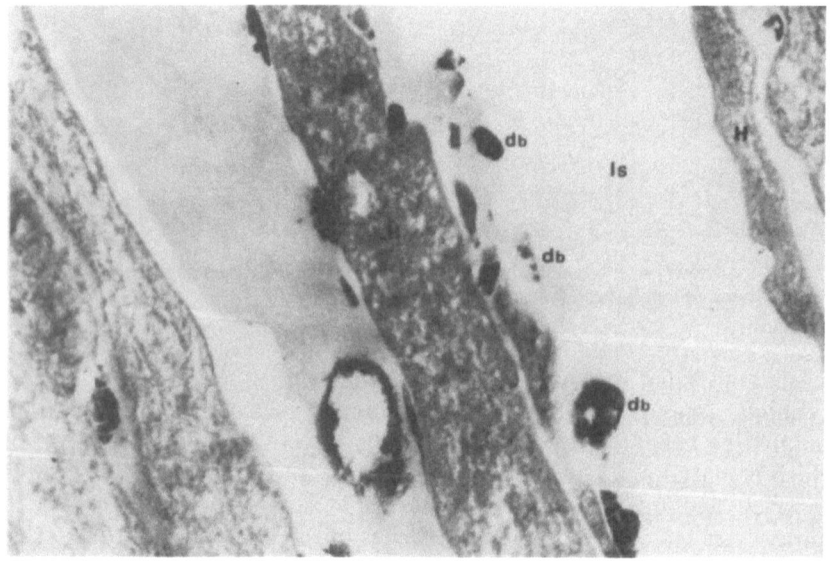

Figure 5. Shows the disorganized keratinocytes at the end of a 4-month course of 13-*cis*-retinoic acid (0.5mg/kg). There is an amorphous material between the keratinocytes and desmosomal bodies (DB) are seen pinched off from their attachment and lying free in the intercellular space (Is). The desmosomal bodies also show vacuolation (×22,500).

with sebum production. There is a two to three log drop in the number of organisms at the end of four months, the drop being a gradual one paralleling clinical improvement and certainly lagging behing the change in sebum excretion (Figure 3). Both King *et al.* and Leyden *et al.* found that the number of organisms was suppressed for 2–3 months after stopping oral therapy but after 4 months or more the bacteria had returned to almost their pre-treatment levels.

We have recently had the opportunity of investigating in 15 patients the effect of 13-*cis*-retinoic acid on ductal flora, and this too shows a significant decrease which parallels the reduction in surface flora (Figure 9). Thus 13-*cis*-retinoic acid does not have a direct effect on bacterial function, but indirectly reduces the bacterial population simply as a result of the change in the microenvironment which now becomes hostile to the growth and function of the organisms, particularly *P. acnes*. Furthermore the marked reduction in the size of the pilosebaceous duct also makes the living accommodation available for the organisms rather cramped.

13-*cis*-Retinoic Acid and Reduction in Inflammation

We have performed few investigations on the anti-inflammatory role of 13-*cis*-retinoic acid. More studies, better controlled, are needed in order to determine whether the decrease in the number and severity of inflamed lesions is a primary effect or simple secondary to the reduction of other aetiological factors. It is just possible that the rate of reduction in the number of lesions could simply represent a natural resolution, there being no stimulus to the genesis of new lesions as the various aetiological factors come under control. Clinically there is a gradual reduction in all forms of inflamed lesions[18,19] (Figure 3), although truncal lesions respond more slowly than facial lesions,[18,19] an observation which is similar to that seen when treating a patient with oral antibiotics and benzoyl peroxide.[24] This gradual reduction in inflamed lesions parallels the reduction in non-inflamed lesions and lags behind the dramatic decrease in sebum production. The reduction in inflamed lesions which parallels the fall in bacterial numbers also supports the idea that much of the improvement in inflammation is more of a secondary rather than a primary event.

Nevertheless there are data suggesting that 13-*cis*-retinoic acid has a significantly primary role in reducing inflammation.[25,26] Plewig and colleagues showed a reduction in the potassium iodide pustular reaction[26] whilst on therapy but one criticism of this study was the lack of an adequate time course study. It would be necessary to carry out this investigation in the first few days of giving the drug – well before other modifying facts come into play. For example, if the potassium iodide test is performed several weeks after starting treatment then it could be argued that the follicular penetration of the potassium iodide is reduced since the follicles become much smaller as therapy progresses. Isotretinoin has been shown to have no effect upon aggregation, chemokinesis or chemotaxis but it profoundly inhibits superoxide anion production and lysosomal enzyme release.[25]

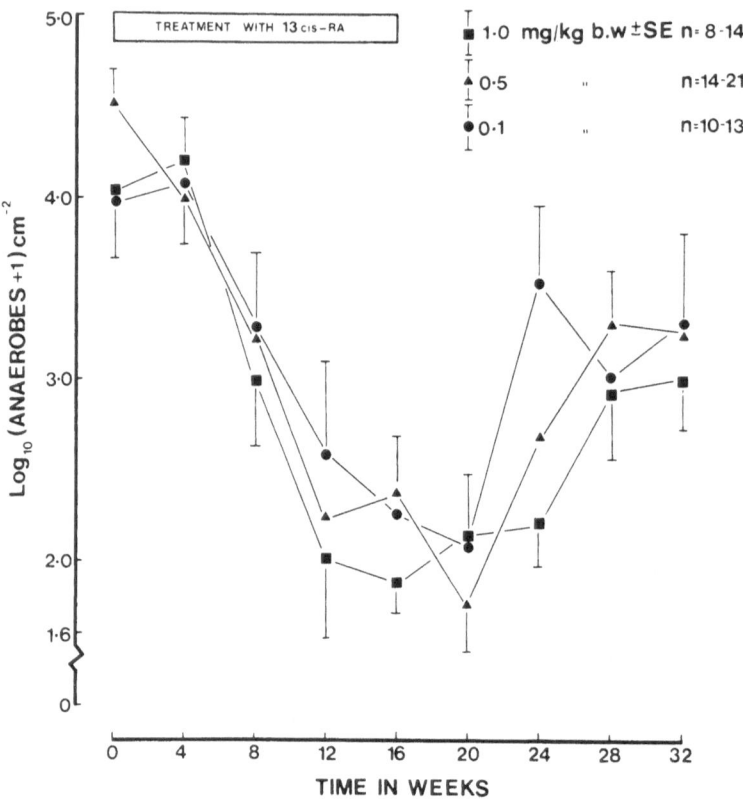

Figure 6. Shows the anaerobic count before, during and after treatment with 13-*cis*-retinoic acid.

Our studies on 13-*cis*-retinoic acid and the immune system suggest the drug has *in vivo* little effect. At the end of 1 month's treatment there is a small but significant increase in T-suppressor cells. The functional significance of this is not clear but may be related to the flare of the acne seen in some patients after 1 month's treatment. The drug has no effect on serum immunoglobulins, nor has it any significant effect on total white count or on the NBT tests. Shalita and colleagues report their own observations indicating a modification of lymphocyte function (Chapter 23).

Contrary to the decrease in acne inflammation seen with 13-*cis*-retinoic acid the drug certainly produces inflammation in its own role.[1,2,3] This is seen clinically as the cheilitis, the facial dermatitis, and the distal dermatitis. The mechanism of this is unclear but no doubt the drug somehow produces some alteration in epidermal structure resulting in the release of inflammatory mediators. Results on the effect of 13-*cis*-retinoic acid on the prostaglandins and leukotrienes are awaited with interest.

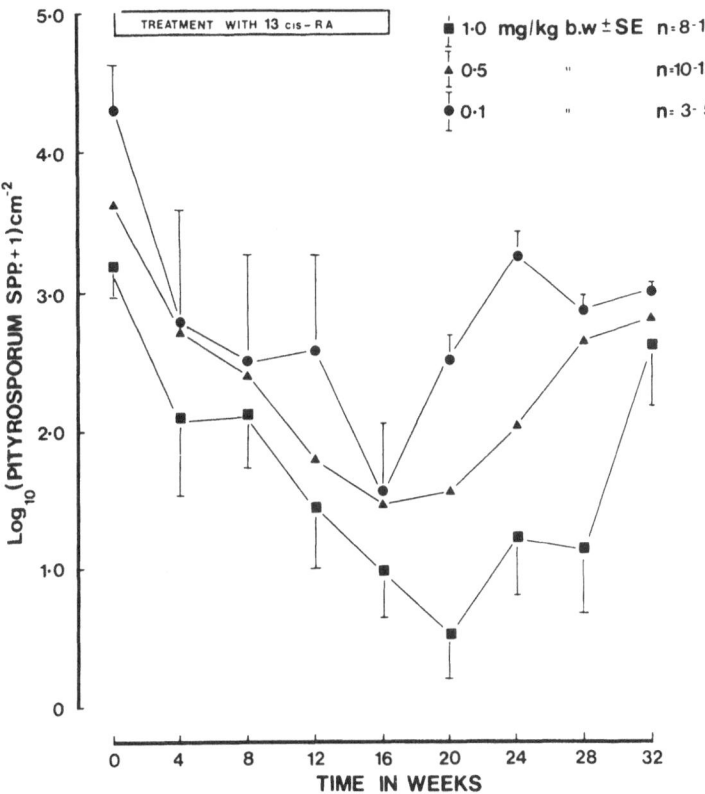

Figure 7. Shows the number of *Pityrosporum* count before, during and after treatment with 13-*cis*-retinoic acid.

Other Functions of 13-*cis*-Retinoic Acid

13-*cis*-retinoic acid could influence the production of vitamin D because of its effect on epidermal lipogenesis. Using UVB as a stimulator of vitamin D synthesis we were unable to detect any alteration in vitamin D production. An aside observation was the increased sensitivity of the skin to UVB whilst on 13-*cis*-retinoic acid and this no doubt could be due to the reduction in sebum excretion, thereby allowing more UVB to penetrate

Table 1. Results (A) "Keratin" coating (mean±SE).

Dose (mg/kg b.w.)	Pre-treatment	Post-treatment	Paired t-test
0.1	1.13±0.22	0.95±0.19	not significant
0.5	1.15±0.20	0.50±0.10	$p < 0.005$
1.0	1.60±0.21	0.67±0.09	$p < 0.005$

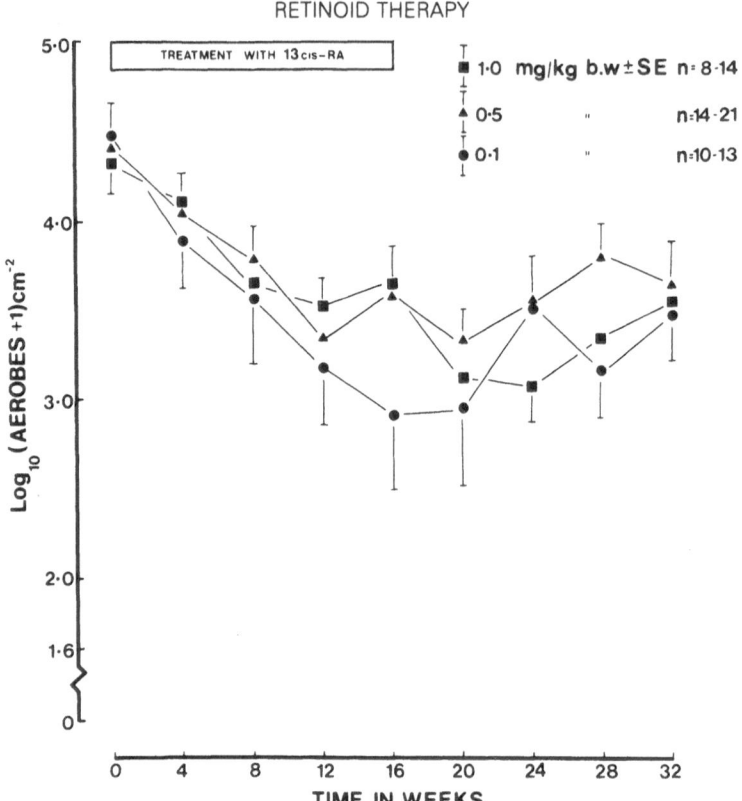

Figure 8. Shows the aerobic count before, during and after treatment with 13-*cis*-retinoic acid.

the epidermis and exhibit its erythrogenic effect. It could be argued that this may increase the risk of cutaneous neoplasms on a long-term basis. Conversely, the drug is known to have an anti-tumour effect, both in animals and in man.[27]

Conclusions

There is no doubt that 13-*cis*-retinoic acid works effectively against the four major aetiological factors involved in the pathogenesis of acne. It will be debated for several years as to whether its prime role is the reduced sebum production or the reduction in ductal hyperkeratization. Nevertheless it does without doubt have a marked effect on these two variables. It also significantly reduces surface and ductal bacteria as a secondary but important event; the drug has no primary effect on the bacteria. Directly and indirectly it influences the mediation of inflammation.

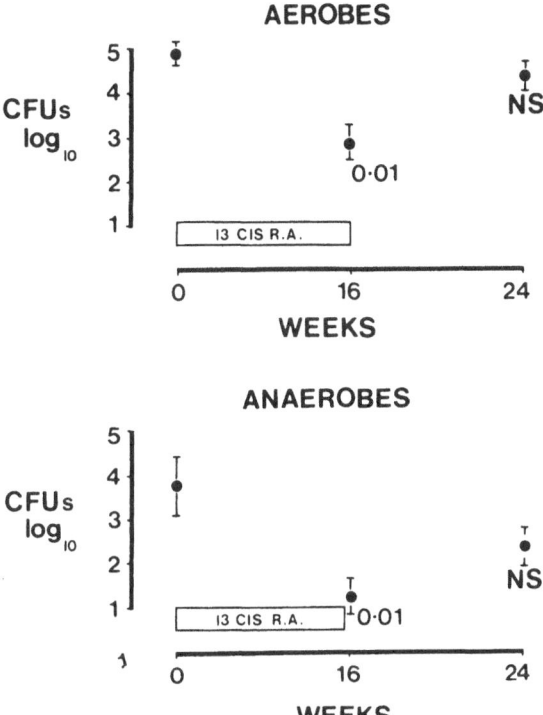

Figure 9. Shows the reduction in aerobic and anaerobic population in the upper part of the pilosebaceous duct during 4-month course of treatment with 13-*cis*-retinoic acid and 8 weeks thereafter ($n = 15$).

Many further studies need to be carried out in order that many of the unanswered questions, in particular those relating to its function at the molecular biological level, can be answered.

References

1. Peck, G.L., Olsen, T.G., Yoder, F.W. *et al.* (1979). Prolonged remission of cystic and conglobate acne with 13 cis retinoic acid. *N. Engl. J. Med.*, **300**, 329
2. Farrell, L.N., Strauss, J.S. and Stranier, A.M. (1980). The treatment of severe cystic acne with 13 cis retinoic acid. *J. Am. Acad. Dermatol.*, **3**, 602
3. Jones, H., Blanc, D. and Cunliffe, W.J. (1980). 13 cis retinoic acid and acne. *Lancet*, **2**, 1048
4. Cunliffe, W.J. and Shuster, S. (1969). The pathogenesis of acne. *Lancet*, **1**, 685
5. Kligman, A.M. and Plewig, G. Acne. (1975). Springer-Verlag, Berlin
6. Lavker, R.M., Leyden, J.J. and McGinley, K.J. (1981). The relationship between bacteria and the abnormal follicular keratinisation in acne vulgaris. *J. Invest. Dermatol.*, **77**, 325

7. Leeming, J.L., Holland, K.T. and Cunliffe, W.J. (1982). Is there a role for bacteria in the initiation of acne vulgaris? Data presented at E.S.D.R., Amsterdam.

8. Strauss, J.S. and Kligman, A.M. (1960). The pathologic dynamics of acne vulgaris. *Arch. Dermatol.*, **82**, 779

9. Scott, D.G., Cunliffe, W.J. and Gowland, G. (1979). Activation of complement – a mechanism for the inflammation in acne. *Br. J. Dermatol.*, **101**, 315

10. Puhvel, M.S. and Sakamoto, M. (1980). Cytotoxin production by comedonal bacteria. *J. Invest. Dermatol.*, **74**, 36

11. Strauss, J.S. and Pochi, P.E. (1961). The quantitative determination of sebum production. *J. Invest. Dermatol.*, **36** 293

12. Cunliffe, W.J. and Shuster, S. (1969). The rate of sebum excretion in man. *Br. J. Dermatol.*, **81**, 697

13. Goldstein, J.A., Socha-Szott, A., Thomsen, R.J., Pochi, P.E., Shalita, A.R. and Strauss, J.S. (1982). Comparative effect of isotretinoin and etretinate on acne and sebaceous gland secretion. *J. Am. Acad. Dermatol.*, **6**, 760

14. Gollnick, H., Meigel, W., Plewig, G. and Wokalek, H. (1983). Oral treatment of conglobate acne with isotretinoin. Co-operative study from 19 departments of dermatology. *J. Invest. Dermatol.*, **80**, 376

15. Sporn, M.B. (1981). Retinoids: new developments in their mechanism of action as related to control of proliferative diseases. In Orfanos, C.E. *et al.* (eds.). *Retinoids: Advances in Basic Research and Therapy.* pp. 73–·76. (Berlin, Heidelberg, New York: Springer-Verlag)

16. Gomez, E.C. (1982). Action of isotretinoin and etretinate on the pilosebaceous unit. *J. Am. Acad. Dermatol.*, **6**, 746

17. Landthaler, M., Kummermehr, J., Wagner, A. and Plewig, G. (1980). Inhibitory effects of 13 cis retinoic acid on human sebaceous glands. *Arch. Dermatol. Res.*, **269**, 29

18. Plewig, G., Wagner, A.N. and Kolowski, J. (1981). Effects of retinoids in animals experiments and after clinical application in acne patients. In Orfanos, C.E. *et al.* (eds.). *Retinoids: Advances in Basic Research and Therapy.* pp. 219–235. (Berlin, Heidelberg, New York: Springer-Verlag)

19. Jones, D.H., King, K., Miller, A.J. and Cunliffe, W.J. (1980). A dose response study of 13 cis retinoic acid in acne vulgaris. *Br. J. Dermatol.*, **108**, 333

20. Marks, R. and Dawber, R.P.R. (1971). Skin surface biopsy: an improved technique for examination of the horny layer. *Br. J. Dermatol.*, **84**, 117

21. Weismann, A., Wagner, A. and Plewig, G. (1981). Reduction of bacterial skin flora during treatment with 13 cis retinoic acid. *Arch. Dermatol. Res.*, **270**, 179

22. King, K., Jones, D.H., Daltrey, D.C. and Cunliffe, W.J. (1980). A double blind study of 13 cis retinoic acid on acne, sebum excretion rate and microbial population. *Br. J. Dermatol.*, **107**, 583

23. Leyden, J.L. and McGinley, K.J. (1982). Effect of 13 cis retinoic acid on sebum production and Propionibacterium acnes in severe nodulo cystic acne. *Arch. Dermatol. Res.*, **272**, 331

24. Greenwood, R., Burke, B. and Cunliffe, W.J. (1983). 425 patients treated in 1 centre. In preparation

25. Camisa, C., Eisenstat, B., Ragaz, A. and Weismann, G. (1982). The effects of retinoids on neutrophil functions in vivo. *J. Am. Acad. Dermatol.*, **6**, 620

26. Plewig, G. and Wagner, A. (1981). Anti-inflammatory effects of 13 cis retinoic acid. An in vivo study. *Arch. Dermatol. Res.*, **270**, 89

27. Peck, G.L., Gross, E.G., Butkus, D. and Dio Giovanna, J.J. (1982). *J. Am. Acad. Dermatol.*, **6**, 815

28
Effect of 13-*cis*-Retinoic Acid and Cyproterone Acetate on Acne Severity, Sebum Excretion Rate, Dermal and Epidermal Lipogenesis, Serum Lipids and Liver Function Tests

.J.R. MARSDEN, S. SHUSTER and F. LYONS

Introduction

The severity of acne is proportional to the amount of sebum produced by the sebaceous glands in the skin[1] and this is probably the primary defect.[2] Reduction of sebum production is, therefore, not only likely to be an effective treatment, but is also likely to be a means of gaining insight into the mechanisms underlying the disease itself and of the drugs being used in therapy. The most logical approach would be to use a topical drug which acts directly on the sebaceous glands to inhibit sebum production but so far this approach has not been successful.[3] Therefore, this study describes the effects of two systemic drugs, each of which is known to powerfully inhibit sebum production. Comparisons have been made between the effects of cyproterone acetate (CPA) and 13-*cis*-retinoic acid (13-*cis*-RA) on sebum excretion rate (SER), acne lesion count and severity, and between their effects on sebaceous lipogenesis as measured by [^{14}C]glucose incorporation, previously shown to correlate well with SER.[4] Measurements have also been made to see whether the drugs act synergistically, and their clinical and biochemical side-effects have been recorded.

Methods

All subjects were males with severe acne aged from 17 to 35 and all were otherwise healthy. Systemic and topical treatments for acne were stopped 3 weeks prior to the study. Duration of treatment with CPA or 13-*cis*-RA was 12 weeks and subjects were divided into five groups. The first three groups received CPA 100mg daily (eight patients), 25mg daily (11 patients) or 5mg daily (eight patients), and groups 4 and 5 received 13-*cis*-RA 0.8mg/kg/day (ten patients) or 0.05mg/kg/day (ten patients). (A further eight patients have received 0.8mg/kg/day 13-*cis*-RA. Whilst data on lipids and liver functions tests are available and are presented here, these patients were not included in the rest of this study.)

Sebum excretion rate was measured using previously described techniques[5] before treatment started and when treatment ended 12 weeks later. At the same intervals the total number of acne lesions was recorded and the severity of acne graded on a 0–4 or 0–10 analogue scale. Measurements of lipogenesis in skin were made in patients receiving 100mg and 25mg/kg/day' CPA and in those receiving 0.8mg/kg/day 13-*cis*-RA; two 4mm punch biopsies were taken from adjacent sites of interscapular skin before and at the end of treatment and the incorporation of [^{14}C]glucose into lipid in dermis and epidermis was measured as described earlier.[4] Lipogenesis is expressed as dpm per total lipid extracted from each biopsy. Furthermore, the total lipid extracted from dermis or epidermis after 100mg CPA and 0.8mg/kg/day 13-*cis*-RA was then separated into its constituent lipids by thin layer chromatography.[4]

Clinical side-effects during treatment were recorded for patients treated with CPA and 13-*cis*-RA and for the latter group the following biochemical measurements were made before and at the end of treatment: levels of serum triglyceride; cholesterol and HDL-cholesterol; liver function tests (bilirubin, alkaline phosphatase, aspartate aminotransferase); γ-glutamyl transpeptidase; serum albumin and total protein. In addition, levels of thyroxine, T_3 uptake, free thyroxine index and TSH were measured in nine patients receiving 0.8mg/kg/day 13-*cis*-RA.

Cholesterol and triglyceride were measured by enzymatic techniques (Technicon Mark II Auto Analyser). HDL-cholesterol was measured after precipitation of other lipoprotein fractions with magnesium phospho-tungstate reagent (Boehringer, Mannheim). Bilirubin and enzymes were measured using a Centrifichem 300 centrifugal fast analyser, protein and albumin with a Technicon Mark II autoanalyser. Thyroxine and T_3 uptake were measured with Amersham RIA and Thyopac 3 kits respectively and TSH by radioimmunoassay.

All statisical comparisons were by Student's *t*-test except for comparisons of acne severity which was by Wilcoxon rank-sum test.

Results

Cyproterone Acetate

In those receiving 100mg daily there was a decrease in sebum excretion rate from $1.50\mu g/cm^2/min \pm 0.16$ SEM before treatment to $0.53\mu g/cm^2/min \pm 0.17$ after treatment ($p<0.005$) compared with a fall from $1.33\mu g/cm^2/min \pm 0.16$ SEM to $0.81\mu g/cm^2/min \pm 0.12$ ($p<0.005$) with a dose of 25mg/day and from $1.67\mu g/cm^2/min \pm 0.20$ SEM to $1.38\mu g/cm^2/min \pm 0.13$ with 5mg CPA daily. Commensurate reductions were seen in lesion count, from 52 ± 4.8 SEM to 14 ± 2.2 ($p<0.001$) with 100mg daily, from 51 ± 7.7 to 28 ± 5.5 ($p<0.001$) with 25mg daily and from 66 ± 7.6 to 57 ± 9 with 5mg daily.

Median severity (scale 0–4) fell from 4 to 1.5 ($p<0.01$ Wilcoxon rank-sum test) with 100mg CPA daily, from 3 to 2 ($p<0.01$ Wilcoxon rank-sum test) with 25mg daily and remained grade 6 (scale 0–10) throughout treatment with 5mg/day CPA.

Lipogenesis was significantly reduced in the dermis following treatment with 100mg daily CPA, although there was considerable variation between the individual results. The pretreatment mean was 8.99×10^4dpm/total lipid extracted (tle) ± 1.36 SEM compared with 5.84×10^4dpm/tle ± 1.09 after treatment ($p<0.05$). There was little difference in dermal lipogenesis following 25mg CPA daily: 5.39×10^4dpm/tle ± 0.55 SEM before treatment compared with 5.93×10^4dpm/tle ± 0.72 after. However, again there were quite large variations in individual responses. Epidermal lipogenesis was also similar before and after treatment with 100mg CPA (5.38×10^3dpm/tle ± 0.59 SEM before compared with 6.08×10^3 dpm/tle ± 0.84 afterwards) and with 25mg CPA (4.70×10^3dpm/tle ± 0.55SEM against 5.32×10^3dpm/tle ± 0.72 at the end of treatment).

There were significant changes in only two of ten component lipids extracted from dermis in seven patients treated with 100mg CPA: a decrease in the percentage of wax diesters (from 7 per cent to 1 per cent, $p<0.05$) and an increase in the percentage of squalene from 11 per cent to 17 per cent ($p<0.01$). Mean levels of the remaining eight lipids changed very little, if at all, with treatment. No significant changes were found in any of the component lipids in epidermis after 100mg CPA, although for technical reasons data were incomplete with the cholesterol and 1,2 diglyceride fractions. Although there was a significant clinical improvement with 100mg and 25mg CPA, 13 out of 27 patients had decreased libido and two were from the 5mg/day CPA group. There were no other side-effects with CPA.

13-*cis*-Retinoic Acid

The effects of treatment with 13-*cis*-RA on SER, lesion count and acne severity are shown in Figure 1. With 0.8mg/kg/day (Figure 1 (a)) SER fell

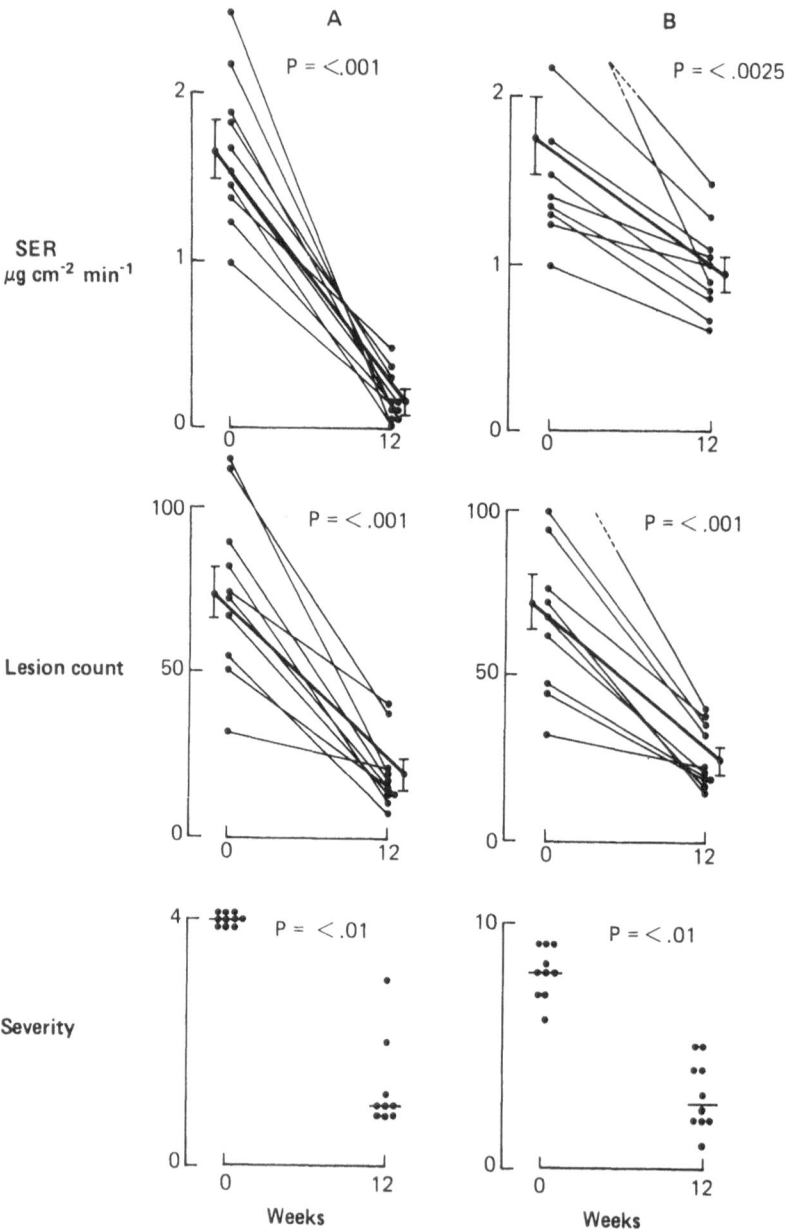

Figure 1. The response of sebum excretion rate (SER), acne lesion count and severity to 0.8mg/kg/day 13-*cis*-RA (A) and 0.05mg/kg/day 13-*cis*-RA (B).

from $1.68\mu g/cm^2/min \pm 0.15$ SEM to $0.18\mu g/cm^2/min \pm 0.05$ ($p<0.001$), lesion count fell from 75 ± 8.02 SEM to 19 ± 3.5 ($p<0.001$) and median severity fell from 4 to 1 (0–4 scale, $p<0.01$, Wilcoxon rank-sum test). Decreases in SER were smaller following 0.05mg/kg/day 13-*cis*-RA falling from a pretreatment mean of $1.78\mu g/cm^2/min \pm 0.20$ SEM to $0.98\mu g/cm^2/min \pm 0.08$ ($p<0.0025$) but there was still a significant therapeutic effect: lesion count decreased from 73 ± 8.9 SEM to 25 ± 2.9 ($p<0.001$) and median severity (0–10 scale) from 8 to 2.5 ($p<0.01$, Wilcoxon rank-sum test, Figure 1 (b)).

There was a profound decrease in dermal lipogenesis following 0.8mg/kg/day 13-*cis*-RA from 7.54×10^4dpm/tle ± 1.75 SEM before treatment to 1.60×10^4dpm/tle ± 0.37 when treatment was finished ($p<0.01$). Despite this, epidermal lipogenesis was significantly increased after treatment (from 4.98×10^3dpm/tle ± 0.44 SEM to 6.39×10^3 dpm/tle ± 0.56 ($p<0.025$), with increased values in seven out of ten subjects.

The percentage of the ten component lipids in dermis measured before and after treatment in nine patients with 0.8mg/kg/day 13-*cis*-RA showed significant changes in eight out of ten lipids, representing a gross disturbance in the overall pattern of sebaceous lipid synthesis in contrast to that found after treatment with 100 mg CPA. Despite the increase in amount of epidermal lipogenesis, the percentage of 1,3 diglyceride was the only difference found in the proportions of epidermal lipids after 13-*cis*-RA, from 6.8 per cent ± 0.8 SEM before treatment to 4.10 per cent ± 0.6 ($p<0.01$) afterwards. Although data were incomplete for the proportions of free fatty acids (six patients), cholesterol (six patients) and 1,2 diglycerides (seven patients) in epidermis, there were no significant differences in any of these measurements.

Biochemical changes after treatment with 13-*cis*-RA are shown in Figure 2. After 0.8mg/kg/day 13-*cis*-RA triglyceride rose from 0.9mmol/l ± 0.1 SEM to 2.2mmol/l ± 0.6 ($p<0.01$) and cholesterol increased from 5.1mmol/l ± 0.2 SEM to 6.1mmol/l ± 0.3 ($p<0.001$) (Figure 2 (a)). HDL-cholesterol fell from 1.1mmol/l ± 0.1 SEM to 0.9mmol/l ± 0.1 ($p<0.001$). Similar but smaller changes were found after 0.05mg/kg/day 13-*cis*-RA (Figure 2 (b)): triglyceride rose from 0.73mmol/l ± 0.07 SEM to 0.96mmol/l ± 0.14 ($p<0.05$) and cholesterol increased from 4.39mmol/l ± 0.30 SEM to 4.73mmol/l ± 0.31 ($p<0.01$). Although HDL-cholesterol levels fell during treatment with the lower dose of 13-*cis*-RA (from 1.09mmol/l ± 0.06 SEM to 1.03mmol/l ± 0.06) this did not reach statistical significance ($t=1.5, p>0.1$). All of these changes had reversed 4 weeks after treatment had stopped and were not significantly different from pretreatment values.

Other changes were found with the higher dose of 13-*cis*-RA (Figure 3). There were decreases in thyroxine (from 98.3nmol/l ± 2.7 SEM to

91.2nmol/l ± 3.6 SEM to 78.2nmol ± 4.7, $p<0.01$). Concentrations of serum albumin fell from 48.9g/l ± 0.7 SEM to 46.6g/l ± 0.5 ($p<0.02$) and levels of γ-glutamyl transferase increased from 13.0 U/l± 1.4 SEM to 21.1U/l± 3.8 ($p<0.01$). With 0.05mg/kg/day 13-*cis*-RA γ-glutamyl transferase increased from 15.9U/l± 2.1 SEM to 19.1U/l ± 2.4 ($p<0.005$) and levels of serum albumin did not change. All of these differences had reversed by 4 weeks after treatment and there were no significant changes in any other biochemical measurements.

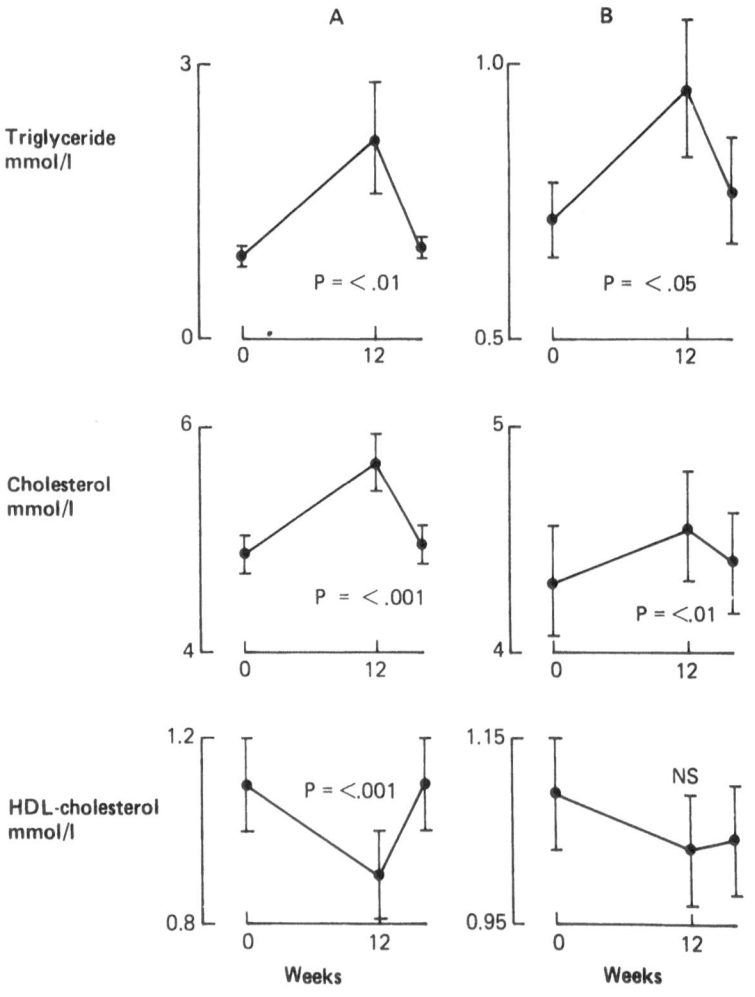

Figure 2. Serum triglyceride, cholesterol and HDL-cholesterol levels before and after treatment with 0.8mg/kg/day 13-*cis*-RA (A) and 0.05mg/kg/day 13-*cis*-RA (B).

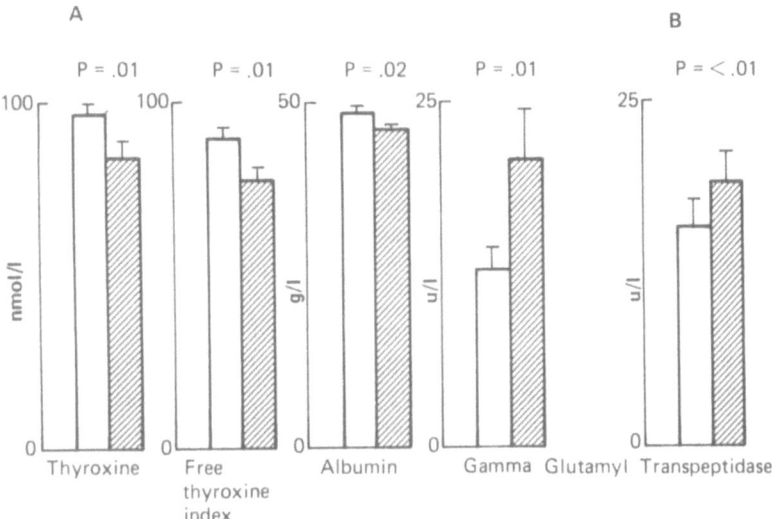

Figure 3. Thyroxine, free thyroxine index, serum albumin and γ-glutamyl transpeptidase levels before (□) and after (■) treatment with 0.8mg/kg/day 13-*cis*-RA (A); changes in γ-glutamyl transpeptidase levels before (□) and after (■) treatment with 0.05mg/kg/day 13-*cis*-RA (B).

Discussion

Our results show that CPA reduces SER, lesion count and acne severity in proportion to the dose given and that only 100mg and 25mg daily are therapeutically effective. However, only 100mg daily CPA significantly reduces dermal (i.e. sebaceous) lipogenesis (by 35 ± 16 per cent SEM) and the largely unchanged pattern of the ten component sebaceous lipids after treatment suggests that this reduction occurs by a general decrease in overall sebaceous lipid synthesis. It is clear that the decrease in libido experienced by half of the patients treated with CPA is not dissociable from the therapeutic effect of the drug and so it is unlikely to be an acceptable treatment for most males with acne.

The greatest reduction in SER (89 ± 4 per cent SEM) was found with 0.8mg/kg/day 13-*cis*-RA. Although the lower dose of 0.05mg/kg/day only reduced SER by 45 ± 9 per cent SEM the decrease in lesion count of 63 ± 10 per cent SEM and severity after 12 weeks was not significantly different from that produced by the higher dose, which agrees with the findings of Jones *et al.*[6] The effect of 13-*cis*-RA on dermal lipogenesis is commensurate with its greater effect on SER, with a 79 ± 23 per cent SEM decrease. The pattern of eight out of ten component sebaceous lipids extracted from dermis after treatment was significantly different suggesting

85.1 nmol/l $\pm$ 5.1, $p<0.01$) and in free thyroxine index (from a qualtitative as well as a quantitative effect on lipid synthesis). These findings, together with the increases of epidermal lipogenesis and serum lipids found with 13-*cis*-RA and absence of anti-androgen effect[7] suggest that its mechanism of action in acne is quite different from that of CPA. However, despite the likelihood that both drugs act differently, and despite using doses of each which fall on the linear part of the dose–SER response curve, we have found that the response to CPA and 13-*cis*-RA in combination is no greater than the response to 13-*cis*-RA alone: SER is reduced by 42 $\pm$ 13 per cent SEM and 45 $\pm$ 9 per cent SEM respectively and decreases in lesion count and severity were similar.

Although 13-*cis*-RA was well tolerated by patients, the changes in serum lipids and liver function tests were present with both doses. As it seems unlikely that 13-*cis*-RA will be effective at doses much below 0.05mg/kg/day then therapeutic effects and these biochemical side-effects are unlikely to be dissociable. Although the relationship between increased triglyceride and coronary artery disease (CAD) is unclear,[8] the association between increased serum cholesterol and CAD is well established. HDL-cholesterol levels also correlate inversely with CAD.[9] The decreases in thyroxine and free thyroxine index were not associated with a change in TSH values and seem too small to be a cause of secondary hyper-lipidaemia.

From these results we conclude that both CPA and 13-*cis*-RA are effective in treating acne and that 13-*cis*-RA is better tolerated. The different effects of the two drugs on the components of sebaceous lipid show that the mechanisms of inhibition of sebaceous lipogenesis are likely to be different. Finally, although combination of 13-*cis*-RA with CPA does not produce synergism, other methods (e.g. topical) of using 13-*cis*-RA ought to be considered as a means of avoiding or reducing the biochemical side-effects.

References

1. Cunliffe, W.J. and Shuster, S. (1969). Pathogenesis of acne. *Lancet*, **1**, 685
2. Shuster, S. (1983). Acne: the ashes of a burnt out controversy. In Epstein, E. (ed.). *Controversies in Dermatology*. In press. (Philadelphia: W.B. Saunders)
3. Archibald, A. and Shuster, S. (1969). The bioassay of androgens and anti-androgens using sebum secretion in the rat. *Proc. R. Soc. Med.*, **62**, 887
4. Cooper, M.F., McGrath, H. and Shuster, S. (1976). Sebaceous lipogenesis in human skin. *Br. J. Dermatol.*, **94**, 165
5. Cunliffe, W.J. and Shuster, S. (1969). The rate of sebum excretion in man. *Br. J. Dermatol.*, **81**, 697
6. Jones, D.H., King, K., Miller, A.J. and Cunliffe, W.J. (1983). A dose-response study of 13-*cis* retinoic acid in acne vulgaris. *Br. J. Dermatol.*, **108**, 333
7. Schill, W.B., Wagner, A., Nikolowski, J. and Plewig, G. (1981). *Aromatic Retinoid and 13-cis Retinoic acid: Spermatological Investigations*. p. 389. (Berlin, Heidelberg, New York: Springer-Verlag)

8. Hulley, S.B., Rosenman, R.H., Bawol, R.D. and Brand, R.J. (1980). Epidemiology as a guide to clinical decisions. The association between triglyceride and coronary heart disease. *N. Engl. J. Med.*, **302**, 1383

9. Miller, G.J. and Miller N.E. (1975). Plasma high density lipoprotein concentrations and development of ischaemic heart disease. *Lancet*, **1**, 16

29
Isotretinoin and Oral Contraceptive Steroids

M. ORME, D.J. BACK, W.J. CUNLIFFE, D.H. JONES, W.L. ALLEN and J. TJIA

Introduction

One of the clinical manifestations of vitamin A deficiency is hyperkeratosis and thus it was natural for synthetic vitamin A derivates to be made and tested in skin disorders where there is a disorder of keratinization. It is now known that at least two retinoids are of value in the treatment of skin diseases: 13-*cis*-retinoic acid (isotretinoin) in acne[1] and etretinate (Tigason) in psoriasis.[2] Both retinoids do have side-effects, however, and in particular teratogenic effects are noted in animals similar to those found in hypervitaminosis A. Hummler and Schupbach[3] found eye abnormalities, cleft palate, craniofacial malformations and defects of the axial and appendicular skeleton in the offspring of rats, rabbits and mice given 2–4mg/kg of etretinate.

Since retinoids, especially isotretinoin, may be given to young girls, it is important that adequate contraceptive precautions are taken by these patients. The oral contraceptive steroids are undoubtedly the most effective method of contraception and the use of these has been recommended in this situation. However, we need to be certain that there is no interaction between retinoids and oral contraceptive steroids that might diminish the efficacy of the contraceptive steroid. We have, therefore, examined the effect of isotretinoin on oral contraceptive steroids in a group of women treated with isotretinoin.

Methods

Patients

Ten women between the ages of 19 and 29 were studied. All patients were suffering from severe pustular acne and had agreed to enter a trial of isotretinoin treatment. As part of that study all patients were taking long-term oral contraceptive steroid therapy and had been receiving this treatment for at least 2 months. Before starting isotretinoin therapy blood samples (20ml) were taken into lithium heparin tubes on days 12, 13, 14 and 15 of the contraceptive cycle (day 1 is the first day of menstrual bleeding) between 22 and 24 h after the previous dose of the contraceptive. In addition blood samples (10ml) were also taken at the same time on days 21 and 23. All blood samples were centrifuged at 2,000 rpm for 10 min and the plasma was pipetted off and stored at $-20°C$ until analysed. The clinical studies were performed in Leeds and the plasma samples dispatched in dry ice to Liverpool.

The oral contraceptives used were Gynovlar (50μg ethinyloestradiol (EE) and 3mg norethisterone (N)) in one patient, Microgynon 30 (30μg EE and 150μg levonorgestrel (Ng)) in three patients, Eugynon 30 (30μg EE and 250μg Ng) in three patients, Ovranette (30μg EE and 150μg Ng) in one patient, Norinyl (Mestranol 50μg and 1mg N) in one patient and Trinordiol in one patient. Trinordiol is a triphasic preparation of EE_2 and Ng.

Two 24-hour urine collections were also made on days 10–11 and 11–12 of the cycle.

Isotretinoin therapy was started on day 23 of the first cycle in a daily dose of 0.5mg/kg such that a women weighing less than 45kg received 2×10mg capsules daily. Patients weighing between 46 and 54 kg received 25mg daily and patients more than 55kg in weight received 30mg/day. The

Table 1. Plasma concentrations of ethinyloestradiol, levonorgestrel and progesterone in the first two patients. Mean ± SE ($n = 3$).

Patient	Control cycle	1st Isotretinoin cycle	2nd Isotretinoin cycle
Plasma ethinyloestradiol concentration (pg/ml)			
V.H.	78 ± 6.8	52 ± 13	28 ± 9.2
N.W.	49 ± 4.9	29*	12*
Plasma levonorgestrel concentration (ng/ml)			
V.H.	0.5 ± 0.3	≤ 0.1	≤ 0.1
N.W.	1.0 ± 0.1	0.9*	≤ 0.1*
Plasma progesterone concentration (pg/ml)			
V.H.	≤ 120	≤ 120	2300 ± 264
N.W.	140 ± 10	≤ 120*	≤ 120*

*Mean of two values

blood and urine sampling was repeated (exactly as in the 1st cycle) in the 2nd cycle of contraceptive use (the first cycle of isotretinoin use) and in the 4th cycle of contraceptive use (the 3rd month of isotretinoin therapy). Isotretinoin therapy was stopped after 3 months. All gave their informed consent to the study which had been approved by the local ethics committee.

Plasma concentrations of ethinyloestradiol were measured by a radio-immunoassay (RIA) that is sensitive to EE in the presence of N or Ng[4]. Plasma concentrations of norethisterone,[5] levonorgestrel,[6] follicle stimu-lating hormone (FSH)[7] and progesterone[8] were also measured by radio-immunoassay. Concentrations of 6β-hydroxycortisol were measured in the 24-hour urine samples by the radioimmunoassay method of Park.[9]

Statistical Methods

The difference between subjects, in the various analyses performed in the control cycle and the isotretinoin cycle were assessed by the use of Student's *t*-test for paired data.

Results

Five patients have completed the study and at the present time the remainder of the patients have been studied over one cycle before isotretinoin therapy and one cycle after starting isotretinoin.

The first patients to be examined in this study (V.H. and N.W.) showed a marked fall in their plasma concentrations of ethinyloestradiol and levonorgestrel during the two isotretinoin cycles as compared to the control value (Table 1). No clinically untoward events were noted and in particular no breakthrough bleeding was seen which might have indicated a failure of contraception. In patient V.H. (see Table 1) there was a significant rise of progesterone during the 3rd isotretinoin cycle but not to levels diagnostic of ovulation. The results of the plasma concentrations of ethinyloestradiol in the five patients who have completed the study are shown in Table 2. Overall there is no significant change in the plasma concentration of ethinyloestradiol during iostretinoin therapy. Patient A.W. had a marked rise in the plasma ethinyloestradiol concentration during the third cycle of isotretinoin therapy.

Table 3 shows the results of the plasma ethinyloestradiol concentrations in the five remaining patients who have so far completed 1 month of isotretinoin therapy. There is no significant change in the plasma con-centration of ethinyloestradiol, being 25 ± 2.7pg/ml in the control cycle and 29.2 ± 6.3pg/ml in the first isotretinoin cycle ($p > 0.1$). If the values for all ten patients are considered, the mean figure in the control cycle is

Table 2. Plasma concentrations of ethinyloestradiol during 3 months of isotretinoin therapy (pg/ml). Mean ± SE (*n* = 3).

Patient	Control	Isotretinoin Cycle 1	Isotretinoin Cycle 3
V.H.	78 ±6.8	52 ± 13	28 ± 9.2
J.S.	43 ± 0.9	43 ± 4.5	26 ± 7.8
T.T.	51 ± 7.7	49 ± 6.6	56 ± 3.8
A.W.	42 ± 3.0	29 ± 6.0	121.5*
N.W.	49 ± 4.9	29*	12*
Mean ± SE *p* ≥ 0.1	52.4 ±6.6	40.4 ± 4.8	48.7 ± 19

*Mean of two values

Table 3. Plasma concentrations of ethinyloestradiol during 1 month of isotretinoin therapy (pg/ml). Mean ± SE (*n* = 3).

Patient	Control	Isotretinoin
B.A.	25 ± 6	53 ±17.2
S.C.	18 ± 2	19 ± 9
K.G.	33 ± 8	22 ± 6
E.N.	30 ± 3.5	31 ± 5.9
M.P.	34 ± 3.8	21 ± 4.5
Mean ± SE *p* ≥ 0.1	25 ± 2.7	29.2 ± 6.3

Table 4. Plasma concentrations of levonorgestrel during isotretinoin therapy (ng/ml). Mean ± SD.

Patient	Control cycle	1st Isotretinoin cycle		3rd Isotretinoin cycle
B.A.	0.6 ±0.1	1.4 ± 0.5		–
S.C.	0.8 ± 0.09	1.03 ± 0.24		–
K.G.	2.5 ± 0.5	1.8 ± 0.5		–
V.H.	0.5 ± 0.3	≤ 0.1		≤ 0.1
E.N.	1.2 ± 0.08	1.1 ± 0.26		–
M.P.	1.4 ± 0.1	0.9 ± 0.1		–
J.S.	0.5 ± 0.1	0.5 ± 0.2		1.3 ± 0.3
T.T.	1.03 ± 0.4	0.83 ± 0.28		1.06 ± 0.37
A.W.	1.2 ± 0.5	≤ 0.1		2.3*
N.W.	1.0 ± 0.1	0.9*		≤ 0.1
Mean ± SE For all ten patients	1.07 ± 0.19	0.87 ± 0.17	*p* ≥ 0.1	–
For five complet- ing study	0.85 ± 0.14	0.68 ± 0.17	*p* ≥ 0.1	0.97 ± 0.41

*Mean of two values

Table 5. Urininary excretion of 6β-hydroxycortisol before (cycle 1) and during (cycle 2) isotretinoin therapy (μg/day). Each value is the mean of two 24-hour urine collections.

Patient	Cycle 1	Cycle 2
B.A.	145	47
S.C.	160	84
K.G.	114	113
V.H.	297	214
E.N.	199	196
M.P.	147	87
J.S.	180	214
T.T.	297	241
N.W.	292	134
Mean ± SE ($p \geqslant 0.025$)	203.4 ± 24.3	147.7 ± 23.3

40.2 ± 5.3pg/ml and 34.8 ± 4.2pg/ml in the first isotretinoin cycle ($p>0.1$). The data for the levonorgestrel plasma concentrations are shown in Table 4. Although plasma concentrations of levonorgestrel fell during isotretinoin therapy in the first two individuals studied (patients V.H. and A.W.) there was no significant change in the group as a whole. The mean plasma levonorgestrel concentrations in the control cycle was 1.07 ± 0.19ng/ml and 0.87 ± 0.17ng/ml in the first isotretinoin cycle ($p>0.1$, $n = 10$). No significant effects have so far been detected in the FSH or progesterone values.

The results of the 6β-hydroxycortisol assays are shown in Table 5 for nine of the ten women. The mean (±SE) 6β-hydroxycortisol excretion in the control cycle was 203.4 ± 24.3μg/day and during the first month of isotretinoin therapy this figure decreased significantly to 147.7 ± 23.3μg/day ($p>0.025$). However, the urine volumes were lower in the isotretinoin cycle (787.0 ± 82ml/day) compared to the control cycle (1008 ± 95.5ml/day, $p>0.01$).

Discussion

The early results from this study suggested that isotretinoin was reducing the efficacy of the combined contraceptive steroids. In patients V.H. and N.W., marked falls in the plasma concentration of ethinyloestradiol and levonorgestrel were noted (see Table 1) and in patient V.H. a rise in the plasma progesterone concentration was seen in the third month of iso-tretinoin therapy. A rise in plasma progesterone concentration is usually taken as evidence of failure of contraception and that a corpus luteum has developed after ovulation. In this case, however, the rise in progesterone was not high enough to reach ovulatory levels (usually $\geqslant$ 20,000pg/ml). Even though the blood samples were not taken at the times of expected progesterone peaks (days 21–22) it seems unlikely that patient V.H. did in fact ovulate. Further studies in all ten patients have not suggested any systematic effect of isotretinoin on ethinyloestradiol kinetics.

A fall in the plasma ethinyloestradiol concentration could be due to a reduced bioavailability of EE caused by isotretinoin. This would be an unusual interaction since EE is well absorbed in women though its mean bioavailability is only about 40 per cent due to first pass metabolism in the gut wall and the liver. To further reduce the bioavailability of EE, the first pass effect would have to be enhanced by isotretinoin and there is no precedent for such an interaction with a drug that is not an enzyme-inducing agent. Enzyme induction could account for the fall in the plasma EE concentration but one of the best indices of enzyme induction is a rise in the urinary excretion of 6β-hydroxycortisol which was not seen in this study. If anything, there was a fall in the 6β-hydroxycortisol excretion during isotretinoin therapy but urine volumes were low during the isotretinoin cycle – sometimes as low as 320ml or 180ml for a complete 24-hour collection. Thus it is difficult to interpret these data with any accuracy but it seems unlikely that enzyme induction had been produced by isotretinoin.

In patient A.W. a rise in the plasma ethinyloestradiol concentration was seen in the third month of isotretinoin therapy. The radioimmunoassay for EE was validated in this study by adding pure isotretinoin to the standard curves and by analysing plasma from male patients known to have taken isotretinoin. No ethinyloestradiol was detected in the male plasma samples but high concentrations of isotretinoin (200–500ng/ml) did displace ethinyloestradiol from its binding to the antibody *in vitro*. When samples, spiked with isotretinoin, were carried through the complete assay for EE there was a slight interference only at the highest isotretinoin concentration used (500ng/ml). This interference would have the effect of producing falsely high concentrations of EE in the plasma and thus the high concentration of EE in patient A.W. could be explained if her isotretinoin concentrations in plasma were unusually high.

The studies to date do not suggest any systematic interaction between isotretinoin and oral contraceptive steroids and our studies on this matter are continuing.

References

1. Peck, G.L., Olsen, T.G., Yoder, F.W., Strauss, J.S., Downing, D.T., Pandya, M., Butkus, D. and Arnaud-Batandier, J. (1979). Prolonged remissions of cystic and conglobate acne with 13-*cis*-retinoic acid. *N. Engl. J. Med.*, **300**, 329

2. Fredriksson, T. and Pettersson, U. (1978). Severe psoriasis – oral therapy with a new retinoid. *Dermatologica*, **157**, 238

3. Hummler, H. and Schupbach, M.E. (1981). Studies in reproductive toxicology and mutagenicity with Ro 10-9359. In Orfanos, C.E. *et al.* (eds.). *Retinoids: Advances in Basic Research and Therapy*. pp. 49–59. (Berlin: Springer-Verlag)

4. Back, D.J., Breckenridge, A.M., Crawford, F.E., MacIver, M., Orme, M.L'E., Rowe, P.H. and Watts, M.J. (1979). An investigation of the pharmacokinetics of ethynylestradiol in women using radioimmunoassay. *Contraception*, **20**, 263

5. Back, D.J., Breckenridge, A.M., Crawford, F.E., MacIver, M., Orme, M.L'E., Rowe, P.H. and Smith, E. (1978). The pharmacokinetics of norethindrone in women 1. Radioimmunoassay and concentrations during multiple dosing. *Clin. Pharmacol. Ther.*, **24**, 439

6. Back, D.J., Bates, M., Breckenridge, A.M., Hall, J.M., MacIver, M., Orme, M.L'E, Park, B.K. and Rowe, P.H. (1981). The pharmacokinetics of levonorgestrel and ethynylestradiol in women. Studies with Ovran and Ovranette. *Contraception*, **23**, 229

7. Wide, L., Nillius, S.J., Gremzell, C. and Roos, P. (1973). Radioimmunosorbent assay of follicle stimulating hormone and luteinizing hormone in serum and urine from men and women. *Acta Endocrinol. Suppl.*, **174**, 1

8. Israel, R., Mishell, D.R., Stone, S.C., Thorneycroft, I.H. and Moyer, D.L. (1971). Single luteal phase progesterone assay as an indicator of ovulation. *Am. J. Obstet. Gynecol.*, **122**, 1043

9. Park, B.K. (1979). A direct radioimmunoassay for 6β-hydroxycortisol in human urine. *J. Steroid Biochem.*, **9**, 963

Section 8

Comparisons of Isotretinoin with other Drugs in the Treatment of Severe Acne

30
Comparison of Isotretinoin and Cyproterone Acetate – a Clinical and Laboratory Study

R. GREENWOOD, D.H. JONES and L. BRUMMITT

Introduction

In 1966 Neumann and Elger[1] first showed that the anti-androgen cyproterone acetate (CPA) reduced the output of the sebaceous glands of mice. This interested those involved in the treatment of acne. The first regime to be used in women was the 'reverse sequential' regime of Hammerstein[2] who gave 100mg of CPA from day 5 to day 15 of the cycle and 50μg of oestrogen from day 5 to day 26. This regime was used to ensure that withdrawal bleeding occurred on completion of the cycle, because of the strong progestrogenic effect, and depot storing of this high dose of CPA. This method of treatment was found to be successful, with rates of response of 70 per cent improvement after 3 months of treatment being claimed. However, because of the potent unphysiological effect of this dose of CPA, a lower dose combination preparation was developed as an oral contraceptive with 2mg of CPA and 50μg of ethinyloestradiol (Diane, Schering).

The first reports of its use in the treatment of acne in women were in 1977 by Breckwoldt et al.[3] as the results of a multicentre study on 514 women. Its efficacy as an oral contraceptive had been proven by its use in many thousands of women-years. This study and subsequent ones such as that of Lachnit-Fixson[4] used subjective methods only for the evaluation of clinical improvement, detailing only good, bad or indifferent responses. A small study[5] on ten patients comparing three oral contraceptives was the first to show a reduction in sebum excretion rate (SER) using the gravimetric technique, rather than only commenting on the subjective fall in seborrhoea.

A recent comparative open study[6] comparing tetracycline and 2mg CPA and 50μg ethinyloestradiol gave encouraging preliminary results for the use of the contraceptive preparation. There have, however, been no double-blind comparisons of conventional acne treatment and the low dose CPA to assess the relative value of this preparation in the treatment of acne, nor has there been any comparison with the more recently introduced 13-*cis*-retinoic acid. With the advent of 13-*cis*-retinoic acid and the reports of its beneficial effect in cystic acne,[7] it has become even more pressing for such work to be undertaken to gain a realistic view of the various therapies to assess their place in the treatment of antibiotic-resistant acne in women.

Patients and Methods

Thirty women between the ages of 16 and 30 with antibiotic-resistant acne were treated, 15 with 0.5mg/kg of isotretinoin and 15 with 2mg CPA and 50μg ethinyloestradiol. All women had been taken off all treatment for at

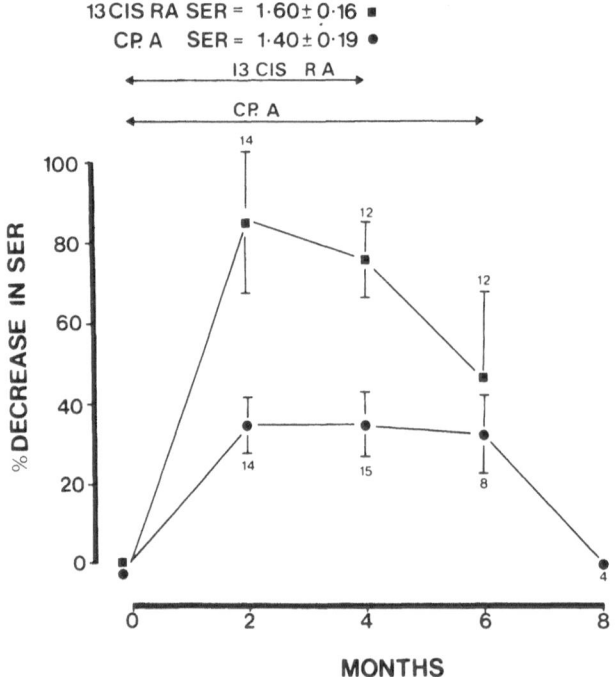

Figure 1. Comparison of decrease in SER.

288

least 1 month prior to starting their treatment, and had had prolonged ineffective courses of oral antibiotics before this. Both groups of women were assessed by means of SER measured by the gravimetric technique of Strauss and Pochi[8], as modified by Cunliffe and Shuster,[9] by clinical assessment of acne grade by the Leeds technique,[10] and by the counting of inflamed acne lesions on the face. All the clinical assessments in each group of women were undertaken by the same observer. Each group of patients was assessed under double-blind conditions as each was part of a larger study undertaken to evaluate the separate treatments. The women receiving isotretinoin were treated for 4 months with a follow-up period of 2 months. Those receiving the CPA were treated for 6 months, with a similar 2 month follow-up period.

Results

The results are shown in Figures 1–4. The mean change in SER, expressed as a percentage fall is shown in Figure 1 at 2, 4 and 6 months, and at 2 months off treatment. The results are significantly different ($p > 0.001$) with isotretinoin causing an 80 per cent fall in SER and CPA a 34 per cent

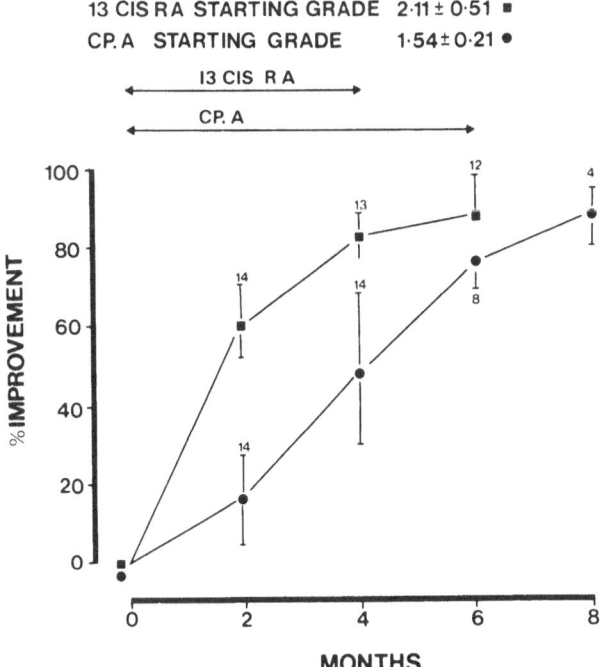

Figure 2. Comparison of improvement in facial acne grade.

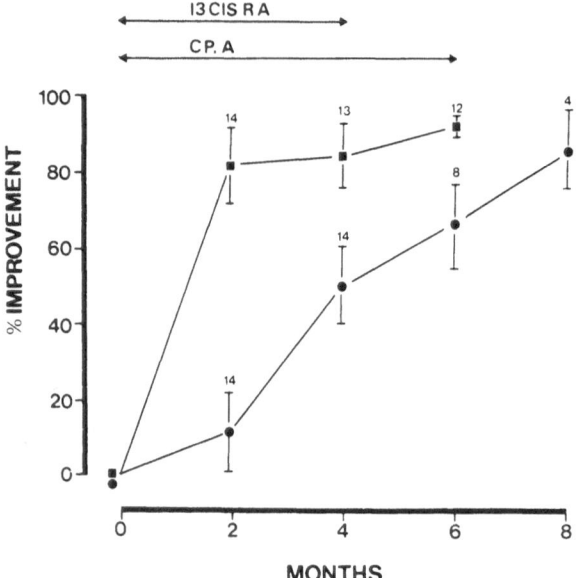

13CIS R A STARTING GRADE 3·91 ± 0·22 ■
C.P. A STARTING GRADE   2·69 ± 0·26 ●

Figure 3. Comparison of improvement in total acne grade.

fall in SER. By the end of the 2-month follow-up period the SER had returned to normal in the CPA group, but only to 54 per cent of normal in the isotretinoin group. This difference is paralleled by the improvement in acne grade (facial and total), Figures 2 and 3, and the lesional count (Figure 4). There was a much slower response to the CPA than the isotretinoin. By the end of the treatment periods the isotretinoin still showed a significantly better response ($p > 0.05$) than the CPA; however, at the end of the follow-up period this difference had been eliminated. This trend was mirrored by the acne-inflamed lesion count.

Discussion

From this comparative study it can be seen that both isotretinoin and CPA are effective at lowering the SER and at improving clinical acne. The optimal length of treatment using the CPA has probably not yet been shown as indicated by the continued improvement of the acne once treatment had been discontinued.

Until the introduction of these two drugs the choice of treatment for this group of antibiotic-resistant women with acne had been limited. An

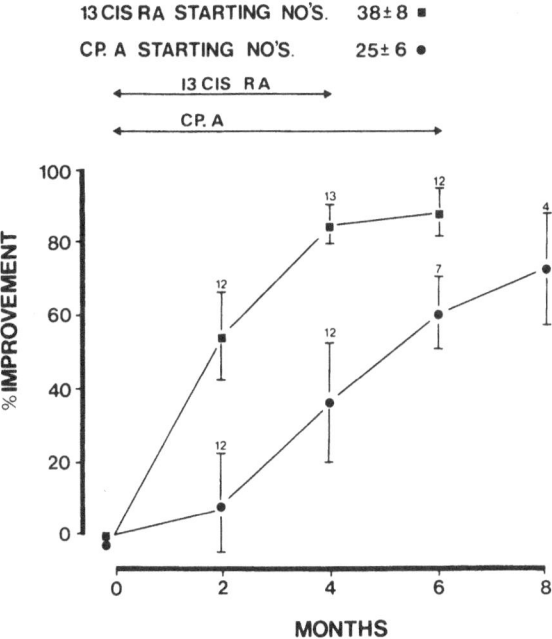

Figure 4. Comparison of improvement in number of inflamed acne lesions on face.

important aetiological factor in acne is the SER[9] and both these drugs lower the SER. It has previously been shown that high dose oestrogens lower the SER and also are useful in the treatment of acne,[11] but the dose of oestrogen required, 100μg, gave an unacceptably high rate of side-effects. Women taking a relatively oestrogenic contraceptive pill have been found to have a statistically significantly lower SER than an age-matched population of women not taking an oral contraceptive.[12] More progestagenic preparations may exacerbate acne. Diane combines a relatively high dose of oestrogen, 50μg of ethinyloestradiol, with an anti-androgenic progestagen.

Many women between the ages of 16 and 30 are taking oral contraceptive preparations and this preparation may, therefore, be highly relevant to such a population who have antibiotic-resistant acne. This preparation does seem to be relatively slow acting, although effective. However, in those women in whom a hormonal preparation is contra-indicated, e.g. high blood pressure, history of thromboembolism, or in whom a more rapid rate of response is required, isotretinoin provides an effective alternative. It is always useful in the clinical situation to have as many options as possible and both these preparations would seem acceptable successful alternatives to antibiotics.

References

1. Neumann, F. and Elger, W. (1966). The effect of a new anti-androgenic steroid 6-chloro-17-hydroxy-1α, 2α-methylenepregna-4,6-diene-3,20-dione acetate (cyproterone acetate) on the sebaceous glands of mice. *J. Invest. Dermatol.*, **40**, 561

2. Hammerstein, J., Meckies, J. and Leo-Rouberg, (1975). Use of cyproterone acetate in the treatment of acne, hirsutism and virilism. *J. Steroid Biochem.*, **6**, 827

3. Breckwoldt, M., Trolp, R., Braendle, W., Roll, H. and Rachel, F. (1977). Anti-androgen oral contraceptives. In Haspels, A.A. and Kay, C.R. (eds.). *International Symposium on Hormonal Contraception.* pp. 81–88. (Amsterdam: Excerpta Medica)

4. Lachnit-Fixson, U. (1979). The development and evaluation of an ovulation inhibitor (Diane) containing an anti-androgen. *Acta Obstet. Gynecol. Scand. Suppl.*, **88**, 33

5. Leis, D. and Clarin, A. (1979). Vergleich der Talgsekrenon der Shernhaut bei Behandlung mit drei Kontrazeptivear Pillen. *Geburtshilfe Frauenheilkd*, **39**, 54

6. Mugglestone, C.J. and Rhodes, E.L. (1982). The treatment of acne with an anti-androgen/oestrogen combination. *Clin. Exp. Dermatol.*, **7**, 593

7. Peck, G.L., Thomas, T.G., Voder, F.W., Strauss, J.S., Downing, D.T., Pandya, M., Butkus, D. and Arnaud-Battandier, J. (1979). Prolonged remissions of cystic and conglobata acne with 13-*cis*-retinoic acid. *N. Engl. J. Med.I*, **300**, 329

8. Strauss, J.S. and Pochi, J.E. (1961). The quantitative gravimetric determination of sebum production. *J. Invest. Dermatol.*, **36**, 293

9. Cunliffe, W.J. and Shuster, S. (1969). The pathogenesis of acne. *Lancet*, **1**, 685

10. Burke, B. and Cunliffe, W.J. (1983). A simple technique for acne grading. (In preparation)

11. Pye, R.J., Meyrick, G., Pye, M.J. and Burton, J.L. (1977). Effect of oral contraceptives on sebum excretion rate. *Br. Med. J.*, **2**, 1581

12. Strauss, J.S. and Pochi, P.E. 1963). The sebaceous gland – regulation by steroidal hormones. *Recent Prog. Horm. Res.*, **19**, 385

31
A Comparative Study of 13-*cis*-Retinoic Acid and Erythromycin Therapy in Severe Acne

D.H. JONES, W.J. CUNLIFFE and A. LÖFFLER

Introduction

13-*cis*-retinoic acid is now accepted as being effective in severe cystic acne[1-4] and has been shown to be superior to both placebo[5] and the aromatic retinoid (etretinate).[6] However, it has not been compared against a conventional regime of antibiotics and topical agents. This study investigates the results of three treatment regimes using 13-*cis*-retinoic acid and oral erythromycin.

Table 1. Patient demography.

Treatment group	13-*cis-retinoic acid*	Combination	Erythromycin
Numbers total	26	24	27
Female	8	7	11
Age (years)	24	24	22
(range)	(14–50)	(16–50)	(14–43)
Duration of disease and range (years)	9.3 (2–30)	10.1 (1–36)	8.1 (2–21)
Acne grade	6.35±0.71	5.28±0.51	6.52±0.78
Acne lesion count	64±9	58±6	76±11
Sebum excretion rate (μg/cm^2/min)	1.80±0.11	1.66±0.13	1.75±0.13

Methods

Ninety patients have been entered into the study but only 77 patients have completed the treatment period (Table 1). All the patients had moderate to severe acne of long duration and had discontinued previous therapy 6 weeks prior to entering the study. The patients were randomly allocated to three treatment groups and the randomization code was stratified to ensure an equal severity of acne in each group. The treatment groups were:

(1)   13-*cis*-retinoic acid active, erythromycin placebo,

(2)   13-*cis*-retinoic acid active, erythromycin active,

(3)   13-*cis*-retinoic acid placebo, erythromycin active.

The dose of 13-*cis*-retinoic acid was 0.5mg/kg body-weight. The dose of erythromycin was 250mg orally four times per day. No other therapy was prescribed. 13-*cis*-retinoic acid was given for 16 weeks and erythromycin for 24 weeks. The study was conducted double-blind.

The following observations have been made on the patients:

(1)   Assessment of acne grade – face, back and chest.

(2)   Count of acne lesions on the face – non -, superficial and deep inflamed.

(3)   Clinical side-effects.

(4)   Liver function tests, fasting plasma lipids, urea and electrolytes and full blood count.

Table 2.   Patient attendance.

Weeks	0	4	8	16	24	32
13-cis-*retinoic acid*						
Attended	26	26	23	23	21	14
Withdrawn	0	0	3	3	4	5
Failed to attend	0	0	0	0	1	2
Total	26	26	26	26	26	21
Combination						
Attended	24	21	21	19	17	13
Withdrawn	0	1	1	1	2	3
Failed to attend	0	2	2	4	5	6
Total	24	24	24	24	24	22
Erythromycin						
Attended	27	26	24	24	16	8
Withdrawn	0	0	1	1	7	12
Failed to attend	0	1	2	2	4	5
Total	27	27	27	27	27	25

(5)   Sebum excretion rate (SER) by the gravimetric method.[7]

(6)   Facial skin microflora.

The observations were made at 0, 4, 8, 16 and 24 weeks. Follow-up has been made at 32, 44 and 52 weeks.

Results

Attendance (Table 2)

Two patients were withdrawn from the 13-*cis*-retinoic acid group because of side-effects (arthralgia and diarrhoea), and one patient because of a failure to adhere to the protocol. Two other patients relapsed requiring further therapy from their 16 and 24 week visits respectively.

In the combination group, one patient was withdrawn because of facial dermatitis at 4 weeks, and another at 23 weeks because of an exacerbation of her diverticulitis. One patient required 13-*cis*-retinoic acid from 24 weeks because of residual lesions.

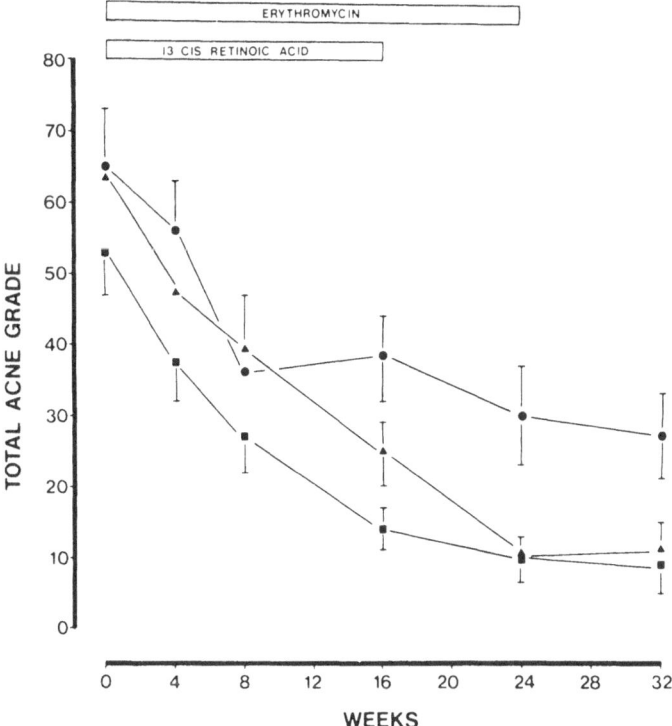

Figure 1.   Response in acne grade vs. time. Key: mean ± SE ●, erythromycin only; ▲, 13-*cis*-RA only; ■, erythromycin ± 13-*cis*-RA.

In the erythromycin group, one patient was withdrawn at 8 weeks because of failure to adhere to the protocol. Six patients were withdrawn from 16 weeks, and a further six after 24 weeks, because of a failure to improve and request for further treatment. They were all placed on active 13-*cis*-retinoic acid.

Acne Grade (Figure 1)

At 16 weeks the greatest improvement was seen in the combination group (73 per cent) and the least improvement was in the erythromycin group (41 per cent). The 13-*cis*-retinoic acid group improved by 62 per cent.

At 24 weeks the combination group had improved further to 81 per cent. The 13-*cis*-retinoic acid group had continued to improve in spite of not being on active therapy and had also achieved an improvement of 83 per cent. The erythromycin group achieved considerably less improvement (54 per cent).

There was no marked relapse of the acne in any of the groups during the 8-week follow-up period.

As in previous studies, the degree of improvement was greater on the face than on the back, and this is especially seen in the erythromycin group (Table 3).

Table 3. Response of difference sites of the acne at 24 weeks (percentage improvement).

Treatment	13-cis-retinoic acid	Combination	Erythromycin
Face	82	90	69
Back	85	76	34
Chest	72	74	30

Acne Lesions (Figure 2)

The pattern of improvement is the same as with the acne grade. The combination group reached a 90 per cent improvement by 16 weeks, which was maintained. The 13-*cis*-retinoic acid group improved to the same extent but more slowly – 76 per cent at 16 weeks and 90 per cent at 24 weeks. The erythromycin group did less well, achieving a 58 per cent and 59 per cent improvement at 16 and 24 weeks respectively.

In the two retinoic acid groups, all lesions were cleared equally well. The erythromycin group did less well, and, interestingly, the antibiotic had far less effect on the non-inflamed lesions (Table 4).

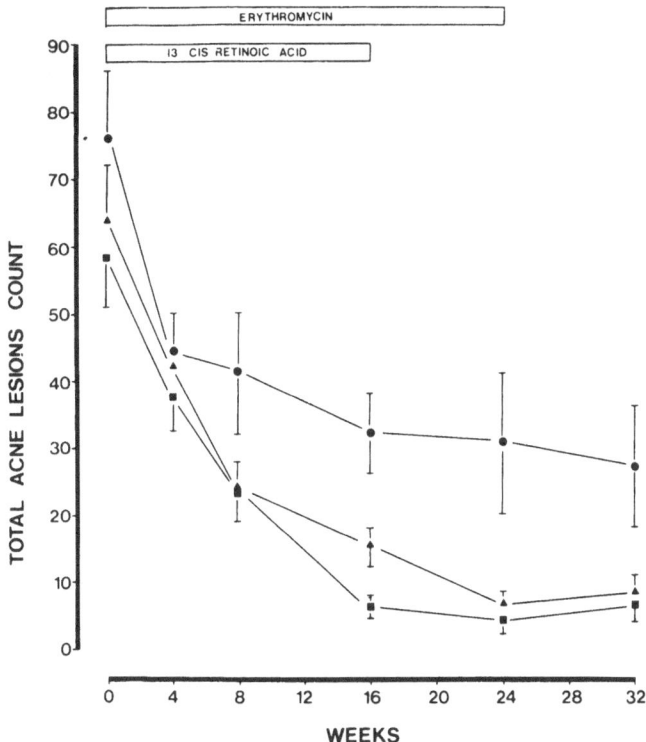

Figure 2. Response in acne lesions vs. time. Key: ●, mean ± SE erythromycin only; ▲, 13-*cis*-RA only; ■, erythromycin ± 13-*cis*-RA.

Table 4. Response of different acne lesions at 24 weeks (percentage improvement).

Treatment	13-cis-*retinoic acid*	Combination	Erythromycin
Non-inflamed	87	85	39
Superficially inflamed	92	95	73
Deep inflamed	90	96	66

Sebum Excretion Rate (Figure 3)

The SER was reduced by 88 and 89 per cent in the two 13-*cis*-retinoic acid groups by 16 weeks, and gradually returned over the next 16 weeks to 40-50 per cent of the pre-treatment levels. There was no change in the erythromycin group. This was the same pattern that we have reported previously.

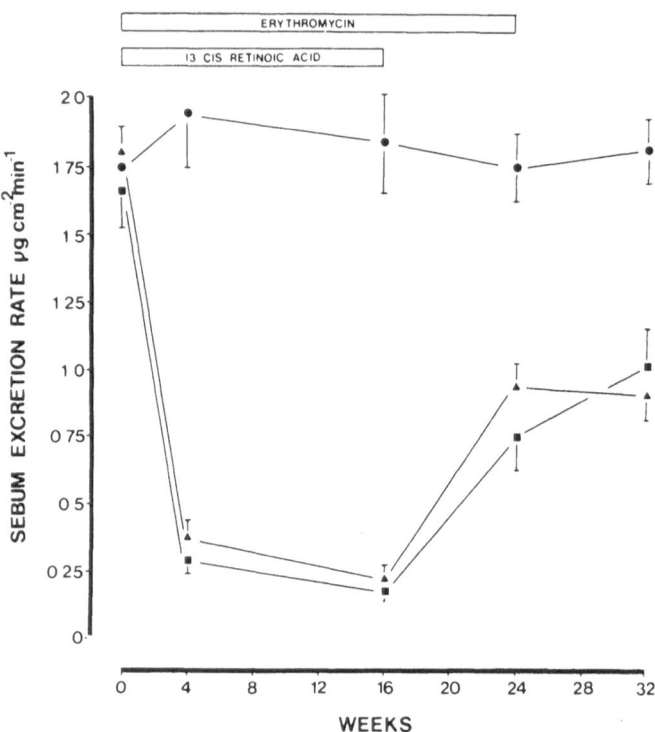

Figure 3. Response of sebum excretion rate vs. time. Key: mean ± SE ●, erythromycin only; ▲, 13-*cis*-RA only; ■, erythromycin ± 13-*cis*-RA.

Side-Effects

Clinical

The range of side-effects seen was the same as in other studies, though the incidence of individual ones varied (Table 5). Epistaxis, arthralgia, desquamation, conjunctivitis and pruritus were all higher in incidence but this was probabaly due, in part, to over-reporting of minor side-effects. There was also variation between the two 13-*cis*-retinoic acid groups in some of the side-effects – facial dermatitis, epistaxis and pruritus.

There was a surprisingly high incidence of side-effects in the erythromycin group suggesting a high placebo effect in terms of the expectation of side-effects.

Biochemical

(1) SGOT. It is interesting to note that the mean levels in all the groups were above the normal range pre-treatment (Figure 4). In the

Table 5. Incidence of clinical side-effects (percentage).

Treatment	13-cis-*retinoic acid*	Combination	Erythromycin
Cheilitis	100	92	66
Facial Dermatitis	96	63	41
Epistaxis	63	38	8
Desquamation	52	42	24
Pruritus	52	38	34
Conjunctivitis	41	29	10
Headaches	37	29	38
Arthralgia	30	29	45
Malaise	19	13	24
Alopecia	7	4	10
Diarrhoea	7	8	21
Thrush	0	4	0

erythromycin group, the level fell steadily during therapy. This presumably represented adherence by the patients to strict injunctures at the start of the trial to avoid alcohol! A rise was seen in the two retinoic acid groups at

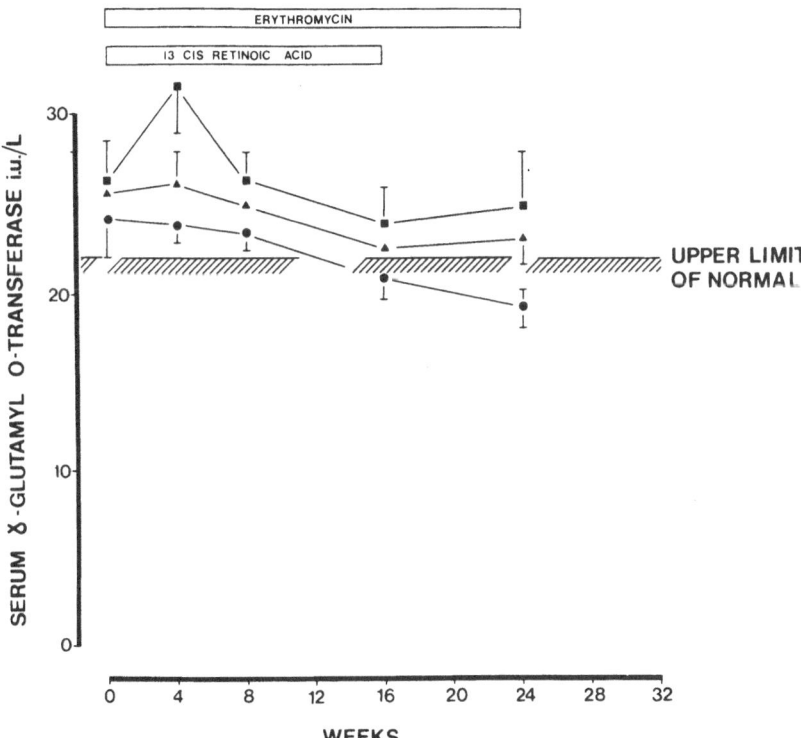

Figure 4. Change of serum γ-glutamyl-*O*-transferase vs. time. Key: mean ± SE ●, erythromycin only; ▲, 13-*cis*-RA only; ■, erythromycin ± 13-*cis*-RA.

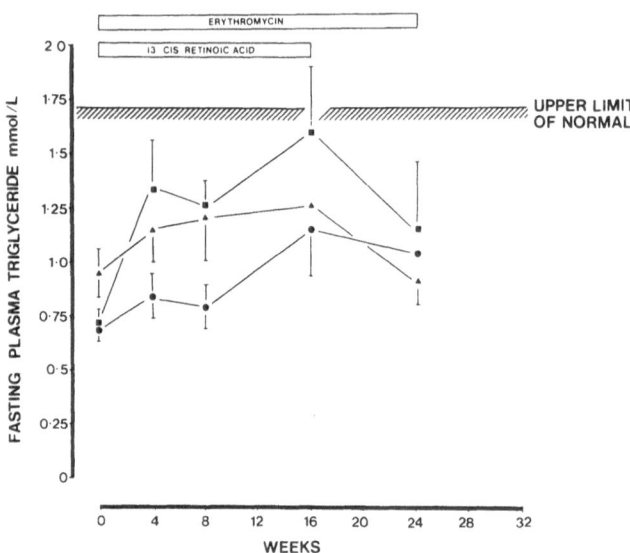

Figure 5. Change of fasting plasma triglycerides vs. time. Key: mean ± SE ●, erythromycin only; ▲, 13-*cis*-RA only; ■, erythromycin ± 13-*cis*-RA.

4 weeks therapy and the levels then settled during therapy. This pattern accorded with the results from our previous study.

(2) Fasting lipids. There was a gradual rise in all groups towards 16 weeks and the levels then settled (Figure 5). None of the mean levels rose above the upper limit of normal. There was the same order of rise in the 13-*cis*-retinoic acid group as in the erythromycin group and a much greater rise in the combination group.

Discussion

This study confirms various observations on antibiotic therapy in acne that other workers have made.

(1) There is a 41 per cent improvement at 4 months.[7] The 54 per cent improvement at 6 months is disappointing but reflects that this is a difficult group of patients, being older and with a longer duration of disease.

(2) Facial acne does much better than truncal acne.[8]

(3) Non-inflamed lesions do not do well with antibiotics.

There are, however, some curious discrepancies – the very high incidence of side-effects, the fall in the SGOT and the rise in fasting lipids.

The latter is particularly important as this has been a major stumbling block in the recommendation for the use of 13-*cis*-retinoic acid.

13-*cis*-retinoic acid has been shown to be much more effective than erythromycin in this study – especially as half the patients in the erythromycin group needed to be placed on active 13-*cis*-retinoic acid by 24 weeks. Though the pattern of improvement in the facial and truncal acne is the same as with erythromycin, 13-*cis*-retinoic acid has produced a much greater improvement in the truncal acne. 13-*cis*-retinoic acid is also more effective in clearing non-inflamed lesions.

One benefit that the combination has is to produce a more rapid rate of improvement, though the final level of improvment is no better than with 13-*cis*-retinoic acid alone.

It would appear, therefore, that 13-*cis*-retinoic acid in this dosage can be routinely used as a single agent and there is no great benefit from combining it with erythromycin. However, it remains to be seen whether the combination produces a lower relapse rate and longer remission period. Another option not yet explored is the benefit of very low doses added to routine antibiotic therapy.

Acknowledgements

We would like to thank Mr R.A. Forster for his technical advice, Mrs J. Mitchell for her technical assistance, Mrs P. Hick for secretarial help and Dr A.J. Miller, Roche Products Ltd. for support.

References

1. Peck, G.L., Olsen, T.G., Yoder, F.W., Strauss, J.S., Downing, D.T., Pandya, M., Butkus, D. and Arnaud-Battandier, J. (1979). Prolonged remissions of cystic and conglobate acne with 13-*cis*-retinoic acid. *N. Engl. J. Med.*, **300**, 329
2. Farrell, L.N., Strauss, J.S. and Stranieri, A.M. (1980). The treatment of severe cystic acne with 13-*cis*-retinoic acid. *J. Am. Acad. Dermatol.*, **3**, 602
3. Jones, D.H., King, K., Miller, A.J. and Cunliffe, W.J. (1983). A dose response study of 13-*cis*-retinoic acid in acne vulgaris. *Br. J. Dermatol.*, **108**, 333
4. Plewig, G., Nikolowski, J. and Wolf, H.H. (1982). Action of isotretinoin in acne rosacea and gram-negative folliculitis. *J. Am. Acad. Dermatol.*, **6**, 766
5. Peck, G.L., Olsen, T.G., Butkus, D., Pandya, M., Arnaud-Battandier, J., Gross, E.G., Windhortst, D.B. and Cheripko, J. (1982). Isotretinion versus placebo in the treatment of cystic acne. *J. Am. Acad. Dermatol.*, **6**, 735
6. Goldstein, J.A., Socha-Szott, A., Thomsen, R.J., Pochi, P.E., Shalita, A.R. and Strauss, J.S. (1982). Comparative effect of isotretinoin and etretinate on acne and sebaceous gland secretion. *J. Am. Acad. Dermatol.*, **6**, 760
7. Greenwood, R. and Cunliffe, W.J. (1982). Rate of response of acne related to sebum excretion rate and antibiotic dosage *Br. J. Dermatol.*, **107**, Suppl. 22, 24
8. Cunliffe, W.J., Clayden, A.D., Gould, D.J. and Simpson, N.B. (1981). Acne vulgaris – its aetiology and treatment. A review. *Clin. Exp. Dermatol.*, **6**, 461

32
Use of Isotretinoin in Severe Cases with Papular Pustular Acne

A. MACK, H. WOKALEK, B. MAAS and R. CÖRLIN

Introduction

The excellent efficacy of 13-*cis*-retinoic acid in cases with conglobate and cystic acne,[1-10] in acne fulminans,[11,12] in severe papular pustular rosacea[13,14] as well as in Gram-negative folliculitis[14,15] is well documented.

Substantial improvement by treatment with orally given 13-*cis*-retinoic acid in dosages of 1–2mg/kg/day has been achieved after a relatively short time even in those patients who have responded poorly to conventional therapy. Although the exact mechanism of action of 13-*cis*-retinoic acid is not yet completely clear, the observed and measured suppression of sebum production is a likely main factor.[16-19] Furthermore, normalization of keratinization of the follicular infundibula has been shown to be an important co-factor.[14,20] The anti-inflammatory and immunomodulating properties of 13-*cis*-retinoic acid has also been considered.[14,21-28] The aim of this study was to investigate the efficacy of 13-*cis*-retinoic acid in low dosages and in a condition closely related to acne conglobata – the severe cases of papular pustular acne which respond poorly to conventional therapy. It is recognized that borderline cases cannot always be precisely defined on the basis of the severity of the skin lesions and the individual psychic reaction of each patient towards his deforming skin disease has to be taken into consideration.

Table 1. Study design - papular pustular acne - 20 weeks.

	0.05mg/kg	No. of patients at each dosage		Total
		0.1mg/kg	0.2mg/kg	
Beginning of therapy	64	62	65	191
Therapy according to protocol	41	54	59	154
Therapy with dose increase	8	2	–	10
Withdrawal due to				
complete remission	–	1	–	1
lack of response	6	2	1	9
Drop-outs not caused by therapy	9	3	5	17

Cases evaluable in efficacy studies = 174
Cases evaluable in studies of side-effects = 191

Patients and Methods

In our study of 14 German dermatology departments of university hospitals 191 patients (148 males, 43 females, mean age 21 years, range 14–24 years) with severe papular pustular acne were treated with 13-*cis*-retinoic acid in a randomized open trial over 20 weeks. At each centre patients were allocated one of the three dosage levels at random, the doses being 0.05, 0.1 and 0.2mg/kg/day.

All acne lesions were counted at the beginning and at regular intervals during therapy. The degree of seborrhoea of skin and hair was graded on a 4 point scale, side-effects were registered, and laboratory values such as leukocytes, alkaline phosphatase, SGPT, SGOT, triglycerides and total cholesterol were repeatedly determined.

Results

191 patients entered the study, the distribution in the three dosage groups being well balanced (Table 1). 154 patients reached the end of the 20 weeks treatment period according to protocol. Ten patients, eight in the 0.05 and two in the 0.1mg/kg/day groups, were given increased dosages, because of poor response. Because of unresponsiveness six patients from the 0.05, two patients from the 0.1 and only one patient from the 0.2mg/kg/day groups had to be withdrawn from the study. 17 patients stopped the study due to reasons not related to treatment. These 17 cases were not evaluated in efficacy studies.

There was a decrease in the average number of non-inflamed lesions – open and closed comedones – in all three dose groups (Figure 1). After 20 weeks the reduction was between 50 per cent in the lowest and 70 per cent in the highest group.

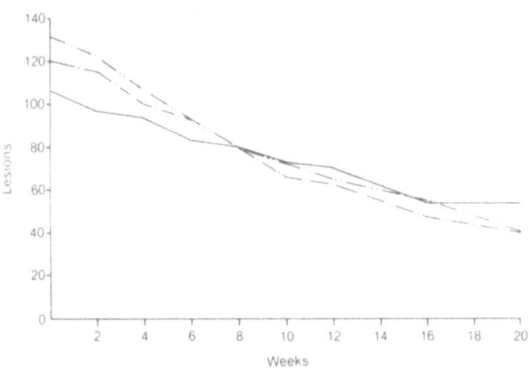

Figure 1. Decrease in non-inflamed lesions (open and closed comedones).
—— 0.05mg/kg; – ·– – 0.1mg/kg; – · · – · · 0.2mg/kg.

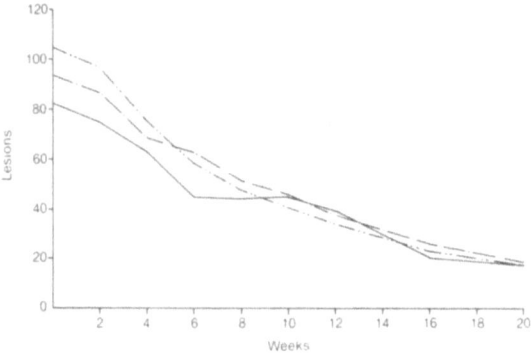

Figure 2. Decrease in inflamed lesions (papules, pustules, nodules). —— 0.05mg/kg;
– · — 0.1mg/kg; – · · – · · 0.2mg/kg.

As in other trials,[6,10] the therapeutic response of the inflamed lesions –
papules, pustules and nodules – occurred more rapidly and more inten-
sively than the non-inflamed lesions (Figure 2). The amount of the
observed decrease, shown in Figure 1 after 12 weeks treatment, occurred 8
weeks earlier for inflamed lesions. An improvement of up to 79 per cent
for the 0.05mg/kg/day dose group and up to 84 per cent for 0.2mg/
kg/day group was achieved after 20 weeks treatment.

treatment.

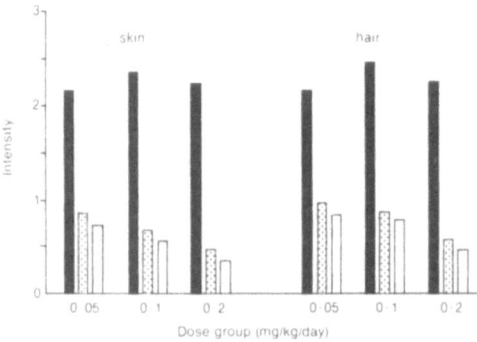

Figure 3. Decrease in seborrhoea (estimated mean intensity, 1 = light, 2 = Moderate, 3 =
Severe). ■ = 0 weeks; ▥ = 12 weeks; □ = 20 weeks.

In all dose schedules a marked decrease of estimated mean intensity of
seborrhoea of the skin and hair was found (Figure 3). Efficacy was more
marked within the first 12 weeks of treatment. The observed decrease in
the following 8 weeks of treatment was slight.

Figure 4 shows the frequency of mucocutaneous side-effects occurring in
more than 20 per cent of the patients. Almost all patients showed a mild to
moderate dryness of lips and up to 70 per cent a light to moderate cheilitis.

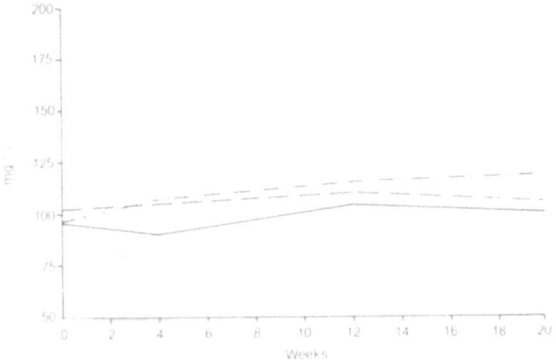

Figure 4. Frequent clinical side-effects (per cent) (> 20 per ent). ■ = 2 weeks; ▨ = 12 weeks; □ = 20 weeks.

Furthermore, facial dermatitis, desquamation of the skin, dry nose and dry mouth occurred in 34–42 per cent of the cases. Most of the observed side-effects were detectable from the second week. Generally, the frequency of side-effects rose within the first months of treatment, but there was no increase of the frequency during the second half of the treatment period. The frequency even decreased in some groups during this time.

Table 2. Uncommon clinical side-effects in all dose groups (percentage) (< 20 per cent).

Side-effect	2 weeks	12 weeks	20 weeks
Skin fragility	0–2	8–10	5–11
Loss of hair	4–9	5–10	5–11
Pruritus	9–12	6–12	0–15
Conjunctivitis	3–6	7–12	4–10
Muscle pain	4–7	5–7	8–10

Figure 5. Triglyceride levels (mean values). —— 0.05mg/kg; – · – · 0.1mg/kg; – · · · – · · 0.2mg/kg.

Uncommon side-effects were observed in less than 20 per cent of patients; they are summarized in Table 2. The overall intensity of all registered side-effects was scaled as light with exception of dry lips and cheilitis. A dose dependency could not be clearly shown. The laboratory data were assessed according to the baseline values used by each trial centre. The measured mean values showed no abnormalities at any dose schedule.

Total cholesterol (Figure 5) and triglyceride (Figure 6) levels showed a slight increase in the 0.2mg/kg/day dose group within the normal range.

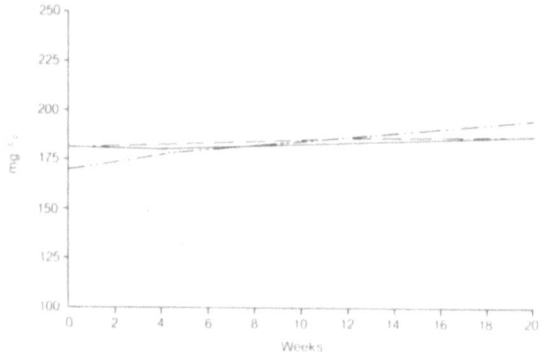

Figure 6. Trigylceride levels (mean values). —— 0.05mg/kg; – · – · 0.1mg/kg; – · · · – · · 0.2mg/kg.

Discussion

Based on the results reported in this paper it can be shown that daily administration of 0.05–0.2mg is able to reduce acne lesions and the accompanying seborrhoea in patients with severe papular pustular acne. This dose regimen is lower than the dosage used so far in acne conglobata. The clinical and laboratory side-effects, especially those of the blood lipids, were of no major importance and less marked than the ones encountered during treatment with higher doses in acne conglobata.[29-32, 34] These results, which were obtained on the basis of a favourable dose–effect relationship, could perhaps lead to a wider use of 13-*cis*-retinoic acid in the management of less severe forms of acne vulgaris. The oral form of medication has its advantages as it is more convenient to use both for the physician and the patient. It should, however, be made clear that the results presented here do not aim to publicize a new indication for 13-*cis*-retinoic acid but merely to elucidate this interesting borderline area of acne conglobata. 13-*cis*-retinoic acid is a very potent compound and undoubtedly represents a major therapeutic breakthrough. Its use, however, is associated with a series of side-effects that cannot be ignored, especially teratogenicity.[33]

We still believe that isotretinoin should continue to be strictly limited to severe cases of acne barely responsive or unresponsive to conventional therapy.

Conclusions

The efficacy of low doses (0.05, 0.1, 0.2mg/kg/day) given over 20 weeks in cases of severe papular pustular acne, which had responded poorly to conventional therapy, was investigated in 174 patients. These patients were recruited from 14 dermatological departments of university hospitals in West Germany. It was shown that:

(1)   Acne lesions were reduced by 49 per cent (non-inflamed lesions) to 84 per cent (inflamed lesions).

(2)   There was a more rapid and more intense response of inflamed lesions compared to non-inflamed lesions.

(3)   A marked decrease in seborrhoea was noted.

(4)   The most frequent common mucocutaneous side-effects were dry lips (up to 100 per cent) and cheilitis (up to 68 per cent). The intensity of all registered adverse effects was low.

(5)   No abnormalities of the mean values of the laboratory tests were recorded, including total cholesterol and triglyceride levels.

(6)   Due to the high rate of drop-out in the 0.05mg/kg/day dose group, the lowest dose limit of satisfactory efficacy of 13-*cis*-retinoic acid in cases of papular pustular acne should be 0.1mg/kg/day.

In view of the high teratogenic potential and the clinical toxicity of 13-*cis*-retinoic acid, the prescription should not be extended to cases with low grade acne treatable by conventional therapy.

References

1.   Farrell, L.N., Strauss, J.S. and Stranieri, A.M. (1980). The treatment of severe cystic acne with 13-*cis*-retinoic acid. *J. Am. Acad. Dermatol.* **3**, 602
2.   Jones, H., Miller, A.J. and Cunliffe, W.J. (1983). A dose-response study of 13-*cis*-retinoic acid in acne vulgaris. *Br. J. Dermatol.*, **108**, 333
3.   Jones, D.H., Cunliffe, W.J. and Cove, J.H. (1981). 13-*cis*-retinoic acid in acne (a double-blind study of dose response). In Orfanos, C.E. *et al.* (eds.). *Retinoids: Advances in Basic Research and Therapy.* pp.255–258. (Berlin, Heidelberg, New York: Springer-Verlag)
4.   Jones, H., Blanc, D. and Cunliffe, W.J. (1980). 13-*cis*-retinoic acid and acne. *Lancet*, **2**, 1048
5.   King, K., Jones, D.H., Daltrey, D.C. and Cunliffe, W.J. (1982). A double-blind study of the effects of 13-*cis*-retinoic acid on acne, sebum excretion rate and microbial population. *Br. J. Dermatol.*, **107**, 583

6. Meigel, W., Gollnick, H., Wokalek, H., Plewig, G. *et al.* (1983). Orale Behandlung der Acne conglobata mit 13-*cis*-Retinsäure. Ergebnisse der deutschen multizentrischen Studie nach Therapieschluss. *Hautarzt.* (In press)

7. Peck, G.L. Olsen, T.G., Yoder, F.W., Strauss, J.S., Dowing, D.T., Pandya, M., Butkus, D. and Arnaud-Battendier, J. (1979). Prolonged remissions of cystic and conglobate acne with 13-*cis*-retinoic acid. *N. Engl. J. Med.*, **300**, 329

8. Peck, G.L., Olsen, T.G., Butkus, D., Pandya, M., Arnaud-Battendier, J., Gross, E.G., Windhorst, D.B. and Cheripko, J. (1982). Isotretinoin versus placebo in the treatment of cystic acne. *J. Am. Acad. Dermatol.*, **6**, 735

9. Plewig, G., Wagner, A. and Braun-Falco, O. (1980). 13-*cis*-Retinsäure. *Münch. Med. Wochenschr.*, **122**, 1287

10. Plewig, G., Gollnick, H., Meigel, W., Wokalek, H. *et al.* (1981). 13-*cis*-Retinsäure zur oralen Behandlung der Acne conglobata. Ergebnisse einer multicentrischen Studie. *Hautarzt*, **32**, 634

11. Plewig, G., Wagner, A. and Braun-Falco, O. (1980). Orale Behandlung schwerster Akneformen mit 13-*cis*-Retinsäure. Klinische Ergebnisse. *Münch. Med. Wochenschr.*, **38**, 1287

12. Wagner, A. and Plewig, G. (1980). 13-*cis*-Retinsäure. *Münch. Med. Wochenschr.*, **122**, 1294

13. Nikolowski, J. and Plewig, G. (1981). Orale Behandlung der Rosacea mit 13-*cis*-Retinsäure. *Hautarzt*, **32**, 575

14. Plewig, G., Nikolowski, J. and Wolff, H.H. (1982). Action of 13-*cis*-retinoic acid (isotretinoin) in acne, rosacea and gramnegative folliculitis. *J. Am. Acad. Dermatol.*, **6**, 766

15. Neubert, U. and Plewig, G. (1980). Gramnegative Follikulitis. Verlaufsbeobachtungen und therapeutische Möglichkeiten. *Zentralbl. Haut. Geschlkr.*, **144**, 38

16. Gomez, E.C. and Moskowitz, R.J. (1980). Effect of 13-*cis*-retinoic acid on the hamster flank organ. *J. Invest. Dermatol.*, **74**, 392

17. Landthaler, M., Kummermehr, J., Wagner, A. and Plewig, G. (1980). Inhibitory effect of 13-*cis*-retinoic acid on human sebaceous glands. *Arch. Dermatol. Res.*, **269**, 297

18. Strauss, J.S., Stranieri, A.M., Farrell, L.N. and Downing, D.T. (1980). The effect of marked inhibition of sebum production with 13-*cis*-retinoic acid on skin surface lipid composition. *J. Invest. Dermatol.*, **74**, 66

19. Strauss, J.S. and Stranieri, A.M. (1982). Changes in long-term sebum production from isotretinoin therapy. *J. Am. Acad. Dermatol.*, **6**, 751

20. Plewig, G., Wagner, A., Nikolowski, J. and Landthaler, M. (1981). Effects of two retinoids in animal experiments and after clinical application in acne patients: 13-*cis*-retinoic acid Ro 4-3780 and aromatic retinoid Ro 10-9359. In Orfanos, C.E. *et al.* (eds.). *Retinoids: Advances in Basic Research and Therapy.* pp. 219–235. (Berlin, Heidelberg, New York: Springer-Verlag)

21. Barnett, J.B. (1982). Immunopotentation of the IgE-antibody reponse by 13-*cis*-retinoic acid. *Int. Arch. Allergy Appl. Immunol.*, **67**, 287

22. Barnett, J.B. (1982). Immunomodulating effects of 13-*cis*-retinoic acid on the IgE-antibody response. *Fed. Proc.*, **41**, 834, Abstr. No. 3300

23. Bauer, R., Gollnick, H., Brand, G. and Orfanos, C.E. (1983). Proliferationskinetik stimulierter Blutlymphozyten unter 13-*cis*-Retinsäure. ADF-abstract. *Arch. Dermatol. Res.*, (In press)

24. Camisa, Ch., Eisenstat, B., Ragaz, A. and Weissmann, G. (1982). The effects of retinoids on neutrophil functions *in vitro. J. Am. Acad. Dermatol.*, **6**, 629

25. Kato, T., Wokalek, H., Ernst, M. and Schöpf, E. (1981). Influence of 13-*cis*-retinoic acid on zymosan-induced chemiluminescence of granulocytes. *Arch. Dermatol. Res.*, **271**, 205

26. Nikolowski, J., Plewig, G. and Hofmann, C. (1982). *In-vivo* Tests zum Nachweis antiinflammatorischen Wirkung der 13-*cis*-Retinsäure. *Dermatol. Monatsschr.*, **168**, 173

27. Plewig, G. and Wagner, A. (1981). Anti-inflammatory effects of 13-*cis*-retinoic acid. *Arch. Dermatol. Res.*, **270**, 89

28. Rhodes, J. and Oliver, S. (1980). Retinoids as regulators of macrophage function. *Immunology*, **40**, 467

29. Gerber, L.E. and Erdman, J.W. (1982). Changes in lipid metabolism during retinoic

administration. *J. Am. Acad. Dermatol.*, **6**, 664

30. Gollnick, H., Schwartzkopff, W., Luley, C. and Orfanos, C.E. (1981). Alterations of lipid metabolism under treatment with oral retinoids (isotretinoin and etretinate). Laboratory monitoring on 46 patients with and without risk factors. Presented at *3rd International Psoriasis Symposium,* July 13–17, Stanford

31. Gollnick, H., Tsambaos, D. and Orfanos, C.E. (1981). Risk factors promote elevations of serum lipids in acne patients under oral 13-*cis*-retinoic acid (isotretinoin). *Arch. Dermatol. Res.*, **271**, 189

32. Gollnick, H., Schwartzkopff, W., Schleising, M. and Orfanos, C.E. (1983). Verhalten der lipolytischen Aktivität des Serums vor und unter 13-*cis*-Retinsäure bei parenteraler Fettbelastung. *Hautarzt* (In press)

33. Kamm, J. and Nutley, N.J. (1982). Toxicology, carcinogenicity, and teratogenicity of some orally administered retinoids. *J. Am. Acad. Dermatol.*, **6**, 652

34. Katz, R.A., Jorgensen, H. and Nigra, T.P. (1980). Elevation of serum triglyceride levels from oral isotretinoin in disorders of keratinization. *Arch. Dermatol.*, **116**, 1369

Section 9

Other Uses of Isotretinoin

33
The Use of Isotretinoin in Rosacea

R.A. FULTON, D.C. DICK and R.M. MACKIE

Introduction

Rosacea is a common skin disorder of unknown aetiology. While it has its own distinctive features, rosacea shares a number of features in common with acne. Both disorders predominantly affect the face, involve pilosebaceous units, and respond to treatment with antibiotics particularly of the tetracycline group. There are important differences between them including the older age of onset, the absence of comedones and the presence of persistent erythema in rosacea. It has also been observed that while the sebum excretion rate tends to be elevated in patients with acne, it is normal in rosacea.[1] The dramatically beneficial effect reported by Peck et al.[2] of isotretinoin treatment of acne prompted us to use the same drug for the treatment of rosacea. We have carried out an open study of the effectiveness of a 6 week course of oral isotretinoin in eight patients with rosacea.

Patients and Methods

Patients were selected for treatment with isotretinoin if they gave informed consent and were inadequately controlled on oral tetracycline. The group consisted of four males and four females, whose ages ranged from 27 to 59 years (median 49) and who have a disease duration from 1 to 20 years (median 5). Patients were excluded who had a history of ischaemic heart disease, liver disease, or who were receiving regular drug therapy for other conditions. The female patients were either post-menopausal or had been previously sterilized.

Isotretinoin was given for 6 weeks in a dose of 0.5mg/kg/day. All other treatment given for rosacea was discontinued 4 weeks before entry into the study although patients who were using topical sulphur or salicylic acid preparations were permitted to continue this treatment throughout the study period.

Patients were assessed clinically at 2-weekly intervals during the treatment period as well as 4 weeks afterwards. The total number of palpable facial lesions (papules and pustules) was counted by the same observer at each visit and patients were asked to mark a 10cm line (visual analogue scale) at a point corresponding to their own assessment of their condition at the time on a continuum between no disease and the most severe they could envisage. They were not permitted to refer to their previous mark when making a new assessment.

Clinical photographs were also taken in standard conditions at each visit. These were assessed by an independent dermatologist who compared pairs of photographs without knowledge of their true temporal sequence. The sebum excretion rate (SER) was measured on the forehead by a gravimetric method before treatment, after 6 weeks and at 10 weeks (i.e. 4 weeks after treatment was stopped). Biochemical liver function tests, cholesterol, triglycerides and full blood count were also measured prior to treatment and after 6 weeks.

Results

Lesion Count

All patients showed a progressive fall in the total number of palpable lesions while on treatment. Four weeks after treatment was stopped six patients still had fewer lesions than on the initial visit while two patients were as bad or worse. When lesions were classed separately as papules or pustules each showed a reduced number after treatment (Table 1) although there was a greater relapse in the number of papules than pustules during the follow-up period.

Table 1. Lesion count before, during and 4 weeks after treatment with isotretinoin. Cumulative total for eight patients.

	Papules	Pustules	Total
Before treatment	76	64	140
After 6 weeks treatment	37	13	50
4 weeks after stopping treatment	84	22	106

Photographic Assessment

Satisfactory photographs for comparisons at 0, 6 and 10 weeks were obtained for seven patients. These were assessed separately for differences in the diffuse erythema component and for differences in focal inflammatory lesions corresponding to well-defined papules and pustules. While there was no consistent change in the erythema component, six patients showed improvement in focal inflammatory lesions and one was

Table 2. Photographic comparison at 6 weeks and 10 weeks with the pre-treatment photographs.

		Improved	Unchanged	Worse
6 weeks	Erythema	2	3	2
	Focal lesions	6	1	0
10 weeks	Erythema	3	3	1
	Focal lesions	6	1	0

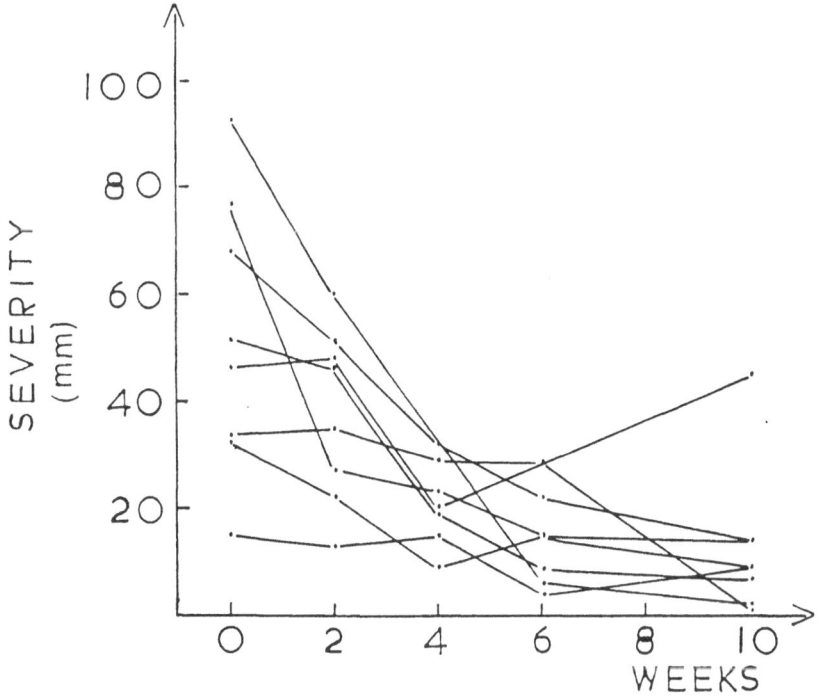

Figure 1. Subjective assessment – visual analogue scale.

317

unchanged after 6 weeks treatment. This improvement was still evident at 10 weeks (Table 2).

Visual Analogue Scale

All patients were improved at 6 weeks and this improvement tended to be maintained during the 4 weeks immediately afterwards (Figure 1).

Sebum Excretion Rate

The mean SER ($\pm$ SE) of the group prior to treatment with isotretinoin was $1.13 \pm 0.21 \mu g \ cm^{-2} \ min^{-1}$. This fell to 0.26 ± 0.14 at 6 weeks and rose slightly to 0.74 ± 0.33 at 10 weeks.

Side-Effects

All patients experienced side-effects although none had to be withdrawn from the study. Eight patients had cheilitis, three had epistaxis, two had conjunctivitis, three had facial dermatitis, one had pruritus and one had raised triglycerides.

Discussion

This study has shown that isotretinoin is an effective treatment for rosacea and confirms the results of Nikolowski and Plewig[3] in a report of 13 patients with severe rosacea treated with isotretinoin for between 12 and 28 weeks. It is doubtful whether the drug has a place in the first-line treatment of the disease because of the high incidence of side-effects compared to the low toxicity of conventional tetracycline therapy. It is worth considering, however, in patients who have responded poorly to antibiotics and are severely affected by the disease.

The mode of action of isotretinoin in rosacea is unknown. In a previous study the authors proposed that the drug was acting primarily as an anti-inflammatory agent.[4] We believe that the action of the drug in rosacea may be consistent with its known property of profoundly suppressing sebaceous gland activity. The development of focal inflammatory lesions is likely to be closely linked with activity of the pilosebaceous unit while the vascular signs of the disease, which do not improve at the same rate as the palpable lesions with isotretinoin, probably have a separate origin. Facial flushing is a feature of rosacea[5] and abnormalities have been sought in the response of facial blood vessels to thermal[6] and other stimuli[7] as an explanation of this phenomenon. Whether these two separate facets of the disease exist in parallel as a result of some fundamental abnormality or whether one arises as a consequence of the other is a matter for speculation.

Acknowledgements

We would like to thank Mr Ian McKie for taking the clinical photographs and Dr R.M. Adams for her assistance with the photographic assessment.

References

1. Burton, J.L., Pye, R.J., Meyrick, G. and Shuster, S. (1975). The sebum excretion rate in rosacea. *Br. J. Dermatol.*, **92**, 541
2. Peck, G.L., Olsen, T.G., Yoder, F.W., Strauss, J.S., Downing, D.T., Pandya, M., Butkus, D. and Arnaud-Battandier, J. (1979). Prolonged remissions of cystic and conglobate acne with 13-*cis*-retinoic acid. *N. Engl. J. Med.*, **300**, 329
3. Nikolowski, J. and Plewig, G. (1981). Orale Behandlung der Rosazea mit 13-*cis*-Retinsäure. *Hautarzt*, **32**, 575
4. Plewig, G., Nikolowski, J. and Wolff, H.H. (1982). Action of isotretinoin in acne rosacea and gram-negative folliculitis. *J. Am. Acad. Dermatol.*, **6**, 766
5. Marks, R. (1968). Concepts in the pathogenesis of rosacea. *Br. J. Dermatol.*, **80**, 170
6. Wilkin, J.A. (1981). Oral thermal-induced flushing in erythematotelangiectatic rosacea. *J. Invest. Dermatol.*, **76**, 15
7. Bernstein, J.E. and Soltani, K. (1982). Alcohol-induced rosacea flushing blocked by naloxone. *Br. J. Dermatol.*, **107**, 59

34
Use of Isotretinoin in the Ichthyoses

W.J. CUNNINGHAM

Introduction

The ichthyoses, in a way, link the past and present in retinoid therapy. Some of the first observations of the effects of deficiency or excess of vitamin A led first to the conclusion that ichthyosis and vitamin A levels were interconnected, and second to the attempts to modify their clinical manifestations with, successively, vitamin A, tretinoin, and 13-*cis*-retinoic acid therapy.

Ichthyosis, with several major types as well as many incidental presentations, is part of the spectrum of the disorders of keratinization, many of which are retinoid therapy responsive. The US experience with this spectrum has included extensive use of 13-*cis*-retinoic acid.

Methods

The methodology of the investigational use of 13-*cis*-retinoic acid in the treatment of 283 patients with disorders of keratinization has been reviewed.[1] Briefly, patients were treated with doses of 0.5–4.0mg/kg/day depending on clinical response and level of side-effects, initially for up to 16 weeks.

After intervening 2 week off-treatment periods, repeated 6 month courses of treatment were allowed with dosage again varying, according to response and side-effects. This design allowed patients, in effect, to act as their own control with relapse during off-treatment periods. Efficacy was measured by an overall (global) rating of −2 to 5 and by a scoring from 1 to 7 of disease parameters of erythema, scaling, induration, and crusting (Table 1).

Table 1. Clinical efficacy measurements.

Global rating	Disease parameter
−2 = worsening	1 = absent
−1 = possibly worse	2 = trace
0 = no change	3 = mild
1 = minimal improvement	4 = mild to moderate
3 = marked improvement	5 = moderate
4 = almost clear	6 = moderate to severe
5 = clear	7 = severe

Safety measurements consisted of clinical observations and laboratory determinations of complete blood count (CBC), urinalysis, and chemical screening including serum triglyceride and cholesterol determinations. Twenty-five of 283 patients left the study because of clinical adverse reactions; 12 left (seven were able to return) because of elevations of triglycerides and one left because of elevations of liver function tests.

Results

A multicentre study evaluated 13-*cis*-retinoic acid therapy of patients with lamellar ichthyosis (59 patients), epidermolytic hyperkeratosis (23 patients), X-linked ichthyosis (five patients), ichthyosis vulgaris (nine patients), and unclassified congenital ichthyosiform erythroderma (four patients).[2]

Table 2. Response of ichthyoses to 13-*cis*-retinoic acid therapy.

Disease	Patients clearly improved/ total treated	Pretreatment	Mean rating	During treatment
Lamellar ichthyosis	57/59	5.9	scaling	2.9
		3.4	erythema	1.8
		2.6	induration	1.3
		1.7	crusting	1.0
Epidermolytic hyperkeratosis	21/23	6.1	scaling	2.8
		3.3	erythema	2.0
		3.2	induration	1.4
		3.1	crusting	1.2
Ichthyosis vulgaris	4/9	4.3	scaling	2.8
X-linked ichthyosis	4/5	4.4	scaling	2.8
Congenital ichthyosiform erythroderma	3/4	7.0	scaling	3.0
		6.2	erythema	3.5
		3.8	induration	1.2

Overall, over 50 per cent of patients with lamellar ichthyosis demonstrated global ratings of definite or better improvement by the 4th week of 13-*cis*-retinoic acid therapy with over 90 per cent similarly responding by the end of the first course of therapy (Table 2). Disease parameters demonstrated marked improvement during therapy with return to pretreatment values after discontinuation of therapy. Additional long-term courses produced similar results.

Epidermolytic hyperkeratosis responded similarly to treatment with 13-*cis*-retinoic acid with global ratings of clear improvement in over 90 per cent of patients treated. Disease parameters in this condition did not show as great a degree of lesion improvement as was noted with lamellar ichthyosis.

Treatment of ichthyosis vulgaris resulted in clear improvement in four of nine patients; of X-linked ichthyosis in four of five patients and of congenital ichthyosiform erythroderma in three of four patients.

In the five types of ichthyosis described, dosage range was 0.5–4mg/kg/day with an overall mean dose of approximately 2mg/kg/day. Total clearing of disease parameters is not to be expected and rapid relapse to near pretreatment status is the rule after discontinuation of 13-*cis*-retinoic acid therapy.

104 patients with Darier's disease were treated with 13-*cis*-retinoic acid in a multicentre study.[3] Within 1–4 weeks 74 per cent of patients were noted to be clearly improving. By 8–16 weeks 85 per cent were clearly improving. Table 3 outlines the response of patients with Darier's disease to treatment with 13-*cis*-retinoic acid. As with nearly all the other disorders of keratinization, relapse is expected after drug discontinuation.

Table 3. Response of Darier's disease to 13-*cis*-retinoic acid therapy.

Patients clearly improving/ total treated	Pretreatment	Mean rating	During treatment
99/104	3.9	erythema	2.1
	4.6	scaling	2.0
	3.5	induration	1.6
	4.1	crusting	1.5

The exception to this rule appears to be 13-*cis*-retinoic acid treatment of pityriasis rubra pilaris where some patients maintain a remission after therapy is discontinued.[4] A study of 45 patients with pityriasis rubra pilaris using mean daily doses of approximately 2.1mg/kg noted clear improvement (definite or better in the global rating) in 28 of 45 patients by week 4, and in 43 of 45 by the end of a first course of therapy. A summary of response data appears in Table 4.

Keratosis palmaris et plantaris is responsive to therapy with 13-*cis*-retinoic acid.[5] A multicentre study using mean doses of 1.95mg/kg/day

Table 4. Response of pityriasis rubra pilaris to 13-*cis*-retinoic acid therapy.

Patients clearly respond- ing/total treated	Pretreatment	Mean rating	During treatment
43/45	5.1	erythema	2.7
	5.2	scaling	2.5
	3.5	induration	1.3

Table 5. Response of keratosis palmaris et plantaris to 13-*cis*-retinoic acid therapy.

Patients clearly respond- ing/total treated	Pretreatment	Mean rating	During treatment
5/6	5.0	scaling	2.7
	4.2	induration	1.7
	3.5	crusting	1.0
	3.2	erythema	1.2

demonstrated definite clearing in five of six patients by the end of a 16-week course of treatment with 13-*cis*-retinoic acid (Table 5).

Side-Effects

The side-effects observed in treatment of cystic acne with 13-*cis*-retinoic acid are not, in general, dissimilar in incidence and severity from those observed in patients treated for disorders of keratinization. There are three exceptions, however. Five patients treated for disorders of keratinization developed corneal opacities while receiving therapy with 13-*cis*-retinoic acid which either tended to clear upon its discontinuation or did not require discontinuation of the drug. Two children treated with 13-*cis*-retinoic acid for disorders of keratinization have been reported to have possible premature closure of an epiphysis.[6] Additionally, for the age group represented, a higher than expected prevalence of spinal hyperostosis has been reported. It must be emphasized that these patients all had a disorder of keratinization and were treated with mean daily doses of 13-*cis*-retinoic acid of approximately 2mg/kg for over 2 years duration. These reported bone abnormalities must interject a note of caution for use of this drug for long-term therapy as it is known that vitamin A itself has profound effects on bone differentiation[7] and that skeletal hyperostosis has been experimentally produced in cats by high dose administration of vitamin A.[8]

Not all patients demonstrating skeletal hyperostosis have been symptomatic and thus, in current clinical investigations, baseline and periodic X-rays of the spine are a protocol requirement for adults. Additionally, periodic bone age determinations in children are required.

Mechanism of Action

The mechanism of retinoid action is far from clear although extensive *in vitro* and *in vivo* experimental data are accumulating.[9] Retinoids affect differentiation of a number of cell types[10] but it is not certain that this directly plays a role in the clinical improvement noted in treatment of disorders of keratinization with 13-*cis*-retinoic acid. Changes in biological membranes have also been noted with retinoid administration and it is perhaps changes in desmosomes, or tonofilaments[11] which may allow desquamation to occur more readily, and thus lead to clinical improvement. Some of the mucocutaneous side-effects might also be explained by these effects which could alter stratum corneum barrier function. As is frequently the case in a developing science, we have more speculations than established facts.

References

1. Windhorst, D.B. (1982). The use of isotretinoin in disorders of keratinization. *J. Am. Acad. Dermatol.*, **6**, 708
2. Baden, H.P., Buxam, M.M., Weinstein, G.D. and Yoder, F.W. (1982). Treatment of ichthyosis with isotretinoin. *J. Am. Acad. Dermatol.*, **6**, 716
3. Dicken, C.H., Bauer, E.A., Hazen, P.G., Krueger, G.G., Marks, Jr., J.G., McGuire, J.S. and Schachner, L.A. (1982). Isotretinoin treatment of Darier's disease. *J. Am. Acad. Dermatol.*, **6**, 721
4. Goldsmith, L.A., Weinrich, A.E. and Shupack, J. (1982). Pityriasis rubra pilaris response to 13-*cis*-retinoic acid (isotretinoin). *J. Am. Acad. Dermatol.*, **6**, 710
5. Bergfeld, W.F., Derbes, V.J., Elias, P.M., Frost, P., Greer, K.E. and Shupack, J.L. (1982). The treatment of keratosis palmaris et plantaris with isotretinoin. *J. Am. Acad. Dermatol.*, **6**, 727
6. Milstone, L.M., McGuire, J. and Ablow, R.C. (1982). Premature epiphyseal closure in a child receiving oral 13-*cis*-retinoic acid. *J. Am. Acad. Dermatol.*, **7**, 663
7. Mandel, H.G. and Cohn, V.H. (1980). Fat-soluble vitamins. Vitamins A, K, and E. In Gilmann, A.G., Goodman L.S. and Gilman A. (eds.). *The Pharmacological Basis of Therapeutics*. 6th Edn., pp. 1583–1601. (New York: Macmillan Publishing Co.)
8. Seawright, A.A. and English, P.B. (1967). Hypervitaminosis A and deforming cervical spondylosis of the cat. *J. Comp. Path.*, **77**, 29
9. Pawson, B.A., Ehmann, C.W., Itri, L.M. and Sherman, M.I. (1982). Retinoids at the threshold: their biological significance and therapeutic potential. *Am. Chem. Soc.*, **25**, 1269
10. Lotan, R. (1980). Effects of vitamin A and its analogs (retinoids) on normal and neoplastic cells. *Biochem. Biophys. Acta,* **605**, 33
11. Blanchet-Bardon, C. and Puissant, A. (1981). Ultrastructural study of the four main types of ichthyosis after one month's treatment with Ro 10-9359. In Orfanos, C.E. *et al.* (eds.). *Retinoids: Advances in Basic Research and Therapy*. pp. 303–306. (Berlin, Heidelberg, New York: Springer-Verlag)

Section 10

New Aspects of Retinoid Therapy

35
Response of Psoriatic Arthropathy to Arotinoid (Ro 13-6298): A Pilot Study

P. FRITSCH, W. RAUSCHMEIER and J. NEUHOFER

Introduction

Arotinoids are third generation synthetic aromatic retinoids under experimental investigation at the present time.[1] The arotinoid Ro 13-6298 (Ar), a compound with high anti-tumour, anti-keratinizing and anti-seborrhoeic activities and of a very favourable therapeutic index in experimental animals,[2] has recently been subjected to clinical trials. From the oral retinoids already introduced into clinical practice it differs in at least two important aspects: its potency (Ar is close to three orders of magnitude more potent than etretinate) and its marked anti-inflammatory and anti-arthritic activity as documented in the experimental Freund's adjuvant arthritis of the rat.[2] The clinical applications of Ar are not yet clearly delineated.

Etretinate has a limited therapeutic effect in psoriatic arthropathy and has been used as an adjuvant treatment modality for several years by other groups[3-6] and by us. In our experience on more than 30 patients with psoriatic arthropathy, unequivocal but partial improvement can be observed in most patients after lag periods of 2–3 months. Improvement is rarely such that administration of analgesics can be stopped. The mechanisms of action are unclear as yet but may be complex: retinoids have been shown to suppress collagenase production in normal and rheumatoid synovial cell cultures;[7,8] they have anti-inflammatory properties in experimental models and may also possess immune regulatory capacities as yet not clearly defined.

Its pronounced anti-inflammatory properties appear to make Ar a promising candidate for application in psoriatic arthropathy. A pilot study on 12 patients, as detailed below, suggests that Ar is in fact an excellent therapeutic modality in this condition.

Patients and Treatment Schedule

12 patients (11 males, 1 female) with moderate to severe psoriatic arthropathy were subjected to Ar treatment. The diagnosis was based on typical history, clinical appearance, negative serological tests for rheumatoid arthritis, X-rays of the affected joints and presence of psoriatic skin lesions. Skin involvement ranged from very slight (two cases) to near erythrodermic (one case); the extent of the skin lesions was not correlated to the severity of joint involvement. The mean age of the patients was 49 years (range 34–62 years), the mean duration of psoriatic arthropathy was 9.5 years (range 0.5–30 years). Five out of 12 patients were positive for HLA B27.

All of the patients had involvement of their interphalangeal joints, the number of affected joints ranging between 3 and 12. Four of 12 patients had also one or more large joints affected (sacroiliacal joints, knees, shoulders). Grossly visible deformities of their fingers were present in five patients.

All but one patient had been extensively treated for their arthropathies for many months up to years. Treatment modalities employed included non-steroidal anti-inflammatory drugs (11/12), oral photochemotherapy (7/12), UV-B (1/12), etretinate (5/11) and methotrexate (1/12). Nine of 12 patients had received several of these modalities concomitantly once or several times during the course of their disease. In all of these patients, the effect of treatment had been only partial and unsatisfactory. At the time of initiation of Ar treatment, 8/12 patients took high daily doses of analgesics and had still highly active arthropathies rendering 7/12 unable to work.

Ar was administered at relatively low daily doses of 0.0005–0.001 mg/kg body-weight. The average maintenance doses were 0.0006–0.0007mg/kg. Slight dose adjustments were only rarely necessary. Prior to treatment, the following laboratory investigations were carried out: blood sedimentation rate, transaminases, alkaline phosphatase, blood urea nitrogen, creatinine, uric acid, bilirubin (total), serum protein, triglycerides, cholesterol, fasting glucose, complete blood count, urinanalysis. In all patients treated the laboratory tests were within normal ranges except the blood sedimentation rates which were moderately to highly elevated in 9/12 patients. Controls were performed at 3-weekly intervals and included clinical examination and determination of the above laboratory tests.

Results

In general, the response of the patients to Ar was excellent in terms of the therapeutic efficacy, incidence and severity of side-effects and patient compliance.

Improvement became apparent after relatively short lag periods of 7–14 days in all but three patients; these latter patients only improved after 3 and 4 weeks, respectively, and their subsequent course was similarly protracted. Improvement was manifest as reduction of swelling and redness of the affected joints, clearing of less inflamed joints, regression or disappearance of morning stiffness and marked improvement of joint motility. There was a significant reduction of joint pains and tenderness, rendering it possible to gradually decrease the daily doses of analgesics and non-steroidal anti-inflammatory agents. Improvement appeared to reach a steady state after 3–4 weeks in 10/12 patients, the slow responders (see above) after 6–8 weeks. At this time, none of the patients took any drugs and were still almost completely free of arthropathic subjective symptoms, the joints showing no signs of active inflammation; pre-existent bone deformities, however, were unchanged. The three slow responders (see above) complained of some residual joint pain and morning stiffness. Three of six patients were continued with oral photochemotherapy for the management of skin lesions.

Ten of the 12 patients are still under Ar treatment at the time of writing, treatment times ranging between 1.5 and 5 months. Two patients (the least severe cases of psoriatic arthropathy in this group) had Ar withdrawn in a completely cleared state after 45 and 60 days, respectively; no relapse has occurred since then (6.5 months) in one patient, the other suffered a complete relapse after a treatment-free interval of 3 months and was subjected to another course of Ar.

Slight fluctuations of residual joint pain were noticed in most patients with subtotal clearing. Interestingly, these episodes were rarely accompanied by objective signs of inflammation. A more substantial relapse of arthropathies despite continued Ar administration was seen only once in a patient with particularly severe manifestations of his condition; in this patient, the relapse was overcome by a temporary increase of the daily doses.

Side-effects were modest: 3/12 patients complained of desquamative cheilitis, only one of them to a substantial degree; one patient had generalized pruritus. Withdrawal of the drug was not necessary in any of these cases; after slight reductions of the daily doses, these minor side-effects became easily tolerable. No other well known dermatological side-effects of etretinate and isotretinoin, such as hair loss or skin fragility, were observed; several patients noticed a clear reduction of sebum production of their scalps and faces. No pathological laboratory values became manifest during treatment, including serum triglycerides and cholesterol levels. On the contrary, the blood sedimentation rates, which were highly elevated in most of the patients prior to Ar treatment, reverted to moderately elevated or normal ranges.

Concomitant skin lesions were largely cleared at about the same time when the maximal effect was achieved on the arthropathy (3–6 weeks after onset). Since most of the patients were subjected to concomitant topical treatment or oral photochemotherapy, the role of Ar in the clearing of skin lesions cannot be unequivocally delimited.

Comment

Important progress has been made in the past decades in the treatment of psoriasis by the introduction of methotrexate,[9] oral photochemotherapy[10] and etretinate.[11] In contrast, psoriatic arthropathy still poses important therapeutic problems. Although all of the treatment modalities cited above do have moderate to partial beneficial effects on this painful and potentially incapacitating manifestation of psoriasis, none of them offers satisfactory relief in reasonable fractions of patients: improvement induced by all of these modalities becomes apparent only after prolonged lag periods, and is only partial in most cases. Therefore, the mainstay of treatment of psoriatic arthropathy is still administration of analgesic and anti-inflammatory drugs and physical therapy.

Our above data seem to indicate that Ar, a new synthetic retinoid, may be capable of filling this therapeutic gap. Ar has potent anti-inflammatory activity which, even in the relatively small doses employed by us in this trial, markedly improves subjective and objective arthropathic symptoms after a very short lag period (1–2 weeks) and leads to subtotal remissions after twice or three times that period. None of the patients, including several severe cases of psoriatic arthropathy, had to continue taking analgesics or other hitherto administered drugs any longer, and joint motility reverted to normal or close to normal ranges if no permanent bone deformities were present at the onset of treatment. Two of the patients, both with less severe manifestations of psoriatic arthropathy, became totally free of objective and subjective symptoms; the duration of total remissions, however, remains to be determined by future experience. The overall efficacy of Ar was thus far higher than that of any other therapeutic modality hitherto employed by us, including etretinate. The same was felt by the patients.

Side-effects were very tolerable and in general less marked than equivalent doses of etretinate and isotretinoin (Accutane). In particular, no alterations of laboratory values were noted (transaminases, triglycerides).

Pending confirmation of our favourable results by trials in larger numbers of patients, we conclude that Ar promises to be an excellent therapeutic aid in psoriatic arthropathy of unprecedented potency.

References

1. Bollag, W. (1981). Arotinoids. A new class of retinoids with activities in oncology and dermatology. *Cancer Chemother. Pharmacol.*, **7**, 27
2. Hofmann-La Roche (1982). *Investigational Drug Brochure.*
3. Rosenthal, M. (1979). Retinoid in der Behandlung von Psoriasis-Arthritis. *Schweiz. Med. Wochenschr.*, **109**, 1912
4. Brackertz, D. and Müller, W. (1979). Die Beeinflussung der Arthropathia psoriatica und der chronischen Polyarthritis durch ein oral wirksames aromatisches Retinoid. *Verh. Dtsch. Ges. Inn. Med.*, **85**, 1343
5. Bahous, J., Bitter, Th. and Rosenthal, M. (1980). Retinoid, Vitamin-A-Säure in der Behandlung der Psoriasis-Arthritis. In *Report 19. Tagung d. dtsch. Ges. für Rheumatologie* 30.9.-4.10.80, Konstanz
6. Stollenwerk, R., Fischer-Hoinkes, H., Komenda, K. and Schilling, F. (1981). Clinical observations on oral retinoid therapy of psoriatic arthropathy (Ro 10-9359). In Orfanos, C.E. *et al.* (eds.). *Retinoids: Advances in Basic Research and Therapy.* pp. 205–209. (Berlin, Heidelberg, New York: Springer-Verlag)
7. Brinckerhoff, C.E., McMillan, R.M., Dayer, J-M. and Harris, E.D. Jr. (1980). Inhibition by retinoic acid of collagenase production in rheumatoid synovial cells. *N. Engl. J. Med.*, **303**, 432
8. Brinckerhoff, C.E., Nagase, H., Nagel, J.E. and Harris, E.D. (1982). Effects on all-*trans*-retinoic acid (retinoic acid) and 4-hydroxyphenylretinamide on synovial cells and articular cartilage. *J. Am. Acad. Dermatol.*, **6**, 591
9. Weinstein, G. and Frost, P. (1971). Methotrexate for psoriasis, a new therapeutic schedule. *Arch. Dermatol.*, **103**, 33
10. Parrish, J.A., Fitzpatrick, T.B., Tanenbaum, L. and Pathak, M.A. (1974). Photochemotherapy of psoriasis with oral methoxsalen and long wave ultraviolet light. *N. Engl. J. Med.*, **291**, 1207
11. Ott, F. *et al.* (1975). Therapie der Psoriasis mit einem oral wirksamen neuen Vitamin-A-Säure Derivat. *Schweiz. Med. Wochenschr.*, **105**, 439

36
Anti-Inflammatory Effects of the Retinoids

D. BRADSHAW, C.H. CASHIN and A.J. KENNEDY

Introduction

Despite the use of retinoids in the treatment of a variety of skin disorders in which inflammation is a significant component, the anti-inflammatory properties of this class of compounds have received little attention. Early studies by Dr. K. Reber (Roche, Basle) demonstrated that retinoic acid and etretinate (Tigason) inhibited inflammation in the developing adjuvant arthritis test. This activity appeared, initially, to be a consequence of an immunosuppressive action since these retinoids were dosed during the early phase of the test and not during the period prior to measurement of inflammation. Moreover, other workers have reported that etretinate and isotretinoin (13-*cis*-retinoic acid, Roaccutane) when dosed throughout the developing adjuvant arthritis test inhibit the immediate paw swelling, induced by the injection of Freunds complete adjuvant, much less than the secondary inflammation that develops as a consequence of the immunological reaction[1] – a profile of activity displayed by some immuno-suppressive agents. Reber also observed, however, that several retinoids dosed to rats with an established arthritis do exert anti-inflammatory activity suggesting a direct anti-phlogistic action. In the present studies we have examined the activity of retinoids in immunological and non-immuno-logical models of inflammation to learn more about the mechanism(s) of their anti-inflammatory actions.

Experimental

Materials

Etretinate, isotretinoin and motretinide (Tasmaderm) were in the form of the pure substances used in commercially available preparations. They were freshly prepared in arachis oil containing 0.05 per cent propyl gallate to optimize absorption and minimize oxidation and were stored in amber glass bottles.

Animals

Male and female outbred MF1 mice were used for the delayed hypersensitivity studies. Female outbred PVG derived hooded rats were used for adjuvant arthritis studies. Female outbred albino rats (Alderley Park Strain 1, Wistar/Charles River derived) were used for pleurisy studies.

Methods and Results

The main tests used for these studies were a delayed hypersensitivity inflammation test in the mouse[2], the adjuvant polyarthritis test in the rat[3] and, for a non-immunological inflammatory model, a carrageenan-induced pleurisy in the rat.[4] These tests will be described in greater detail below. Some additional studies have also been carried out to provide a more complete profile of the potential antirheumatic activities of particular retinoids.

Sensitization (day 0) of mice with methylated bovine serum albumin (MBSA) instigates a cell-mediated immune reaction. Mice are subsequently challenged with the same antigen by injecting it into a hind paw. This provokes a delayed hypersensitivity inflammatory reaction which is quantitated by measuring the degree of paw swelling 24 h after challenge. Immunosuppressive and some anti-inflammatory drugs inhibit the swelling.[2] Isotretinoin, etretinate and motretinide were administered orally on days 0–4 of the test. Motretinide showed greatest activity in this test reducing inflammation by more than 50 per cent at a dose of 10mg/kg. Subsequent studies showed that significant activity was observed[5] at 3mg/kg. Etretinate also displayed considerable activity in this test but isotretinoin did not significantly reduce the inflammatory response (Table 1).

These same retinoids were examined in the developing adjuvant arthritis test in the rat. In this test rats are injected into one hind paw with a suspension in mineral oil of heat-killed *Mycobacterium tuberculosis*. This evokes an inflammatory swelling in the injected paw (1° lesion). From about 12 days after sensitization a secondary inflammation develops in both hind and fore paws as a consequence of an immunologically mediated

Table 1. Activity of retinoids in the MBSA delayed hypersensitivity test in mice.

Treatment	Dose (mg/kg) p.o.	Per cent reduction 24 h paw volume
Isotretinoin	100	25
	30	21
Etretinate	30	43*
	10	42*
Motretinide	30	58†
	10	56†

Retinoids were dosed orally on days 0–4, day 0 being the day of sensitization of mice with MBSA. Mice were challenged on day 9 and paw inflammation measured 24 h later. Student's two-tailed t-test was used to determine the significance of differences in values between the treated and control groups. *$p<0.05$;   †$p<0.01$.

systemic disease (2° lesion). Isotretinoin, etretinate and motretinide were dosed throughout the test by the oral route (Table 2). The three retinoids all showed significant activity in the test. The 1° paw inflammation measured over the initial 5 days was not significantly reduced whereas all aspects of the secondary response were inhibited. However, examination of the primary swelling after 7 days showed small but significant reductions of inflammation with all three compounds, indicative of a delayed onset of action. Isotretinoin markedly inhibited 2° lesion inflammation at 100mg/kg and motretinide modestly inhibited this parameter at 30mg/kg.[7] Etretinate significantly inhibited 2° lesion inflammation at 30 and 10mg/kg and showed a dose-related effect at these two dose levels. These anti-inflammatory effects were accompanied by evidence of protection of rats from other disease-associated lesions and an improvement in the ankle joint mobility was observed. However, whereas these activities were associated with an improvement in weight gain in rats dosed with isotretinoin, neither etretinate nor motretinide afforded significant gains in body-weight. This difference may reflect the relative potencies of the compounds in the induction of hypervitaminosis A in the rat.

Injection of 1 per cent lambda-carrageenan into the pleural cavity of the rat evokes an acute oedematous inflammatory reaction. This is quantitated by measuring, after 4 h, the volume of inflammatory exudate and by counting the number of infiltrating leukocytes. Differential counts for polymorphonuclear cells (PMN) and mononuclear cells (MN) are also carried out. Etretinate and isotretinoin were examined in this test. Each retinoid was dosed orally for 10 days prior to the instigation of pleural inflammation. The results obtained are shown in Tables 3 and 4. Etretinate

Table 2. Activity of retinoids in the developing adjuvant arthritis test.

Treatment	Dose (mg/kg) p.o.	Per cent reduction of paw volume				Ankle joint mobility (°)‡	Lesion score**	Body-weight cf. control (Δg)
		Injected paw			Non-injected paw			
		0–5 day*	7 day†	7–16 days*	7–16 days*			
Isotretinoin	100	10	26††	44††	93††	66††	71††	+14
	30	1	11	20	37	15	16	+4
Etretinate	30	14	32††	67††	100††	67††	86††	0
	10	14	10	34††	53††	30	48††	−6
Motretinide	30	3	13††	16††	53	35	35	−1
	10	−4	−5	10††	9	−19	2	−3

*Per cent reduction calculated from integrated paw volume over stated time period.

†Per cent reduction calculated on day 7 only.

‡Per cent reduction calculated from angle of ankle joint rotation between flexion and extension.

**Per cent reduction calculated from lesion score (0–3 scale) on paws, nose, ears and tail.

††Values significantly different from controls at $p < 0.05$ by Student's t-test (2-tailed) or Wilcoxon rank-sum test (2-tailed) for lesion score.

Table 3. Effect of etretinate on a 4-hour lambda-carrageenan pleurisy.

Treatment	n	Exudate volume		Total cell count		Total PMN		Total MN	
		(ml)	Per cent change	(× 10⁶)	Per cent change	(× 10⁶)	Per cent change	(× 10⁶)	Per cent change
Arachis oil (5mg/kg/day)	8	1.43 ± 0.11		129.8 ± 9.7		117.0 ± 8.9		12.8 ± 0.9	
Etretinate (45mg/kg/day)	5	0.94 ± 0.19	−34†	65.7 ± 14.5	−49‡	55.2 ±12.4	−53‡	10.4 ± 2.1	−19*
Etretinate (15mg/kg/day)	8	1.05 ±0.12	−27†	92.7 ± 6.0	−29‡	79.7 ± 5.2	−32‡	13.1 ± 1.0	+2*
Etretinate (5mg/kg/day)	8	1.13 ± 0.09	−21*	89.3 ± 8.4	−31‡	79.2 ± 7.9	−32‡	10.0 ± 1.1	−22*

*Not significant; †$p<0.05$; ‡$p<0.01$. Statistical analyses were performed using Student's t-test (two-tailed); n = number of animals in the group. Etretinate was administered daily for 10 days and the pleurisy was induced 1 h after the last dose.

Table 4. Effect of isotretinoin on a 4-hour lambda-carrageenan pleurisy.

Treatment	n	Exudate volume (ml)	Exudate volume Per cent change	Total cell count (× 10⁶)	Total cell count Per cent change	Total PMN (× 10⁶)	Total PMN Per cent change	Total MN (× 10⁶)	Total MN Per cent change
Arachis oil (5mg/kg/day)	8	1.25 ± 0.12		77.1 ± 8.0		68.8 ± 7.0		8.3 ± 1.0	
Isotretinoin (135mg/kg–day)	7	0.99 ± 0.14	−21*	50.4 ± 6.5	−35†	45.2 ±5.8	−34†	5.2 ± 0.8	−37†
Isotretinoin (45mg/kg/day)	8	0.74 ± 0.07	−41‡	57.0 ± 9.5	−26*	51.1 ± 8.9	−26*	5.8 ± 0.7	−30*
Isotretinoin (15mg/kg/day)	8	0.73 ± 0.07	−42‡	58.7 ± 6.7	−24*	51.5 ÷ 6.0	−25*	7.2 ±0.8	−13*
Isotretinoin (5mg/kg/day)	8	1.04 ± 0.14	−17*	67.9 ± 9.9	−12*	59.3 ± 8.5	−14*	8.2 ± 1.2	−1*

*Not significant;† $p < 0.05$; ‡ $p < 0.01$. Statistical analyses were performed using Student's t-test (two-tailed); n = number of animals in the group. Isotretinoin was administered daily for 10 days and the pleurisy was induced 1h after the last dose.

dosed at 5, 15 and 45mg/kg caused a dose-dependent inhibition of exudate formation (34 per cent, $p<0.05$ at 45mg/kg). A significant inhibition of PMN infiltration was measured at doses of 5, 15 and 45mg/kg. MN infiltration, however, was not significantly changed. The weight gain of rats dosed at 45 mg/kg was significantly lower than that of the arachis oil treated control group. Isotretinoin dosed at 5, 15, 45 and 135mg/kg inhibited the volume of exudate (41 per cent at 45mg/kg, $p<0.01$). A dose-dependent inhibition of PMN and MN accumulation was measured which was statistically significant only at the highest dose (PMN 34 per cent, $p<0.05$; MN 37 per cent, $p<0.05$). Isotretinoin did not impair weight gain in this test.

Discussion

The present studies show clearly that retinoids display anti-inflammatory activity in animal models of inflammation. A direct anti-inflammatory activity of isotretinoin has also been previously demonstrated in man,[6] when marked inhibition of inflammation resulting from the application of a potassium iodide patch to the skin was observed.

Species differences in absorption and metabolism of retinoids complicate a simple comparison of the activity of the three retinoids in the three inflammation tests studied. Etretinate showed significant activity in all three tests. Isotretinoin did not display significant activity in the MBSA test but this may be due to a relatively poor absorption in mice compared with rats. Marked anti-inflammatory activity was measured for isotretinoin in this test when a longer (10 day) dosing regime was employed. The pleural inflammation test provided direct evidence for an anti-inflammatory activity of etretinate and isotretinoin as distinct from an anti-inflammatory effect resulting from modulation of an underlying immunological mechanism. It is tempting therefore to conclude that the anti-inflammatory activity observed for the three retinoids in the immune inflammation tests was a consequence of anti-phlogistic activity.

It has been apparent to us that retinoid anti-inflammatory activity is delayed in onset. It is not observed after administration of single doses nor in the first days after induction of the 1° lesion paw swelling in the adjuvant rat. Moreover, following repeated dosing of the retinoids, their anti-inflammatory activity is readily detected for many days following cessation of dosing. Whilst pharmacokinetic reasons may be advanced to explain these observations, some studies we have carried out employing time-dependent dosing raise the possibility that activity may be indirect and result from a progressive induction of metabolic or tissue changes.

The observation that etretinate reduced PMN infiltration is in accord with the findings of Dubertret et al.[7] who noted inhibition of neutrophil migration into skin chambers in orally dosed human volunteers. The difference in activities of etretinate and isotretinoin on the type of cell infiltrating the pleural cavity were of note and caution against the assumption that both compounds share a single mode of action. The clinical activities of these two agents are also evidently distinctive.

The mechanism(s) of action of the retinoids in reducing inflammation is not clear. This class of compounds is capable of exerting a wide range of biological activities several of which might be pertinent. The ability of retinoic acid to inhibit collagenase production in rheumatoid synovial cells has been described.[8] However, isotretinoin and etretinate did not reduce collagenolytic activity in the inflamed paws of adjuvant arthritic rats.[1] Though retinoids clearly can exert anti-inflammatory activity in a non-immunological inflammation, the well-documented immunomodulatory actions of these compounds may also significantly contribute to the overall response in immune inflammatory disorders. For example, we have observed a striking exacerbation of inflammation in an established model of arthritis in the rat instigated by sensitizing animals with Type 2 collagen. The three retinoids tested here all shared this pro-inflammatory action in this assay which may *inter alia* have resulted from immunomodulatory actions. This activity has previously been observed for isotretinoin by others.[9]

In conclusion, the anti-inflammatory activities observed for isotretinoin, etretinate and motretinide in these studies may represent an interesting lead for the development of novel therapeutic agents. These activities may contribute to the efficacy of these retinoids in some inflammatory skin disorders. The elucidation of the mechanisms underlying these anti-phlogistic actions may further the selection of more effective anti-inflammatory retinoids. Progression of this lead to other therapeutic fields such as the rheumatic diseases will demand the careful monitoring of the hyper-vitaminosis A activity of successor retinoids since the capacity of vitamin A to induce bone fragility and cartilage changes is documented.[10]

Acknowledgements

The authors would like to acknowledge the skilled contributions to this work of Mr B.B. Dodge, Mr P.H. Franz, Miss S.A. Jones and Mr E.J. Lewis.

References

1. Coffey, J.W., Baruth, H., Nemzek, R., Salvador, R.A. and Sullivan, A.C. (1981). Comparative effects of two retinoids and 2-[4-(p-chlorophenyl)- benzoyloxyl]2-methylpropionic acid (CLOZIC) on the levels of inflammation and collagenolytic activity (CLA) in paws from adjuvant treated rats. *Fed. Proc.*, **40**, 1814

2. Cashin, C.H., Jones, S.A., Gill, J. and Kennedy, A.J. (1979). An assessment of the delayed hypersensitivity reaction to methylated bovine serum albumin in the mouse and its use in the evaluation of drug effects on cell mediated immune reactions. *Agents Actions*, **9**, 553
3. Newbould, B.B. (1963). Studies on adjuvant arthritis in rats. *Br. J. Pharmacol.*, **21**, 127
4. Di Rosa, M., Giroud, J.P. and Willoughby, D.A. (1971). Studies of the mediators of the acute inflammatory response induced in rats in different sites by carrageenan and turpentine. *J. Pathol.*, **104**, 15
5. Jones, S.A. and Kennedy, A.J. (1983). Activity of a retinoid Ro 11-1430 (motretinide) in some immunological models. *Br. J. Pharmacol.*, **78**, 57P
6. Plewig, G. and Wagner, A. (1981). Anti-inflammatory effects of 13-*cis*-retinoic acid. *Arch. Dermatol. Res.*, **270**, 89
7. Dubertret, L., Lebreton, C. and Touraine, R. (1982). Inhibition of neutrophil migration by etretinate and its main metabolite. *Br. J. Dermatol.*, **107**, 681
8. Brinckerhoff, C.E., McMillan, R.M., Dayer, J.M. and Harris, E.D. (1980). Inhibition by retinoic acid of collagenase production in rheumatoid synovial cells. *N. Engl. J. Med.*, **303**, 432
9. Trentham, D.E. and Brinckerhoff, C.E. (1982). Augmentation of collagen arthritis by synthetic analogues of retinoic acid. *J. Immunol.*, **129**, 2668
10. Lotan, R. (1980). Effects of vitamin A and its analogues (retinoids) on normal and neoplastic cells. *Biochim. Biophys. Acta*, **605**, 33

37
No Influence of Three Synthetic Retinoids (Ro 10-1670, Ro 4-3780. Ro 13-6298) on Lipoxygenase Activity in Two *in Vitro* Systems

I. KNIPPEL, R. BAUER and C.E. ORFANOS

Introduction

The directional migration of periphral blood PMNs generally occurs in response to some chemotactic gradient. Three main chemotactic stimuli may be responsible for directional cell migration: (a) the complement-component C5a, (b) a tripetide of the amino acids formylmethionine, leucine and phenylalanine, and (c) the leukotriene B4 (LTB4), which obviously exerts the strongest chemotactic properties.

In recent experiments we investigated the ability of various synthetic retinoids to inhibit lipoxygenase activity as a key enzyme of leukotriene biosynthesis using two different assay systems. The oxygenation of arachidonic acid by soybean lipoxygenase was determined by a spectro-photometric and by a selective solvent extraction technique.

Material and Methods

Spectrophotometric assay

Arachidonic acid, 1mmol (99 per cent pure, Sigma Comp., St Louis, Mo., USA) first was dissolved in 0.1ml ethanol and 0.2mol/l borate buffer pH 9.0 was slowly added with continuous stirring until a final volume of 30ml was reached. This substrate solution remained optically clear at room temperature and was used within 30min (solution A). Lipoxygenase (soybean lipoxygenase EC 1.13.11.12, spec. act. 150 IU/μg protein, Sigma Comp.) was dissolved in cold borate buffer (0.2mol/l, pH 9.0) at a concentr-ation of 10^4 IU/ml (solution B).

2ml of substrate solution A and 1ml of borate buffer and 0.01ml of test compounds dissolved in dimethylsulphoxide (DMSO) were pipetted into silica cuvettes (1cm lightpath). Fatty acid peroxidation was started by the addition of 0.05ml of solution B. Each assay contained 65.8μmoles of arachidonic acid, 500IU lipoxygenase, less than 0.3 per cent DMSO and varying amounts of test compounds in a final volume of 3.06ml. All experiments were performed in triplicate for each concentration of test compound whereby blanks containing buffer instead of enzyme and controls containing pure DMSO were always run through the same procedure simultaneously. 1-Phenyl-3-pyrazolidone (phenidone) and nordihydroguaiaretic acid (NDHG) served as standard inhibitors of the lipoxygenase pathway.[1,2]

The time-dependent increase of absorbance was monitored at ambient temperature in a Gilford 250 spectrophotometer at 234nm for 10 min and specific enzyme activities were calculated from the mean maximal changes in absorbance/min between the 1–4 min intervals.

Selective Solvent Extraction Technique

Lipoxygenase inhibitors decrease the total formation of the peroxidation products 15-HPETE and 15-HETE[3] from a fixed amount of arachidonic acid (AA) which can be accurately measured after selective solvent extraction of the ^{14}C-labelled precursor as previously reported.[4]

[1-^{14}C]Arachidonic acid (spec. act. 56Ci/mol, ^{14}C-AA) was provided by the Radiochemical Centre, Amersham, UK.

The influence of synthetic retinoids on fatty acid lipoxygenation was carried out at 25°C for 10min in a mixture containing 0.05mol/l potassium phosphate buffer pH 8.0, [1-^{14}C]arachidonic acid (38nCi, 2.5 μmol/l), 1 per cent ethanol to dissolve AA, 750IU soybean lipoxgenase (spec. act. 1501 V/μg protein) and varying amounts of retinoids or known lipoxygenase inhibitors in a final volume of 0.3ml. Retinoids were predissolved, if necessary, in a small volume of acetone or ethanol, final solvent concentrations did not exceed 3 per cent. Test drugs and enzyme were preincubated for 10min at ambient temperature before the lipoxygenation was started by the addition of [^{14}C]AA. After incubation for 10 min at 25°C product formation was complete and the reaction was terminated by the addition of 2.5vols (0.75ml) of n-hexane. The remaining AA was selectively extracted into the organic solvent using an Eppendorf Mixer 5432 for 1 min. After centrifugation at 10000×g for 1 min (Eppendorf Centrifuge 5414) the organic phase was disgarded and the extraction procedure was repeated twice. After addition of 0.5vols (0.15ml) of ethanol to the remaining buffer phase containing the labelled lipoxygenation products, the lipocygenase activity was quantified by liquid scintillation counting of an aliquot (0.3ml) of the ethanolic buffer phase in 10ml scintillation fluid (Pico Fluor 15, Packard Instr.) in a Beckman Model 2800 LS counter.

Inhibition of lipoxygenase activity by test compounds was calculated by comparison of the individual total product yield to the non-inhibited peroxidation reaction. All experiments included controls containing buffer and corresponding amounts of solvent (ethanol or acetone) instead of test drugs, blanks with heat-inactivated lipoxygenase and varying concentrations (10^{-3}–10^{-6}mol/l) of the reference inhibitors phenidone or NDHG. All enzyme activities measured were the mean of at least four separate observations, the IC_{50}-values were derived from three concentration–response curves.

Results

The retinoid compounds Ro 4-3780, Ro 10-1670, and Ro 13-6298 were tested against soybean lipoxygenase dependent oxygenation of arachidonic acid at concentrations of 60μg/ml (200μmol/l), 30μg/ml (100μmol/l), 10μg/ml (33μmol/l), 3μg/ml (10μmol/l) and 1μg/ml (3.3μmol/l). The IC_{50}-values of the standard lipoxygenase inhibitors were 50 ± 3μmol/l (phenidone) and 70 ± 2mol/l (NDHG).

We found that soybean lipoxygenase activity could not be inhibited by any of the retinoid compounds investigated in this study. Non-significant alterations of the increase in absorbance at 234nm and uninhibited yield of [^{14}C]lipoxygenation products were measured in all experiments at all ranges of concentration.

These results indicate that the responsiveness of PMNs to various stimuli is rather influenced by a direct effect of synthetic retinoids on the cells themselves; whereas the synthesis of chemotactic active mono- and di-HETES is not suppressed by these agents *in vitro*.

References

1. Blackwell, G.J. and Flower, R.J. (1978). 1-Phenyl-3-pyrazolidone: an inhibitor of cyclo-oxygenase and lipoxygenase pathways in lung and platelets. *Prostaglandins*, **16**, 417
2. Hamberg, M. (1976). On the formation of thromboxane B₂ and 12 L-hydroxy-5,8,10,14-eicosatetraenoic acid (12 ho-20:4) in tissues from the guinea pig. *Biochim. Biophys. Acta*, **431**, 651
3. Hamberg, M. and Samuelsson, B. (1967). Oxygenation of unsaturated fatty acids by vesicular gland of sheep. *J. Biol. Chem.*, **242**, 5329
4. Knippel, I., Baumann, J., von Bruchhausen, F. and Wurm, G. (1981). Interactions of sulfhydryl agents and soybean lipoxygenase inhibitors. *Biochem. Pharmacol.*, **30**, 1677

38
The Management of Cystic, Conglobate and Severe Acne Irresponsive to Systemic Antibiotics with Roaccutane

A. J. MILLER & W. J. CUNLIFFE

Introduction

At the London Retinoid Symposium, May 1983, several speakers with considerable experience of treating severe acne in clinical trials in the UK, USA and Germany, discussed their views on the management of severe acne with this drug.

Although there were some differences, particularly in the dosage used, between the USA and Europe, it was possible to gain a concensus view of the management of these patients.

This final chapter attempts to put concisely that view for the benefit of those less experienced in using the drug. In no way can this be said to be definitive, but hopefully it reflects the state of the art at time of writing.

The first section contains six examples with short case histories of typical cases of severe acne unresponsive to conventional therapy, that serve to elucidate the efficacy and duration of effect of Roaccutane.

The first four are examples of severe facial acne treated by Dr W. J. Cunliffe at Leeds General Infirmary, England, and the last two are cases of severe truncal acne treated by dermatologists in the USA. It will be seen that there are considerable differences in dosages used between these two groups. This will be discussed in the second section.

The second section, as implied, is concerned with appropriate dosage according to the severity and distribution of the acne. Criteria for modification of dosage during therapy are defined to contend with either of two situations; lack of efficacy or intolerance to the drug.

The third section describes some of the common and not so common clinical side-effects that have been described in the literature and some that have been first described at the symposium.

Finally and appropriately, the reader is reminded of the precautions the manufacturer has made on the prescribing of Roaccutane and of the conditions of supply of the drug, properly imposed by the Committee on Safety of Medicines, in the UK.

Section 1   Examples of Efficacy

Six examples (with short case histories) of the efficacy of Roaccutane in severe acne are now given. The acne in the four patients (Case Histories A, B, C and D) was graded on the Leeds Scale for each of the three areas, face, back and chest making a maximum grade of 30. The last two patients (E and F) were not graded according to this system, but an approximate grade has been included for comparison.

Case History A

Top: *Pre-treatment. Grade 6.0 acne.*
Bottom: *Post-treatment after 16 weeks with 1.0mg/kg body-weight/day Roaccutane. Grade 0.75 acne.*

Mr P. L. is a 14-year-old schoolboy with a history of acne of 5 years duration. He had been treated with erythromycin 1g daily continuously for 2 years.

On first being seen he presented with a total acne grade of 3.5 in June 1976. Despite conventional therapy his acne worsened to a total grade of 7.0 in December 1978 and just prior to commencing Roaccutane his acne grade was 13.5

After 16 weeks therapy his acne grade fell to 4.25 and by 32 and 44 weeks was 2.0 and 0.5 respectively.

The adverse reactions that he experienced were cheilitis, facial and peripheral dermatitis and malaise and these were well tolerated.

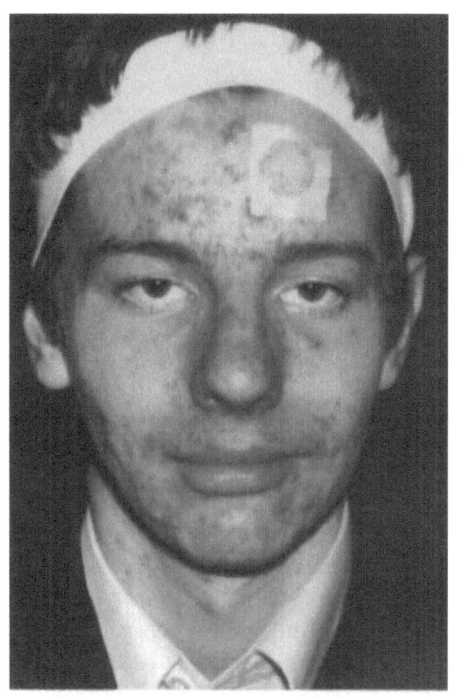

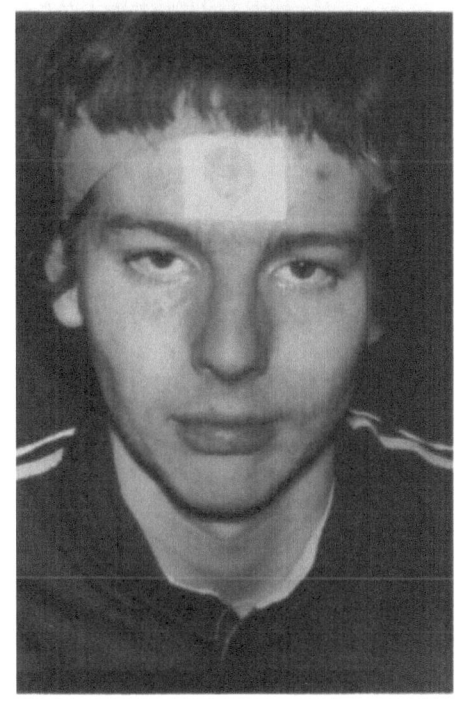

351

Case History B

Top: *Pre-treatment. Grade 6.0 acne.*

Bottom: *Post-treatment after 16 weeks therapy with 0.5mg/kg body-weight/day Roaccutane. Grade 1.0 acne.*

Mr A. M. is a 16-year-old schoolboy with a 2 year history of acne.

He was referred from another centre in the same region where he had received in the course of 2 years Deteclo, tetracycline and dapsone. Despite this his acne grade in January 1981 was 7.0.

After 16 weeks therapy his acne grade fell to 1.0 which was confined to the face. He continued to improve off therapy and at 32 and 44 weeks his acne grade was further improved to 0.5 and 0.25 respectively.

To date he remains clear of acne.

His only adverse reaction was cheilitis.

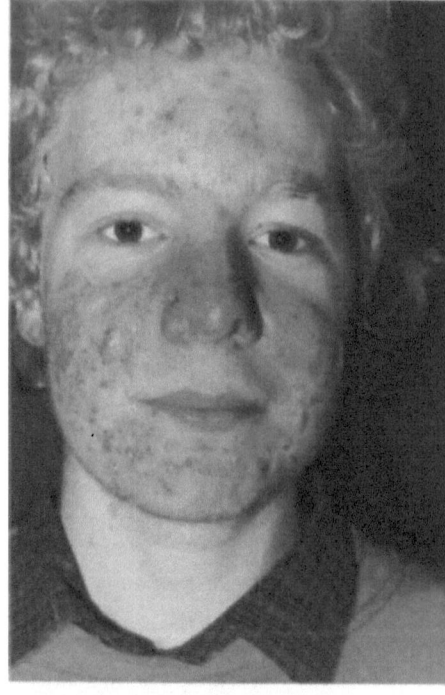

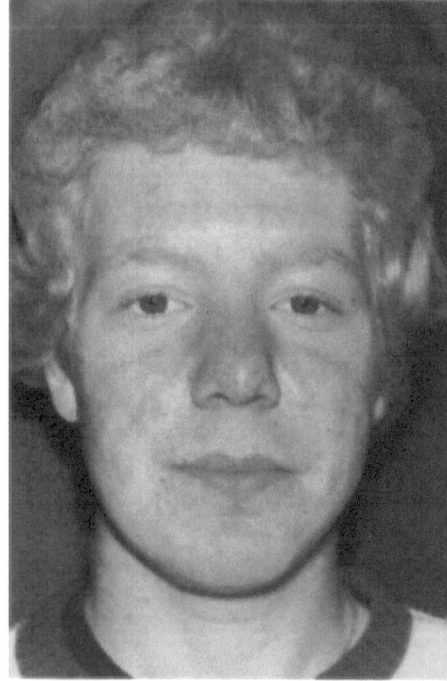

Case History C

Top: Pre-treatment. Grade 6.0
        acne.
Bottom: Post-treatment after 16 weeks
        with 0.5mg/kg body-weight/
        day Roaccutane. Grade 0.5
        acne.

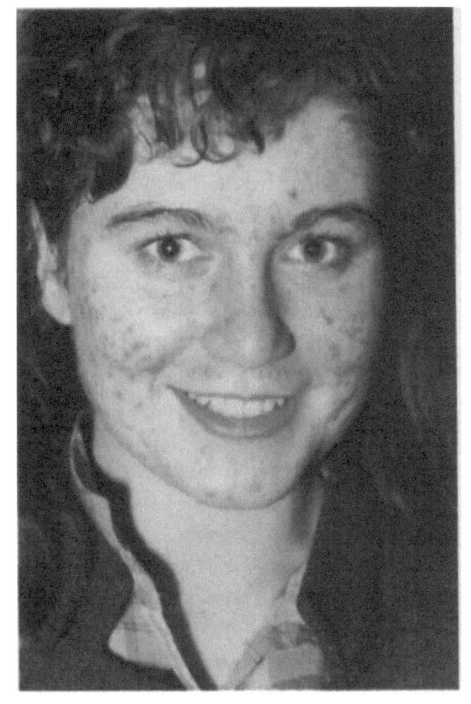

Miss A. M. G. is a 19-year-old student,
who at commencement of Roaccutane
therapy had a history of acne of 9 years
duration. For 8 of these years she had
had continuous antibiotic therapy with
tetracyclines and clindamycin. She was
referred from another region and on
presentation in January 1981 had an
acne grade of 8.0.

    After 16 weeks therapy her total acne
grade fell to 1.75. Off therapy she
continued to improve and had no acne at
32 and 44 weeks.

    The only adverse reactions
experienced with cheilitis and fragile
skin.

    Now clear of acne she has remarked
that her life was revolutionized.

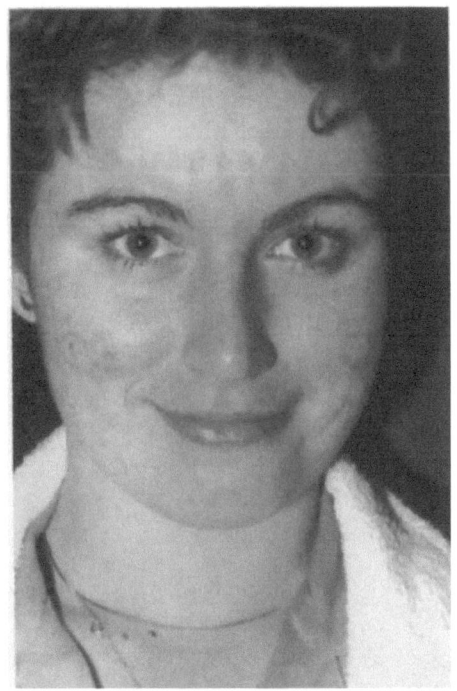

Case History D

Top: *Pre-treatment. Grade 2.0
           acne.*
Bottom: *Post-treatment after 16 weeks
          with 0.1mg/kg body-weight/
          day Roaccutane. Grade 0.25
          acne.*

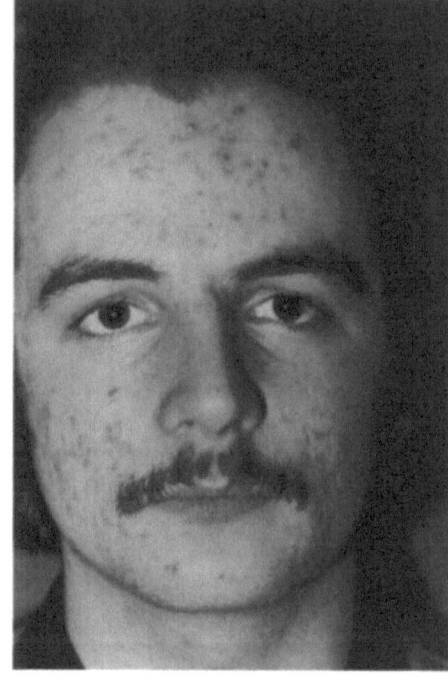

*Mr D. R. is a 19-year-old student. He
was a regular patient of the department
for 5 years and had had acne for 6 years.
During this time he was treated with
oxytetracycline, erythromycin and
septrin. His acne became unresponsive
to the latter therapy and in fact worsened
despite Septrin three times daily. At that
stage his acne grade was 2.75.*

*After 16 weeks therapy his acne grade
fell to 0.35. At 32 weeks his acne was
mild (Grade 0.35) and confined now to
his face. By 44 weeks there was a slight
relapse of the face and return of his
truncal acne. His acne grade was then
0.75. He was treated with topical
benzoyl peroxide 5% gel. From time to
time his acne recurred but each
recurrence was now well controlled with
short courses of Septrin.*

*His only adverse reaction was
cheilitis.*

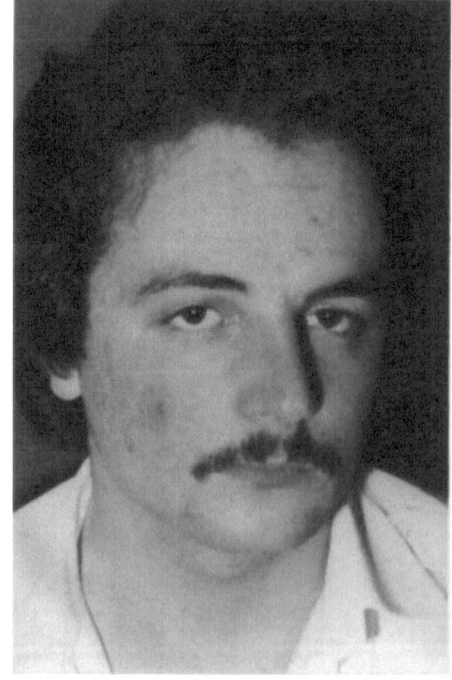

Case History E

Mr. L. H. is a 19-year-old male caucasian who weighed 69 kg. He had prior to starting Roaccutane therapy a 7 year history of scarring cystic acne. Whilst he was not graded according to the Leeds scale, his acne was clearly grade 7–8 on that scale.

His three older brothers had less severe forms of acne.

In the past he was treated with oral and topical antibiotics, topical steroids, topical vitamin A acid, ultraviolet light and surgical drainage.

He was prescribed 70mg b.i.d. Roaccutane (2.0mg/kg body-weight/ day) for the first week and 30mg b.i.d. (0.86mg/kg body-weight/day) for the remainder of the 20 week course.

At the end of therapy and at all post- therapy evaluations by both physician and patient the disease was rated as almost clear (i.e. < 0.25 Leeds grading).

No clinical adverse reactions were reported. However plasma triglyceride and LDH levels were elevated during Roaccutane therapy, while HDL levels were decreased.

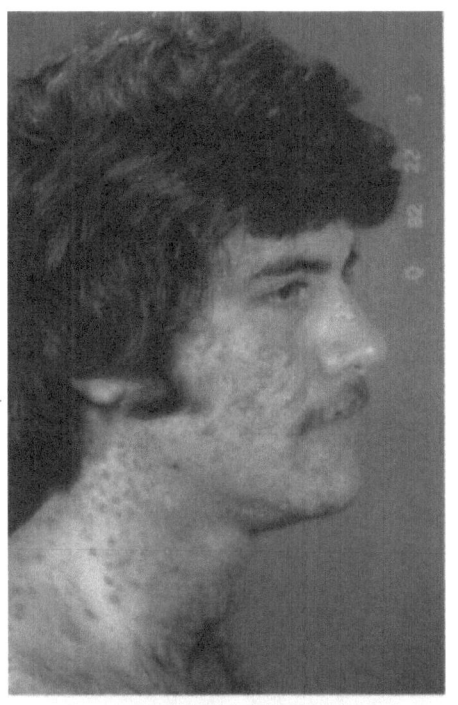

Case History E (Pre-treatment)

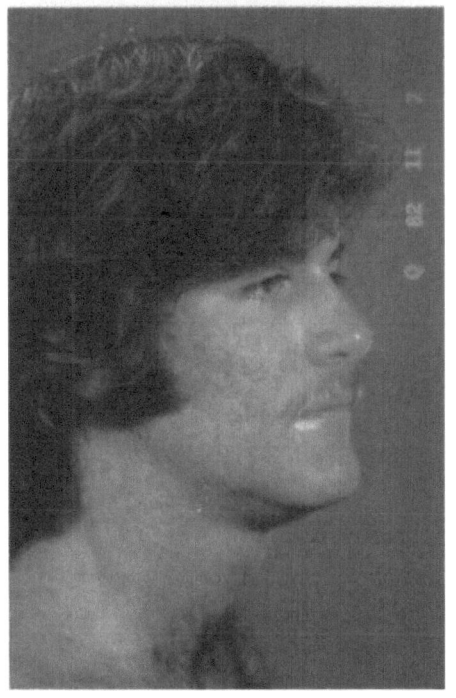

Continued on next page

355

Case History E (Post-treatment)

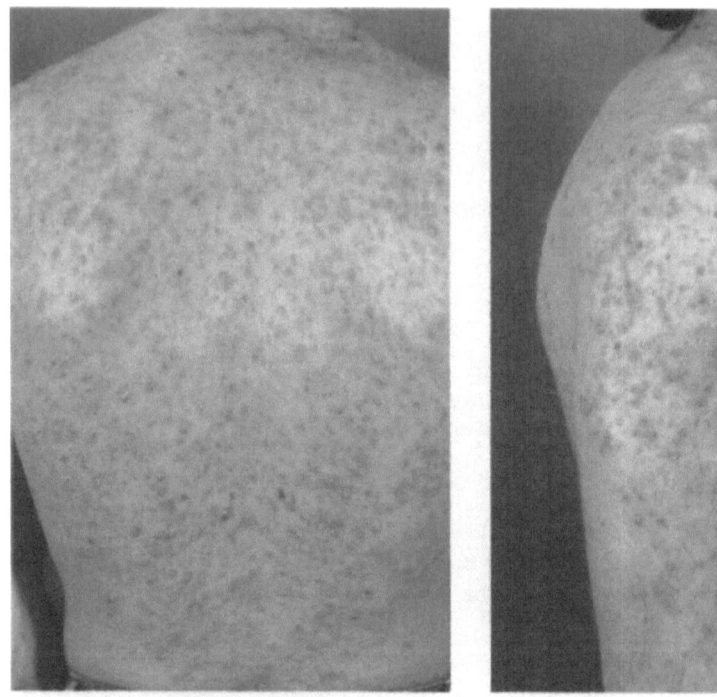

Case History E (Pre-treatment)

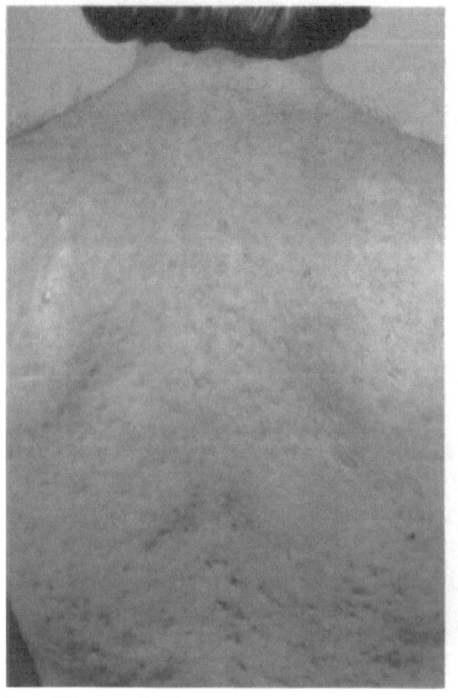
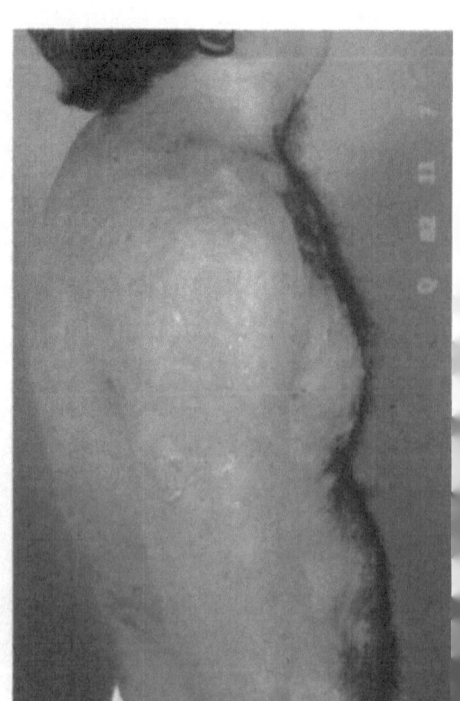

Case History E (Post-treatment)

Case History F

Mr J. F. is a 21-year-old male caucasian who weighed 60 kg. Prior to entering the study he had a 4 year history of cystic acne (6–7 Leeds grading).

One brother had less severe inflammatory acne. Prior to receiving Roaccutane he had been treated with topical and oral antibiotics, topical benzoyl peroxide, topical vitamin A acid, oral steroids, ultraviolet light and surgical drainage.

He was prescribed 60mg b.i.d. Roaccutane (2mg/kg body-weight/day) for the first week and 30mg b.i.d. (1mg/ kg body-weight/day) for the remainder of the 20 week course.

There was marked improvement in the disease after 1 and 2 months therapy. At the end of therapy the physician and patient reported the condition to be almost clear.

At the post-therapy evaluation both physician and patient rated the disease as clear.

No clinical adverse reactions were reported. A mild increase in LDH was reported at the end of the study; however, the investigator believed this to be non-specific and inconsequential.

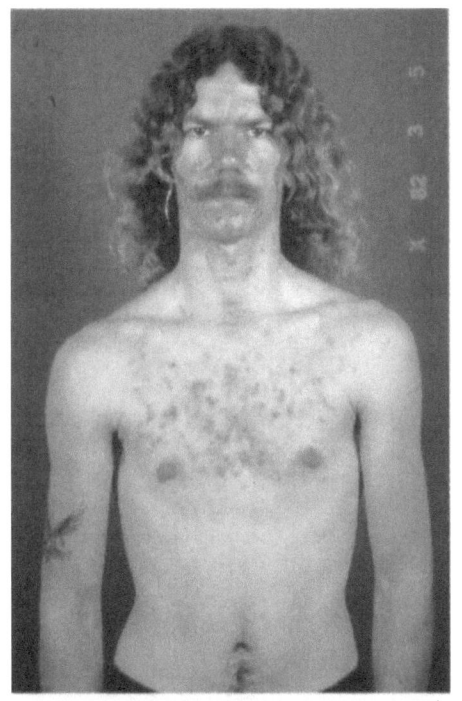

Case History F (Pre-treatment)

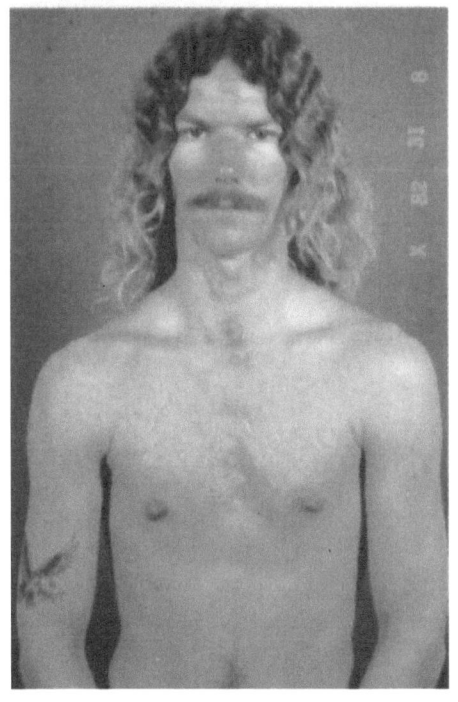

Case History F (Post-treatment)

Continued on next page

357

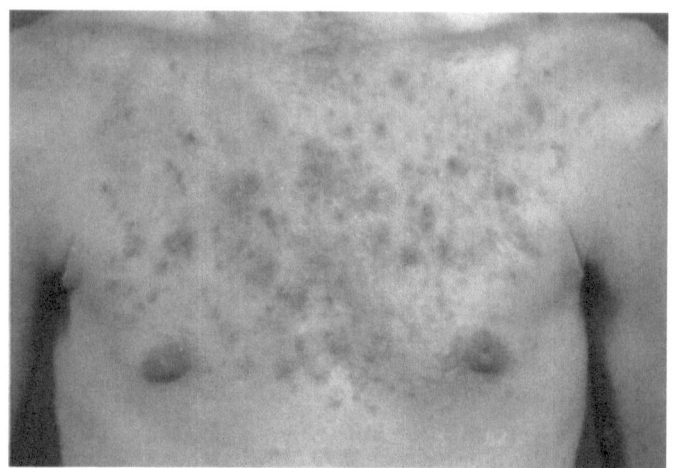

Case History F (Pre-treatment)

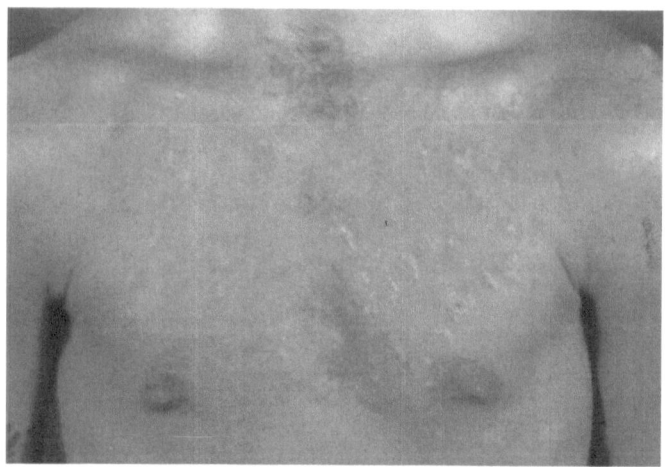

Case History F (Post-treatment)

Section 2   Dosage
and Duration of Dosage

It can be seen from the examples that there is considerable variation in dosage, ranging from 0.1 to 2.0mg/kg/day. In the UK the Committee on Safety of Medicines has approved dosage recommendations from 0.1 to 1.0mg/kg/day for 12–16 weeks whereas the FDA in the USA has approved 1.0–2.0mg/kg/day for 15–20 weeks. These variations reflect experiences resulting from differing clinical trial designs, in that generally lower dosages had been used in Europe (including the UK); possibly patients treated in trials in the USA had somewhat severer acne; and also, it is now generally accepted that severe truncal acne requires higher, and probably more prolonged dosage than facial acne.

The manufacturer's advice to commence with 0.5mg/kg/day for a duration of 12–16 weeks agrees with most European investigators' experiences for acne of grade 2–7 for the face and 2–5 for the back. If at 4 weeks, the response is poor, the dose should be increased to 1.0mg/kg/day. However, if intolerance to the drug (*vide infra*) should occur, dosage will need to be reduced to 0.5 or even 0.1mg/kg/day or to a level previously known to be tolerated.

Several truncal acne (grades 5–10) associated with or without facial involvement has, contrariwise, been shown to require a high dosage from the outset and often a more prolonged treatment. It is recommended that 1.0mg/kg/day, if tolerated, be given throughout the course of therapy.

If after 16 weeks of any regime therapy there has been a good result but there is also a considerable degree of acne still present, therapy should be prolonged for a further month. It is important to point out here that in many cases improvement, off drug, will continue so that complete clearance of all acne lesions should not be regarded as the end-point of treatment.

Repeat courses are not generally recommended. However, it has been given in many cases with clearing of acne after the second or even third course of Roaccutane. Continuous therapy for years should not be given (*vide infra*).

Section 3   Side-effects

The common side-effects of Roaccutane are well known and in the case of cheilitis almost universal. These will not be described in detail, but some will be illustrated in the following examples with advice on management, while still continuing therapy. A few uncommon side-effects, and two, so far unreported until the Symposium will be shown and accompanied again with advice on management.

The first two (Figures 1 & 2) cases illustrate cheilitis and facial dermatitis.

Management:

Cheilitis – Initially use an 'over-the-counter' (OTC) lip salve progressing onto 1% hydrocortisone ointment or even a medium strength steroid ointment should it be deemed necessary.

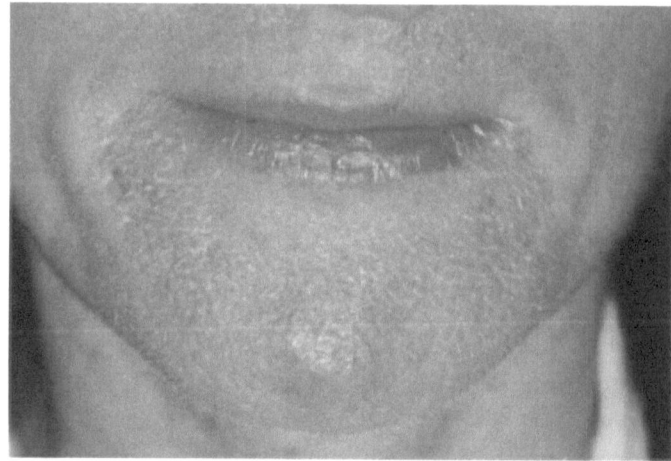

Figure 1

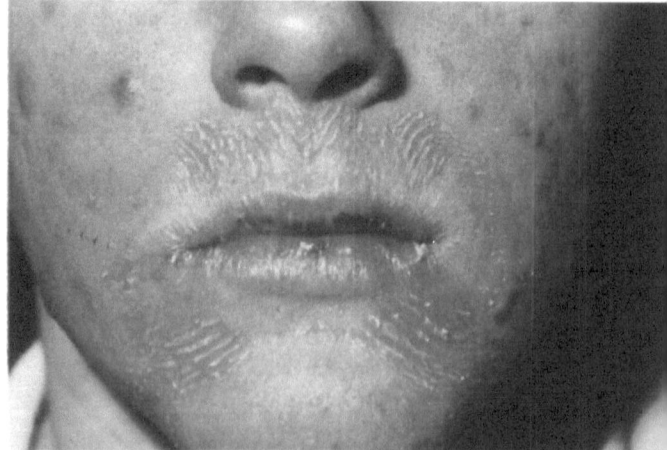

Figure 2

Facial dermatitis – An OTC emollient such as "Nivea" or "Oil of Ulay" will suffice in most cases. Very occasionally in others 1% hydrocortisone ointment will be required.

Occasionally an irritant, eczema craquelle-like, dermatitis of the rest of the body (Figure 3) occurs, which responds to oilated bath oil. If necessary 1% hydrocortisone ointment may be used.

Nasal mucosal drying and cracking may lead to nose bleeds (Figure 4) which are not profuse and dribble rather than frankly bleed. This is more of a problem if there is a concurrent coryzal inflammation. Most often the nares are blocked with crusts. Apply Unguentum Merck daily. Should pain occur there may well be a *Staph. aureus* cellulitis. Swabs should be taken for bacterial culture and 7 days treatment with an oral antibiotic such as erythromycin 250mg q.i.d.

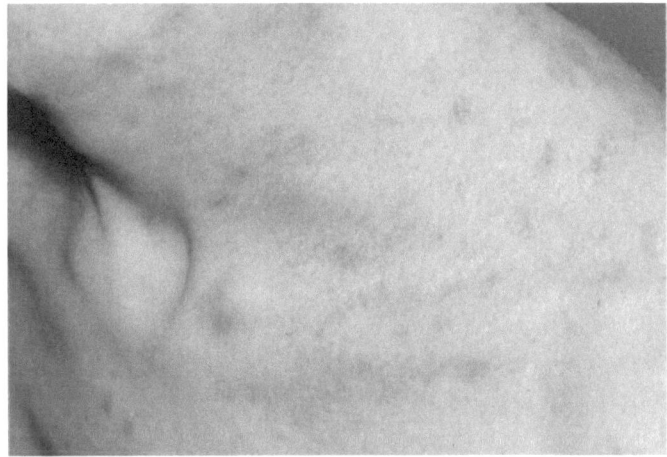

Figure 3

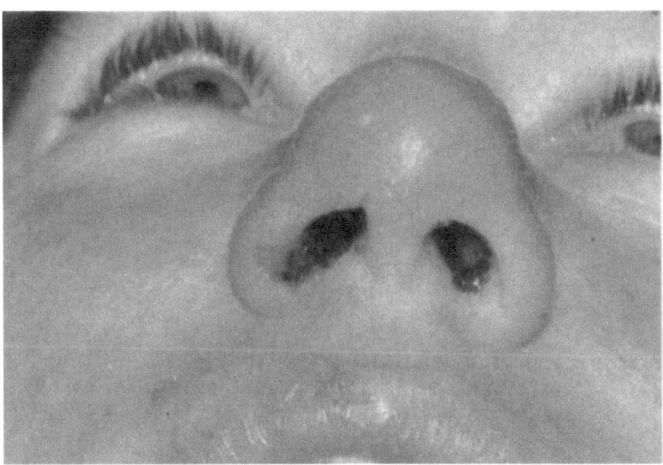

Figure 4

commenced. Topically, Naseptin is of help.

Far less common are scalp folliculitis (Figure 5) and pyogenic granuloma (Figures 6, 7 and 8).

Scalp folliculitis is mainly seen on stopping treatment but can be seen during therapy. *Staph. aureus* is often grown on culture. The condition responds to systemic erythromycin plus Naseptin ointment topically and cetrimide shampoo but the condition may be recurrent.

Pyogenic granuloma is a rare but sometimes spectacular side-effect of healing truncal acne. Three examples are shown. Cracks should be soaked off with Eusol daily and silver nitrate applied with a stick twice weekly. Therapy with Roaccutane should continue.

Other unwanted side-effects include skin fragility due to epidermal thinning (n.b. not dermal) and arthralgia. The latter responds to analgesics and non-steroidal anti-inflammatory drugs.

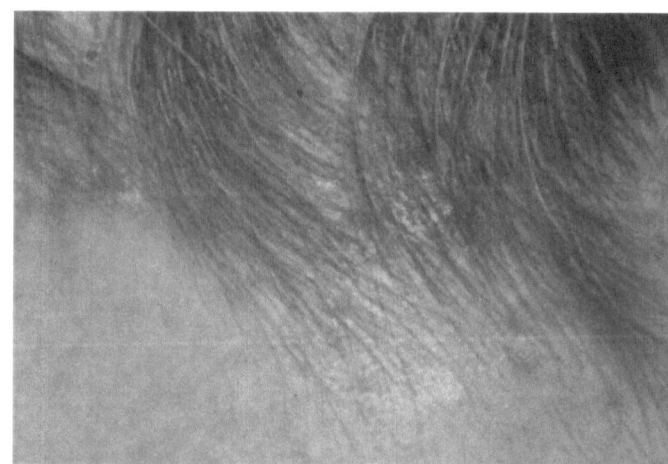

Figure 5

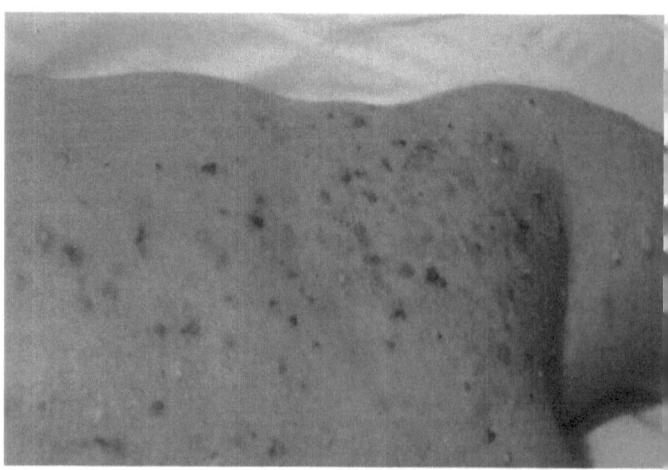

Figure 6

Therapy rarely needs to be discontinued. Epidermal thinning may give rise to some soreness especially if exposed to strong sunlight. A good sun cream is recommended.

Finally, acne may flare during the second to sixth week of therapy to a degree worse than that seen immediately pretreatment. This flare has always settled down and not affected the eventual outcome with continuing therapy.[2]

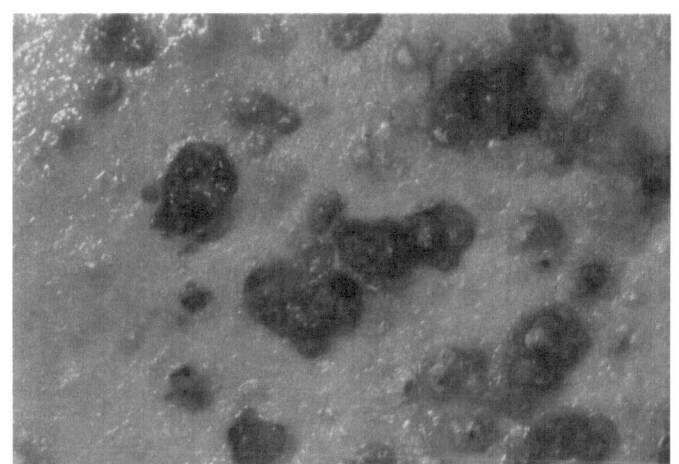

Figure 7

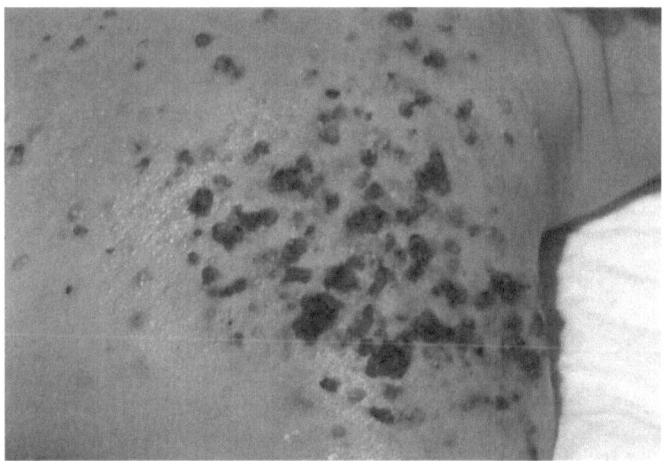

Figure 8

Section 4   Precautions

It is always necessary to remind prescribers that Roaccutane is teratogenic and major foetal abnormalities have been reported in five acne patients in the USA.[3] Only one of the patients had been taking contraceptive precautions and in this case conception occurred within a few days of removal of her IUD and starting oral contraception, i.e. a period when reliable contraception could not be expected. There have been no reports of similar tragedies from the UK or continental Europe. It is important to note that no cases of oral contraceptive failure have been identified, as predicted by the study of M. Orme *et al.* (p.277). It remains of the utmost importance for dermatologists to advise their female patients of the urgency of using effective contraceptive precautions.

Prolonged continuous therapy is not recommended as there are reports of diffuse idiopathic skeletal hyperdystrophy (DISH) in patients receiving high dosages of Roaccutane (3–4g/kg/day) for 2–6 years continuously for the treatment of inherited disorders of keratinization.[4]

It has not been thought necessary to detail the patient management with regards laboratory changes as these have been adequately described in the manufacturer's literature and elsewhere.

Roaccutane is now widely recognized as an important advance in the successful management of severe recalcitrant acne. In the UK the drug has been properly restricted to the specialist supervision of dermatologists. It is hoped that these notes will be of help to dermatologists in confident prescribing to suitable patients.

References

1. Cunliffe, W. J. (1981). Acne. *Update Postgraduate Centre Series*
2. Katz, R. A. *et al.* (1983). *J. Am. Acad. Dermatol.*, **8**, 132
3. Rosa, F. W. (1983). *Lancet,* **ii,** 513
4. Pittsley, K. A. and Yoder, F. W. (1983). *N. Engl. J. Med.*, **308,** 1072

Index

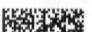